The Comprehensive School Health Challenge

The Comprehensive School Health Challenge

Promoting Health Through Education

Volume One

Peter Cortese, DrPH, CHES, and
Kathleen Middleton, MS, CHES, Eds.

ETR ASSOCIATES
Santa Cruz, California
1994

ETR Associates (Education, Training and Research) is a non-profit organization committed to fostering the health, well-being and cultural diversity of individuals, families, schools and communities. The publishing program of ETR Associates provides books and materials that empower young people and adults with the skills to make positive health choices. We invite health professionals to learn more about our high-quality publishing, training and research programs by contacting us at P.O. Box 1830, Santa Cruz, CA 95061-1830.

Published by ETR Associates, P.O. Box 1830, Santa Cruz, California 95061-1830

Printed in the United States of America
9 8 7 6 5 4 3 2 1

Cover design by Ann Smiley
Text design by Cliff Warner
Title No. 573

Library of Congress Cataloging-in-Publication Data

The Comprehensive school health challenge : promoting health
  through education / Peter Cortese and Kathleen Middleton,
  editors.
      p. cm.
    Includes bibliographical references (p.)
    ISBN 1-56071-344-5
    1. Health education—United States. 3. School hygiene—
United States. 3. Students—Health and hygiene—United States.
I. Cortese, Peter. II. Middleton, Kathleen.
LB1588.U6C587   1994
371.7'0973—dc20   93-24711

Dedication

To Dr. Elena Sliepcevich, whose vision of the possibilities in comprehensive school health continues to light the way.

Contents

Volume One

Comprehensive Health Education for Tomorrow

Programmatic Issues

Content Issues

Foreword

In 1987, after 26 years of practice as a pediatrician and specialist in endocrinology, I was approached by then-Governor Bill Clinton with an intriguing offer—to serve as director of the Arkansas Department of Health. It was an offer I couldn't refuse. One of my earliest tasks was to learn more about the status of children's health in Arkansas and the nation. Even after a lifetime of pediatric practice, I was shocked by what I learned. Most disturbing to me was the fact that teenagers were the only population group in the nation experiencing a rising mortality rate. And these children were *having* children at alarming rates, creating the hub in the cycle of American poverty. These facts propelled me into a campaign to increase public awareness and action regarding the health needs of children and youth.

It has been said that you can't educate a child who isn't healthy and you can't keep a child healthy who isn't educated. I think that statement succinctly states the challenge before all of us who want to improve the health and educational status of our children. Clearly, poor health in all its dimensions adversely affects school performance. And, increasingly, the threats to the health of our children are not biomedical in origin. Injuries, homicide, suicide, pregnancy and substance use are experienced by American youth at alarming rates. These contemporary morbidities are primarily the result of social environment and behavior.

We *must* give greater priority to policies and programs that advance preventive health care practices. At issue is whether we want to invest now or pay later. We can invest in strategies that make a positive difference in our children's health and future, or we can continue to pay for costly intervention and treatment of preventable problems. I think the most promising strategy we can invest in is comprehensive school-based health education.

The chapters in this book cover a continuum of issues within today's school health education challenge: a review of the past, a vision of the future, the nuts and bolts of curriculum content and implementation, key concerns within health education research, and the growing need for partnerships. The chapters challenge us to use our scientific knowledge, professional skill, individual commitment, community support and political will to protect and improve the health of all school-age children through education. With a consensus of values and a collaboration of effort, it's a challenge I know we can meet.

M. Joycelyn Elders, MD

Preface

Comprehensive school health is a concept whose time has truly come. The major health risks children and youth face today can be reduced or minimized by effective prevention methods. Never before has this concept been so universally embraced. The Youth Risk Behavior Surveillance System (YRBSS) recently established by the U.S. Centers for Disease Control and Prevention (CDC) has provided strong evidence of the existence of these risk behaviors among our youth. We know that most of the health problems teenagers experience are caused by a relatively small number of behaviors, such as drinking and driving and sexual intercourse at a young age.

Every year, 1 million unintended pregnancies occur among teenagers in the United States. This group also experiences 2.5 million cases of sexually transmitted disease each year. In the United States, nearly 70 percent of all deaths in young people ages one through twenty-four result from the following four causes:

- motor vehicle crashes—33 percent
- other unintentional injuries—15 percent
- homicides—10 percent
- suicides—10 percent

Acute and chronic morbidity also result from these causes.

Sixty percent of all deaths among all age groups in the United States are due to heart disease and cancer. Tobacco use, consumption of excessive fat, and lack of physical activity play a major role in these diseases. These behaviors are frequently established during youth. With proper educational intervention, the health problems caused by these behaviors can be prevented or minimized.

In 1988, CDC began to monitor these risky behaviors through cooperative agreements with state education agencies. As the years go by, these periodic surveys provide us with data about how we are progressing in our efforts to change the behavior of our school-age children and youth.

Schools include many health-related components in their programs. For several years, many leaders in the school health education field have proposed that these elements should work in concert to improve the health of students, faculty and staff. Health education alone cannot do the job. We need coordinated efforts among those who manage or provide the following health-related components.

- health education
- school lunch programs
- guidance and counseling
- physical education
- school health services
- school health environment
- schoolsite health promotion program for faculty and staff

Those who provide these components must also work with individuals and groups in the community as well as parents. A coordinated effort is an essential aspect of a comprehensive school health program.

The first National Education Goal in *America 2000*, a report of the U.S. Department of Education, calls for every child in America to start school ready to learn. A quality school health program should be designed to help students maintain such a healthy start. In addition, a good comprehensive school health program can be a great help toward the nation's attainment of the goals delineated in the U.S. Public Health Service's document *Healthy People 2000*.

The authors of the chapters in *The Comprehensive School Health Challenge: Promoting Health Through Education* are all recognized leaders in the areas about which they write. The work is presented in two volumes and is designed to give you the impressions of leaders based upon their extensive experience. Volume One, the first eighteen chapters, addresses issues of goal-setting, coordination of programs, skill development and content guidelines. The fourteen chapters in Volume Two focus on research and evaluation, restructuring health education programs to meet "real life" education challenges, preparation of educators, and community linkages.

We hope this approach will be helpful to those planning to implement comprehensive school health programs, to those studying to be professionals in one of the component areas of a comprehensive school health program and to those wanting to improve their programs. Leaders developing policy related to school health programs can use this book as a tool for preparing advocacy speeches or documents. Community members and parents who want to learn more about what a health program can accomplish in a school can use this book as a guide.

All too frequently health programs are planned and implemented in a noncoordinated way. We hope this book will help convince you that a total comprehensive approach is the answer to a successful program—a program that will help to reduce illness, disease and infirmity among our citizens.

Acknowledgments

The efforts of numerous individuals in the development and production of this publication must be acknowledged. First, we would like to thank the contributors. Throughout this project, we had the great pleasure of working with dedicated and talented professionals. We are truly grateful for the time and energy given to this project by some of the busiest people we know.

We specifically want to acknowledge Dr. Wanda Jubb for her support of this project. She was involved in conceptualizing the framework of the book and the development of specific chapters.

Staff in ETR Associates' Editorial and Prepress departments deserve special acknowledgment. We feel fortunate to have had such capable people on the team for this project.

Finally, we wish to acknowledge Mary Nelson, publisher at ETR Associates. This project could not have happened without her leadership. She developed the prototype book in ETR Associates' "Challenge" series and continues to support the development of professional yet practical materials for health education.

*Comprehensive
Health Education
for Tomorrow*

Chapter 1

School Health Education: What Are the Possibilities?

Marian V. Hamburg, EdD, CHES

Proponents of school health education are thoroughly familiar with the "ideal program." They can state its rationale, diagram its components, provide a model for its curriculum, describe its teaching methodologies and materials, identify the roles of personnel involved in its delivery and provide evaluation tools. Everything needed to put comprehensive school health education in place is available. That the ideal has never been fully achieved does not seem to dampen optimism that some day it will be. Its promoters are convinced of the theoretical soundness of its design and feel that its widespread adoption awaits only "the right time."

For years, the health education profession has led the promotion of an ideal health education program, in the hope that policy makers in the public and private sectors would recognize its value and take vigorous action toward its establishment. Throughout this time, school leaders have always agreed on the importance of education for health, but have been slow in effecting change in schools. Why?

Perhaps the time has not yet been just right. Public concern about health has not been high enough. The pressure exerted on schools by the health professions has not been sufficiently strengthened by parents and other voters. Or maybe it is simply resistance to change. The long tradition has been to focus on certain academic subjects such as reading, science and mathematics. These conditions, however, seem to be changing, and there may well be good reason for optimism that comprehensive school health education now has its golden opportunity.

The enormous health problems of young people can no longer be ignored. Today, for the first time in the history of our country, young people are less healthy and less prepared to take their places in society than were their parents (National Commission on the Role of the School and Community, 1990). They are at serious risk of being damaged by drugs, alcohol, poor nutrition, teen pregnancy, sexually transmitted disease, violence and injuries—problems that have their roots in behavior. Although it is true that children from poor families are at greater risk, adequate income and high social status provide no immunity to falling prey to dangerous practices that can lead to permanent damage or death. The situation in the United States has reached crisis proportions.

An alarm has been sounded by important groups. The Children's Defense Fund (1990) signals: "SOS America!...The mounting crisis of our children and families is a rebuke to everything America professes to be." Some staggering statistics are provided:

- Every 67 seconds an American teenager has a baby (472,623 in 1987).
- Every seven minutes, an American youth is arrested for a drug offense (76,986 a year).
- Every thirty minutes, an American youth is arrested for drunken driving (17,674 a year).

The Carnegie Corporation's Task Force on Education of Young Adolescents (1989) estimates that "seven million young people—one in four adolescents—are extremely vulnerable to multiple high risk behaviors and school failure, and another million may be at moderate risk, but remain a cause for serious concern."

A Code Blue alert, a call for extraordinary action in a life-threatening emergency, has been issued by the National Commission on the Role of the School and the Community in Improving Adolescent Health (1990). It calls upon the nation to collectively demonstrate the political will to respond to the serious health problems growing at a frightening pace among our young people. Specifically, "schools should offer students a new type of health education that provides honest, relevant information and teaches skills and strategies to make wise decisions and develop positive values."

The challenges that young people face in their growing years have not changed. But our society has. Today, children are faced with unprecedented choices and pressures and are surrounded by temptations of all kinds of high-risk behaviors, including use of tobacco, alcohol and other drugs, and sexual activity. They get conflicting messages from the adult world about most of these things. And many lack the support of a stable family where they can count on receiving love and guidance to help them make decisions that will increase their chances for healthful, fulfilling lives. Their world is far different than their parents' was. Their schools must be different too.

There is every indication that schools will change. Schools are also in a crisis situation, suffering pressures from a frustrated society to improve student performance. People are calling for schools to provide more with less: more choice, more services, more achievement and more graduates with less money, less parental involvement and less community support. A national reform movement is under way in education; the system is in for a major restructuring. In this climate, health education can scarcely be ignored. The stepchild of academic offerings may finally attain a new legitimacy in elementary and secondary schools.

Where Are We Today?

In spite of the fact that health education has never been a school priority, the link between learning and health has always been well understood by educators. They know that children who are sick, malnourished, or impaired by drugs, neglect or emotional problems cannot benefit fully from schooling. As children's health problems have become more severe and more prevalent and as school dropout rates have soared, there has been a growing acceptance of the necessity for schools to play a more prominent role in prevention. The home, even with the support of religious institutions and community agencies, cannot do the job alone, as was once believed.

Schools have been pushed to accept more significant responsibility for students' general well-being. Many have greatly expanded and improved their health education offerings by adopting a comprehensive approach—sequential broad-based teaching that progresses from kindergarten through high school. This is a radical change from the disconnected, piecemeal approach motivated by disease-of-the-month campaigns.

Today, well over half of all schools provide comprehensive school health education. In a recent national survey, 67 percent of the teachers questioned reported that their schools have comprehensive programs in place. Eighty-two percent of the school children reported that they had had health education as a separate school subject; 52 percent of these had health in more than two grades (Louis Harris and Associates, 1989).

Several factors are contributing to this development in comprehensive school health education. First, a philosophical statement that provides some basic guidelines has been put forward (A Point of View, 1992). School health education should:

- emphasize "broad-based constructive action in the shaping and reshaping of human lives for better health, rather than...the acquisition of knowledge about health"
- display a "broad curricular scope and methodological diversity, rather than...focus on narrow topical coverage or limited methodology"
- be "dynamic and evolving, not static and fixed"
- have flexibility for altering structure "as experiences and research point out improved ways to accomplish the goal"
- invite "participation in design and delivery from all actors in the school and community, including students, employees and citizens"

Second, current information about the major health problems of children is immediately available to help schools plan curricula and keep them up to date and relevant. In this age of technology, there are many sources of general and specific health information. One of the most widely used is *Healthy People 2000* (1991), a publication of the U.S. Public Health Service that provides a health profile of children and youth based on more than the usual morbidity and mortality data. Included are children's emotional, psychological and learning problems as well as the social and environmental risks to which these are related.

The *National Adolescent Student Health Survey* (ASHA, AAHE and SOPHE, 1989) sponsored by three national professional health education organizations is also an important information source for schools because it gives insights on what our nation's teenagers know and how they act concerning eight health topic areas: AIDS, injury prevention, violence, suicide, alcohol, drug and tobacco use, sexually transmitted disease, consumer health and nutrition.

Third, goal setting for health education has been made easier. The Health Objectives for the Nation (U.S. Department of Health and Human Services, 1990) provide a model for establishing goals and action plans for schools. School policy makers have taken good advantage of the pattern. The American Association of School Administrators presents its plan in *Healthy Kids for the Year 2000* (1990). The approach of the National School Boards Association can be found in its manual *School Health: Helping Children Learn* (1991).

Recently, the American Cancer Society used the national health objectives as the basis for an invitational workshop of national organization representatives to develop a collaborative plan to institutionalize comprehensive school health education for all school-age children (American Cancer Society, 1992). Reasonable, measurable goals for schools consistent with national objectives sharpen the focus of health education and greatly facilitate accountability.

Replicable models for comprehensive school health education programs have been identified. Metropolitan Life has led the way. Its "Healthy Me" program, designed to promote excellence in school health education by recognizing and rewarding exemplary programs, made more than 150 awards over a period of five years. A compendium of these winning programs has been widely distributed to spread the word about high-quality comprehensive health education as encouragement to schools throughout the nation to implement similar efforts. No school has to start from scratch.

Excellent curriculum guides and other teaching materials are now available. Most state education departments provide curriculum outlines, and there are many sources of free and inexpensive supplementary teaching materials. The past decade, however, has seen a great increase in school district adoption and purchase of fully developed curricula, several of which have been nationally validated. *Growing Healthy* and *Know Your Body* are two examples of widely used elementary school curricula that have an additional feature of teacher training. *Teenage Health Teaching Modules* are very popular with high school teachers. ETR Associates publishes the *Contemporary Health Series*, which includes *Actions for Health* for kindergarten through grade six, *Into Adolescence* for middle school students and *Entering Adulthood* for high school students. Teacher training is also available for the series.

In addition to such multitopic curricula, other teaching materials, such as *Here's Looking at You 2000*, address specific topic areas of concern such as alcohol and drug use, sex education or nutrition. School districts no longer have to create their own curricula or develop their own teaching aids unless they choose to do so.

Standards for teacher preparation have also improved. Several factors, all of them related to the professionalization of the field of health education, are responsible. The most basic was a study conducted to determine the role of generic health educators by defining their responsibilities and the competencies needed to carry them out. This Role Delineation Study (National Conference for Institutions Preparing Health Educators, 1981) provided the basis for a new Framework (National Task Force on the Preparation and Practice of Health Educators, 1985) for programs of professional preparation, which was promulgated to the 275 or more institutions offering health education specialization. The study also made it possible for national health education organizations to introduce an Approval Process for such baccalaureate programs (SOPHE/AAHE Joint Committee on Health Education Undergraduate Program Approval, 1985) and for the Association for the Advancement of Health Education to assist the National Commission for the Accreditation of Teacher Education in improving the standards for health education that are used in assessing institutions for accreditation.

Concurrently, a national competency-based credentialing process for individual health education practitioners, including teachers, was established. It is administered by the National Commission for Health Education Credentialing, which sets standards for attaining and maintaining certification. School districts can have more assurance than ever before that the teachers they employ are well prepared to provide the quality of leadership demanded for comprehensive school health programs.

There are new mechanisms to facilitate cooperation and coordination among the many groups and sectors involved in school health. National organizations have banded together to share resources, coordinate program efforts and provide single sources of multiple resources to schools. The National School Boards Association organized a National Consortium to Foster Comprehensive School Health Programs in the Public Schools. The National School Health Education Coalition promotes health in schools by providing strong leadership in advocacy. A newly formed Comprehensive School Health Education Network provides technical assistance and training through centers that now exist in every state in the union. Support from the Centers for Disease Control and Prevention has greatly assisted these activities.

In addition to the coalitions that support school health broadly, there are those that focus on a single topic area. A National Coalition to Support Sexuality Education helps schools deal with issues that may be controversial and also provides guidelines for curriculum development. National cooperative mechanisms have provided the model for numerous state and local coalitions, councils and committees to effect intersectoral cooperation that could not be easily achieved otherwise.

There is evidence that comprehensive school health education works. Some of the most compelling data come from an evaluation of comprehensive school health education in American public schools conducted by Louis Harris and Associates with the sponsorship of the Metropolitan Life Foundation (1989). A comparison between schools with comprehensive programs and a national cross-section of schools where health education is taught on a limited basis or not at all showed that students in schools with comprehensive programs have more knowledge and better health-related attitudes and behaviors than students with no exposure to health classes. In addition, the study revealed a linear trend of increase in health-related knowledge and behavior as the number of years of health classes increased for students in the national cross-section. Such data have helped to convince school policy makers that only continuous health education over several years influences health behavior patterns.

To sum up where we are today: Most schools do offer at least some health education, and more of them than ever before have comprehensive programs. All of the elements for continued momentum toward comprehensive school health education seem to be in place:
- an established need
- a heightened public awareness
- national health objectives
- a philosophical basis for health education
- program guidelines and replicable models
- high-quality curriculum materials
- prepared teachers
- tools for evaluation
- evidence that comprehensive school health education works

Where Could We Be in the Year 2000?

Imagine it is the year 2000. The results of a national survey on school health education have just been released. Here are some highlights.

Comprehensive School Health Education

- 70% of teachers report their school has comprehensive school health
- 90% of students have had health as a separate subject
- 57% of students have had health for more than two years
- 53% of parents report that they know what's being taught in health
- 31% of parents have become involved in their child's program in some way

Student Knowledge and Practice

HIV/AIDS—95% of junior high students know the facts about HIV and how to reduce their risk of getting it

Cigarette smoking—96% of high school students are non-smokers

Alcohol use—87% of high school students are non-drinkers

Drug use—92% of junior high and high school students report never using such drugs as marijuana, crack, speed or downers

Nutrition
- 93% of all students can identify less nutritional foods
- 16% of junior high and high school students think about the health consequences of the foods they choose
- 83% almost always eat breakfast

Safety
- 53% of high school students never drive after drinking
- 40% of junior high and high school students never ride with a driver who has been drinking
- 38% of all students regularly wear a safety belt
- 5% of student bicyclists regularly wear a helmet

A positive picture of school health in the year 2000? Yes! It may, in fact, be too optimistic, because each reported item shows a 10 percent improvement over a similar survey completed just over a decade earlier (Louis Harris and Associates, 1989).

Should we be satisfied with such improvement? Absolutely not! Only percentages much closer to 100 percent, with the implications for the health of the nation that accompany such scores, can bring any real pride of achievement.

After all, our imaginary year 2000 survey indicates that 13 percent of high school students drink regularly, 8 percent have used drugs and 4 percent smoke on a regular basis. An overwhelming majority (95 percent) do not wear bicycle helmets and 62 percent do not use safety belts. And even though knowledge about HIV/AIDS is at a high level (95 percent), there is no way of knowing whether that knowledge is being put into practice for reducing the risk of getting infected. If knowledge about nutrition and its effect on making food choices is any indicator, the gap between knowing and doing is probably wide.

Teaching to reinforce positive health practices and change negative ones has always been a great challenge for health educators. Knowledge, important as it is, does not necessarily lead to practice. Nor does all the teaching about health emanate from schools.

What Are the Obstacles?

With so much going for health education in schools, why aren't excellent programs more widespread? What are the obstacles? Three are critical.

The first is lack of support. Some school policy makers do not view health education as important. They give it much lower priority than other subjects, particularly language, math and science, and are satisfied with the outdated tradition of teaching health as a part of physical education. Resistance to comprehensive health education can be found at both state and local levels.

State education departments vary in their recommendations

concerning the teaching of health, and there are few mandates. Where mandates do exist, they are more likely to address single topics only, such as HIV/AIDS, drugs, alcohol or smoking, which serves to reinforce the idea of a limited, fragmented curriculum.

Even when mandates call for comprehensive health education, they are ineffective if school boards and administrators are weak in their support of such programs. Local districts can and do meet the letter of the law without fulfilling its intent. Some of their reluctance to making change is undoubtedly due to practical problems such as where to find time in the curriculum, how to develop a curriculum, and where to find teachers within budget constraints. However, the strong support of comprehensive school health being given by the Council of Chief State School Officers, the National School Boards Association and the American Association of School Administrators is an indicator that this barrier is being lowered.

Lack of teacher training is the second major obstacle. Elementary classroom teachers lack adequate preparation in health education, yet are expected to teach the subject. Rarely does their preservice preparation program include more than one or two courses related to health. This means that they must depend upon the availability of inservice offerings if they are to gain the skill and knowledge that a modern approach to the teaching of health education requires. It is common for voluntary health agencies, local colleges and other community groups to sponsor inservice courses, but these opportunities cannot be counted on to reach all teachers with the depth or breadth needed to do the job well.

In recent years, the training offered in connection with school districts' adoptions of comprehensive curricula has alleviated this situation greatly. However, teacher preparation for health should not have to depend on a school district's purchase of curriculum materials. Until teacher education programs are modified to provide better preservice preparation, we cannot expect the quality of elementary health education to improve.

There is no lack of professionally prepared health educators for teaching positions in secondary schools, but there is sometimes a problem with the quality of teaching at this level. This problem results from the practice of assigning specialists in other subjects to teach health. A myth believed by some school administrators is that "anyone can teach health." The inevitable result when "anyone" is assigned to do so is pedestrian teaching, disinterested students and poor results.

The third obstacle is that no one is in charge. Comprehensive health education differs from other school subjects because it is interdisciplinary in nature and must be linked not only to other subjects in the curriculum but also to the community in which it exists. Parents need to be encouraged to participate in their children's program because of the home's significant influence on health attitudes and practices. Students need to gain an understanding of health in its larger social context by being exposed to local, state, national and even international concerns. Many excellent resources are to be found in the public, private and professional organizations of the community. Schools need to reach out; communities need to contribute. Working together can provide the dynamic, relevant curricula envisioned for comprehensive health education programs. Such collaboration requires leadership beyond the classroom. Someone needs to be in charge. Often no one is.

Designating or employing a health coordinator is recommended by some state education departments and used successfully by some school districts. The job often includes leadership of a school/community council or advisory committee. The spread of such appointments has been slow, primarily for economic reasons. In times of tight school budgets, it is hard to justify support of a school health coordinator. New ways of dealing with the need for intersectoral collaboration must be found.

What Are the Possibilities?

Can these barriers to progress be overcome? What are some realistic possibilities for school health programs of the future?

The National Association of State Boards of Education has put forward the view that the current education reform movement provides an extraordinary opportunity for gaining wider acceptance of school health education. The potential for success, however, is greatly dependent on the extent to which those concerned with school health take leadership in working with education reformers in the development of new strategies for integrating health into education. Health education professionals need to join the movement, not remain separate from it. Successful advocacy for school health education requires flexibility, not rigidity; open mindedness, not being closed to new ideas; and the skillful use of cooperation and collaboration.

Policy makers can be expected to become more supportive of school health education when they are convinced that health outcomes belong in the goals for education and when they can envision reasonable ways to achieve them. Teacher training institutions can be expected to find new ways to strengthen the preparation of elementary school teachers when they become familiar with current innovative health education curricula that can be used to develop teacher competencies which can be generalized to other subject areas.

School administrators who have opportunities to experience the excitement that comes from opening school doors to community people who can relate health teaching to real situations can be expected to actively seek ways to make new and better things happen in their schools.

Those who form the architectural teams for the basic remodeling of our schools will determine the new infrastructure. This time it won't be just patchwork or add-ons. The new look will be more than cosmetic change. Will the planners include health education proponents? If so, the possibilities for comprehensive school health education to be built into the very foundations of education, where it belongs, have never been better.

References

American Association of School Administrators. 1990. *Healthy kids for the year 2000: An action plan for schools.* Arlington, VA.

American Cancer Society. 1992. National Action Plan for Comprehensive School Health Education. Phoenix, Arizona, June 1992.

American School Health Association, Association for the Advancement of Health Education and Society for Public Health Education. 1989. *National adolescent student health survey: A report on the health of America's youth.* Oakland, CA: Third Party Press.

A point of view for health education. 1992. *Journal of Health Education* 23 (1): 4-6.

Carnegie Council on Adolescent Development. 1989. *Turning points: Preparing American youth for the 21st century.* Report of the Task Force on Education of Young Adolescents. Washington, DC.

Children's Defense Fund. 1990. *Children 1990: A report card, briefing book and action primer.* Washington, DC.

Council of Chief State School Officers. 1991. *Beyond the health room.* Washington, DC: Resource Center on Educational Equity.

Joint Committee on Health Education Undergraduate Program Approval. 1985. Draft program review procedures for baccalaureate programs in health education. Association for the Advancement of Health Education, Reston, Virginia, and the Society for Public Health Education, Berkeley, California.

Louis Harris and Associates. 1989. *Health—You've got to be taught: An evaluation of comprehensive health education in American public schools.* New York: Metropolitan Life Foundation.

Metropolitan Life Foundation. 1990. *Healthy Me initiative to promote excellence in school health education: A compendium of award winning programs 1985-1989.* New York.

Sullivan, C., and J. F. Bogden. 1993. Today's education policy environment. *Journal of School Health* 63 (1): 28-32.

National Commission on the Role of the School and the Community in Improving Adolescent Health. 1990. *Code blue: Uniting for healthier youth.* Alexandria, VA: National Association of State Boards of Education.

National Conference for Institutions Preparing Health Educators. 1981. *Proceedings.* DHHS Publication No. 81-50171. Washington, DC.

National School Boards Association. 1991. *School health: Helping children learn.* Arlington, VA.

National Task Force on the Preparation and Practice of Health Educators. 1985. *A framework for the development of competency-based curricula for entry-level health educators.* New York: National Commission for Health Education Credentialing.

U.S. Department of Health and Human Services, Public Health Service. 1991. *Healthy people 2000: National health promotion and disease prevention objectives.* DHHS Publication No. (PHS) 91-50212. Washington, DC.

Curricula Resources

Contemporary Health Series. A comprehensive health education program for grades K-12, with three components: *Actions for Health* for grades K-6; *Into Adolescence* for grades 5-8; and *Entering Adulthood* for grades 9-12. ETR Associates, P.O. Box 1830, Santa Cruz, California 95061-1830.

Growing Healthy. A comprehensive health education program for grades K-6. National Center for Health Education, 72 Spring Street, New York, New York 10012.

Here's Looking at You, 2000. A K-12 curriculum for drug education. Comprehensive Health Education Foundation, 22323 Pacific Highway S., Seattle, Washington 98198.

Know Your Body. A comprehensive elementary school health education program. American Health Foundation, 320 East 43rd Street, New York, New York 10017.

Teenage Health Teaching Modules. A comprehensive health education curriculum for grades 7–12. Education Development Center, Inc., 55 Chapel Street, Newton, Massachusetts 02160.

Resources

Comprehensive School Health Education Network. Education Development Center, Inc., 55 Chapel Street, Newton, Massachusetts 02160.

National Coalition to Support Sexuality Education. Sex Information and Education Council of the United States, 130 West 42nd Street, New York, New York 10036.

National Commission for Health Education Credentialing, Inc., 475 Riverside Drive, New York, New York 10115.

National Consortium to Foster Comprehensive School Health Programs in the Public Schools. National School Boards Association, 1680 Duke Street, Alexandria, Virginia 22314.

National School Health Education Coalition, 100 Vermont Avenue NW, Washington, D.C. 20005.

Chapter 2

School Health Education Today: Highlights and Milestones

Ann E. Nolte, PhD, CHES

Many forces and factors influence health education in the public schools today. These include the preparation of teachers, local and national health problems, school finances, controversy regarding health education in general and specific topics in the curriculum, and values and religious beliefs of various communities.

Today, more and more educators recognize that for health education to be effective, it needs to be initiated at the elementary level. Health behavior is based not only in knowledge but in values and attitudes, and the foundation for these develop at the elementary ages. If health education is to begin at the elementary level, however, changes need to occur in several areas. First, there has to be a demand for it. Demand can come from professional organizations, parents, school administrators, state departments of education and state legislatures. Second, the preparation of elementary teachers needs to change.

At the secondary level, changes have already occurred in professional certification requirements. More health education teachers are being prepared to teach health education specifically, as opposed to dual preparation. However, there is also a growing need for continuing education in health education. The rapid expansion of knowledge and technology are increasing the need for inservice for teachers to remain competent professionals. (See Chapter 30 for a discussion of credentialing and certification.)

The health profiles of the nation and the individual community influence health education—not only the health topics taught in the classroom but also the techniques, resources and materials used. The financial base for schools also affects the quality of a health education program. Adequate funding will mean qualified teachers; up-to-date library and audiovisual materials, texts and curriculum materials; and funding for field trips. The financial base for programs often depends upon administrators having adequate knowledge about programs. Administrators must be kept informed of the progress and needs of the program.

Two other influencing factors are very much interrelated—the values of the community and potential areas of controversy springing from these values. Several actions can help control these factors, including:
• getting to know the community through its residents
• developing a profile of the community and using it as you interact with the population
• understanding the religious background of the community

Certain areas of the health curriculum touch upon very sensitive issues. As the curriculum is developed for the school year, health educators must keep families informed about topics and activities in the classroom and encourage techniques for involving families in the lessons.

The factors mentioned here influence the success of a health education program today. All of these influencing factors are interrelated and require new responses as they change. With thoughtful study and communication, however, they can be approached in ways that will have a positive influence and further the goals of the program.

Highlights of the Past

The early history of the United States reflects a situation similar to what we face today. The country was attempting to establish a system of government that would provide a direction toward the future. Challenges included numerous immigrants and many health problems. Regulations and laws were established; schools were constructed; churches were built. A system of order was developed.

Disease and health problems took their toll as the new settlers attempted to carve out an existence in this country. Poor sanitation was thought to be the cause of health problems, so sanitary commissions were established in larger communities. Physicians and others trained in these areas attempted to ferret out causes of epidemics and identify methods of controlling or preventing them. Some communities prohibited spitting in the street.

In 1850, Lemuel Shattuck wrote a *Report of the Sanitary Commission of Massachusetts*. The report stated that "it has recently been recommended that the science of physiology be taught in the public schools; and the recommendation should be universally approved and carried into effect as soon as persons can be found capable of teaching it." This was one of the first recommendations in the United States for teaching about health (i.e., physiology, hygiene).

The temperance movement that occurred during the 1800s

also influenced the teaching of health in the public schools. The American Society for the Promotion of Temperance had more than one million members. In 1874 the Women's Christian Temperance Union (WCTU) was organized. The WCTU was very influential in getting information about the effects of alcohol, tobacco and narcotics into textbooks. Physiology books used in the public schools often included a statement indicating that the book had been approved by the WCTU because it had a section on the evils of alcohol, tobacco and narcotics. This crusade resulted in the passage of legislation in 1890 requiring the teaching of physiology and hygiene in 38 states.

Along with the WCTU, other organizations related to health developed, including the American Medical Association, the American Public Health Association and the American Association for the Advancement of Physical Education. They all had a concern for and vested interest in health. The journal of the American Association for the Advancement of Physical Education frequently had articles on the teaching of hygiene.

At the turn of the century, many voluntary health organizations originated. The National Tuberculosis Association (now the American Lung Association) promoted open-air schools and developed materials for classroom teachers. Other health organizations that arose at this time were the American Cancer Society, the Society for Mental Hygiene and the National Safety Council.

One of the most significant organizations for health education to develop during this time was the Joint Committee on Health Problems in Education of the National Education Association (NEA) and the American Medical Association (AMA). This committee existed from 1911 until 1975. The Joint Committee was initiated by leaders of the AMA, who talked with some leaders of the NEA. The AMA leaders were concerned about the health subject matter being taught in schools; the NEA was concerned about the physical health status of school children. The Joint Committee was chaired by Thomas Wood, MD, a professor at Columbia University. Under Dr. Wood's leadership, the Joint Committee moved toward the development of a focus on health instruction, health services and healthful environment. Materials were developed expressing the viewpoints of both medicine and education on rural schools, health examinations and sanitation in the schools. These materials were widely distributed.

In 1924, the Joint Committee published its first book. *Health Education: A Program for Public Schools and Teacher Training Institutions* detailed the following concerns:
- the aims of health education
- the problems of health in the United States
- what the schools could do
- the subject matter for the teacher
- educational problems
- suggestions for courses of study in health education (inclusive of K-12)
- measurement of results
- training of teachers

This comprehensive document set the standard for the future. It was revised periodically over the years to update the substance. The Joint Committee also developed recommendations regarding health instruction, health problems of school children, environmental conditions in schools, and physical education activities. The committee kept a watchful eye on the education of children and made recommendations to significant people when necessary.

At the time of the Second World War, the same conditions existed as were apparent at the beginning of the First World War. Recruits and enlistees were not in good physical condition, and the finger of blame was pointed at the schools. As a result, health and physical education were again targeted for emphasis. Health and physical education were taught by a teacher prepared in both subjects, and the time allotted for teaching was limited in both areas. Health education was often taught only on days when the physical education classes could not be outside for activity.

This method of organizing for health instruction continued through the 1940s and into the 1950s. In the fifties, there was a surge in the field of science. Russia had launched a rocket, and the United States was fearful of being in second place. Blame was again directed at the schools. Students were not being prepared in the sciences and, therefore, the United States did not have trained scientists able to keep pace with the Russians. This concern launched a movement of curriculum reform in the schools.

Interestingly enough, the Joint Committee was still in existence and meeting regularly. Toward the end of the fifties, a recommendation was made to evaluate nationally what was occurring in health education, with the expectation that the results might demonstrate a need for curriculum reform.

Milestones in School Health Education

School health education has existed to some degree in the public schools of the United States since the mid-1800s. Each decade has fostered activities that focus on the relationship of education and health. Most of these activities have been crisis oriented and have not generated a quality of change that is effective over time. The early years of health education reflected the belief that knowledge about the "evils" would change actions and promote health. Since that time, research has indicated that cognitive skills are only part of changing behavior.

The following activities, with one exception, have occurred since 1960. They have been organized with a focus on long-term change and have involved leaders in health, education, government, and social, professional and voluntary agencies. The activities attempt to target specific audiences. These audiences are then cultivated and encouraged to bring about change in public schools for improved health education. Each activity or organization illustrates a structure and an action focused on change. School health education in the year 2000 will illustrate the effectiveness of these activities and organizations.

Health Education Terminology

Terminology in health education has evolved over the past 58 years through the efforts of the Association for the Advancement of Health Education. The rationale for defining terminology was to enable members of the profession of health education to communicate more effectively. Five different committees met during this period to consider terminology unique to health education. Reports of these committees were published in 1934, 1951, 1963, 1973 and 1991. Figure 1 summarizes the terms defined by each committee.

Each committee established its own procedures for arriving at final definitions. The 1934 committee prepared a list of common terms with definitions, then circulated them to people in the profession for their comments and suggestions. The committee developed definitions for ten terms (Committee Report of the Health Education Section of the APEA, 1934).

The 1951 committee limited terminology definitions to terms commonly used in school health (Committee on Terminology in School Health, 1951). Definitions were developed for these terms and submitted to a representative group of school health educators for their comments. These comments were then utilized in refining the terms.

The scope of terminology in 1963 was broadened to include

public health education and related terms in order to foster and improve understanding on the part of both school and public health educators (Committee on Terminology in School Health, 1963). This was accomplished by including representatives from organizations representing public health. After consideration of more than 150 terms, the 1963 committee developed definitions for 23 of them.

In 1973, the Committee on Health Education Terminology identified health education terms and agreed on the most common terms used by school and community health educators. After the terms were selected and definitions developed, the terms were reviewed by corresponding members and selected reviewers. Following the review, the terms were revised and refined into a final report.

The most recent compilation of terminology was published in 1991 (Report of the 1990 Joint Committee on Health Education Terminology, 1991). Committee members consisted of the delegates from the Coalition of National Health Education Organizations, a coalition of all of the professional associations with a direct concern for health education, plus a representative of the American Academy of Pediatrics.

A draft document was developed and circulated to a select number of outside reviewers for comment. The final report of terminology was organized around four categories: contextual definitions, primary health education definitions, definitions related to community settings, and definitions related to educational settings. (See Appendix B for the full text of the report.)

Health education terminology has evolved with the profession, and a study of the terms reveals not only the specific definitions but also the changing context of the profession. Each committee has expanded participation of organizations in the process, and the terminology has moved from a primary focus on school health to a much broader view of health education.

Figure 1
Health Education Terminology

1934
- health education
- school health education
- public health education
- hygiene
- sanitation

- health
- health instruction
- health service
- healthful school living
- health examination

1951
- school health program
- school health services
- health appraisal
- school health counseling
- school health education

- healthful school living
- health coordination
- school health council
- school health educator

1963
- dental examination
- dental inspection
- health appraisal
- health observation
- medical examination
- screening test
- cumulative school health record
- school health educator
- school health program
- healthful school living
- healthful school environment

- health science instruction
- school health services
- school health coordination
- school health nurse
- public health educator
- school medical advisor
- private health agency
- public health agency
- professional health agency
- school health education
- safety education
- health counseling

1973
- health education
- health science instruction
- community health education
- mass communications (in health)

- community organization (for health)
- patient education
- consumer participation (in health planning)

(continued)

Figure 1 (continued)

1973 (continued)

- private health agency
- public health agency
- group process
  (in health education)
- public (community) health
  educator
- health education of the public
- school health education
- health education program
- school health education
  curriculum guides
- health education resources

- school health education
  curriculum
- health environment
- health information
- school health educator
- health instruction
- school health program
- health science
- school health services
- health science educator
- voluntary health agency

1991

Contextual Definitions

- health
- health promotion and disease
  prevention
- healthy lifestyle

- official health agency
- voluntary health organization
- private health agency

Primary Health Education Definitions

- health education field
- health education process
- health education program
- health educator
- Certified Health Education
  Specialist (CHES)

- health education coordinator
- health education administrator
- health information
- health literacy
- health advising

Definitions Related to Community Settings

- community health education

- community health educator

Definitions Related to Educational Settings

- comprehensive school health
  program
- school health education
- school health services
- school health educator

- comprehensive school health
  instruction
- post-secondary health
  education program

School Health Education Study

The School Health Education Study (SHES) began in September 1961 with a grant from the Samuel Bronfman Foundation of New York City. The impetus for the study came from the efforts of Granville Larimore, MD, first deputy commissioner of the State Department of Health of New York; Herman Hilliboe, MD, professor and head of public health practice, Columbia University; and three educators working in school and college health education. This task force developed a proposal and presented it to the foundation.

As a result of the funding, Dr. Elena M. Sliepcevich was selected as the director of the study. Support from the foundation continued through the first year and was extended through 1965. The 3M Company provided financial support from 1966 until the conclusion of the project. An advisory committee was established. A larger committee of 16 individuals representing public health, medicine, school and college health education, and educational administration was then identified to offer expert guidance for the project's development.

From its inception to its conclusion in 1973, the School Health Education Study accomplished four major tasks:

1. The development of the book *Synthesis of Research in Selected Areas of Health Instruction* (1963), a summary of studies conducted from 1920 to 1963 in 14 areas related to health instruction.
2. A nationwide study of instructional practices in health education in public schools and a study of health behavior (knowledge, attitudes and practices) of students (elementary and secondary). This study is reported in *School Health Education Study: A Summary Report* (1964).
3. The selection of a writing group of eight people to develop and refine the philosophy of the conceptual approach to health

education, the development and testing of experimental curriculum materials in two areas, and the publication of *Health Education: A Conceptual Approach to Curriculum Design* (1967).
4. The writing and publication of curriculum materials not previously developed.

SHES was recognized as one of the leading curriculum projects in education. It included all of the processes deemed appropriate for curriculum development. SHES was one of many curricula developed during the education curriculum reform movement that began in 1956. The results of this study can still be observed in school health education today—in support for health education in kindergarten through grade 12; in support for a comprehensive, sequential curriculum; and in a focus on attitudes and practices as well as knowledge.

President's Committee on Health Education
President Richard Nixon's health message to Congress in February 1971 indicated that an individual has the major responsibility for her or his health, but little attention had been given to the health education of people. "There is no national instrument, no central force to stimulate and coordinate a comprehensive health education program," Nixon said. Nixon then established a Committee on Health Education in September 1971. Nineteen people, representing a variety of businesses and public interests, were selected for the committee. The charge to the committee was as follows (Department of Health, Education and Welfare, 1972):
• Describe the "state of the art" in health education of the public in the United States today.
• Define the nation's need for health education programs, and their basic characteristics, in terms of major groupings of health consumers.

- Establish goals, priorities, and immediate and long range objectives of a comprehensive, nationwide effort to raise the level of "health consumer citizenship."
- Propose the most appropriate scope, function, structure, organization, and financing of such an effort, possibly in the form of a "National Health Education Foundation."
- Develop a plan for the implementation of its recommendations.

A staff, staff assistants, staff council and consultants facilitated the numerous activities of the committee. The committee held eight public hearings in major cities, at which many hours of testimony were taken. Forty-seven states and Puerto Rico were represented in the testimony. Directors of 22 neighborhood health centers talked with the committee. Producers of health education materials and programs shared their successes and failures with materials. Papers were commissioned on such topics as motivation and behavior, school health, health education programs in hospitals, and cost effectiveness of health education programs in industry.

Many other data-gathering activities were conducted over a period of a year and a half to respond to the five goals. A report released in 1972 contained findings and recommendations. The findings were reported in the following areas:

- health problems and health education
- age groups and health education
- the health care delivery system and health education
- schools and colleges and health education
- employment and health education
- health education services
- leadership for health education

Significant to school health education were the recommendations that:
- Health education be explored for preschool children.
- Model state laws for school health education be developed and adopted.
- Feasibility of matching state funds with federal funds be explored to support school health education.
- Periodic surveys to determine health education needs and interests be administered to children and youth preschool through college.
- The Department of Health, Education and Welfare (now Health and Human Services) and/or its Office of Education initiate research and evaluation in school health education.

Another major recommendation was to establish a National Center for Health Education in the private sector of society. This recommendation was described in detail and, as a result, the National Center was established in 1975. Also as a result of a committee recommendation, the federal government provided a focus on school health education in the Office of Disease Prevention and Health Promotion in 1974. This then provided action in the public sector of society.

Coalition of National Health Education Organizations
The Coalition of National Health Education Organizations was formally established in 1972. Currently, this coalition consists of representation from the following organizations:
- Association for the Advancement of Health Education (AAHE)
- American College Health Association
- American Public Health Association, through its Public Health Education and School Health Education and Services sections
- American School Health Association

- Conference of State and Territorial Directors of Public Health Education
- Society for Public Health Education
- Society of State Directors of Health, Physical Education and Recreation

Feasibility studies for the coalition were initiated by the School Health Section (currently AAHE) of the American Association for Health, Physical Education and Recreation (currently AAHPERD) in 1971. After three meetings to explore a rationale and establish an agreement to provide structure and function, all of the organizations signed a working agreement.

The focus of the coalition is to mobilize resources of the health education profession to expand and improve health education in the United States (Cauffman, 1982). The five purposes are as follows:

1. Facilitate national-level coordination, collaboration and communication among the member organizations.
2. Provide a forum for the identification and discussion of health education issues.
3. Formulate recommendations and take appropriate action on issues affecting the member interests.
4. Serve as a communication and advisory resource for agencies, organizations and persons in the public and private sectors concerning health education issues.
5. Serve as a focus for the collaborative exploration and resolution of issues pertinent to professional health educators.

The coalition is in its twenty-first year of existence and has functioned extensively within the five purposes. Meetings have focused on federal legislation in health education, credentialing mechanisms for health education, and the development of position statements on critical issues, such as the need for health instruction in the elementary school and the need to establish health education as a basic subject in school. The coalition has been a forum for the profession and, through its collective strength, has made a difference in the arena of health education.

National Commission for Health Education Credentialing

Activities leading to the establishment of the National Commission for Health Education Credentialing in 1988 began in 1978. Representatives included:
- Health Education Section of the American College Health Association
- Public Health Education and School Health Education and Services sections of the American Public Health Association
- American School Health Association
- Association for the Advancement of Health Education
- Society for Public Health Education
- Society of State Directors of Health, Physical Education and Recreation
- State and Territorial Directors of Public Health Education

These representatives organized a conference of health educators from a variety of practice settings. The two purposes of the conference were to analyze the commonalities and differences that existed in the preparation of health educators for different practice settings and to determine the potential for developing acceptable guidelines for professional preparation that would include all practice settings of health educators. The conference, entitled "Preparation and Practice of Community, Patient, and School Health Educators," was sponsored by the Bureau of Health Professions of the Health Resources Administration of the Department of Health, Education and Welfare (now the Health Resources and Services Administration of the Department of Health and Human Services).

The National Task Force on the Preparation and Practice of Health Educators was formed at this conference. The task force was instructed by a consensus of the participants to pursue the development of a credentialing system for the health education profession. A five-step process was developed to provide direction for the accomplishment of the task. The process was to

1. delineate the role
2. verify and refine the role
3. prepare an educational resource document for professional preparation programs
4. develop a self-assessment instrument for practitioners
5. prepare materials and develop programs to ensure continuing competencies through continuing education

This process took nine years to develop. Very careful and extensive procedures were used to establish the framework of responsibilities and competencies that define the practice of health education and to establish criteria for certification. Professionals from throughout the United States and all settings of health education practice were employed in the process. Involvement of practitioners was important to achieve acceptance by the profession.

In 1988, the National Task Force moved to a more permanent status by incorporating and becoming the National Commission for Health Education Credentialing, a nonprofit agency supported by fees for service. The commission consists of nine commissioners who establish policy and three division boards to implement the three major purposes:

1. development and administration of a national competency-based examination
2. development and promulgation of standards of professional education
3. professional development through continuing education programs

Each division board is composed of seven members, all of whom are Certified Health Education Specialists (CHES), as are the members of the board of commissioners. The CHES designation assures employers and consumers that these educators have met national standards as health education professionals and are expanding their skills and knowledge through continuing education.

During an initial time period (October 1988 through April 1989), health educators could submit their professional credentials for evaluation according to specific criteria. If these criteria were fulfilled, the health educator became charter certified. The certification examination was initiated in 1990, and the current requirements for becoming certified include:

- completion of a professional program of study in the field of health education at the bachelor's degree level or above
- passing the certification examination

This activity of the National Commission for Health Education Credentialing helps strengthen health education as an established profession.

Michigan Model for Comprehensive School Health Education

The Michigan Model for Comprehensive School Health Education illustrates the process of combining the efforts of several state agencies to achieve comprehensive health education. The state has instituted a health education curriculum consisting of ten topics addressed at each grade level. The curriculum was created through the efforts of the departments of education, health, social services and mental health and the offices of substance abuse services, health and medical affairs, and highway safety planning. It allows for sequencing of topics and age-appropriate materials.

The Michigan Model, as it is known, was officially begun in 1984; however, much background work preceded that time (Association for the Advancement of Health Education and the American College of Preventive Medicine, 1985). Cooperative efforts of the state health and education departments initiated the actions. Involvement of many people, many agencies and the state legislature finally gave birth to the idea. From that point, curriculum materials were developed, teacher inservice was organized and classroom materials and evaluation procedures were developed.

Implementation has been gradual, starting with lower elementary grades and moving to upper level grades as materials have been developed. Evaluation of materials, students and teachers has provided information for refining materials and techniques.

The Michigan Model has been carefully planned, and implementation strategies have been characterized by the use of leaders at the local level. Even with excellent planning, however, problems arise. The planners and implementers of the Michigan Model have had to address the kind of controversy that surrounds health education information on human sexuality, substance use and values, to name a few. Other problems have included funding through the state legislature. These problems can be planned for and approached in numerous ways, and the Michigan Model is exemplary.

Seaside Health Education Conference
The Seaside Health Education Conference, which was initiated in 1977 in Seaside, Oregon, was the result of a needs assessment conducted by the health education specialist of the Oregon Department of Education, Len Tritsch. The assessment indicated that health educators in Oregon needed skills to become change agents within their communities if health education was to prosper.

The first Seaside Conference theme was "Health Education at the Crossroads." There were 152 people registered. One of the goals was to create a health education network throughout the state. Other goals included:
- Assess the effectiveness of health education in Oregon schools.
- Share successful health education techniques with others.
- Analyze personal practices of daily eating, drinking and exercise.
- Participate in experiences that enhance positive feelings about the participants themselves and their profession.

This conference led to annual conferences in Oregon and ultimately to conferences of a similar nature in 25 states. Two factors have contributed to the success of these conferences. The first has been the requirement of team participation. Districts send administrators, teachers, staff and community members to attend the conferences together. The second has been the requirement that the team attend the entire conference. Team meetings are scheduled, and objectives of the teams are developed and achieved. In effect, success is built into the conference structure.

Many people and agencies have been involved in the fifteen years of these conferences. Those concerned with school health education have set up displays with materials appropriate to conference themes. The name of the conference was changed to Seaside Health Promotion Conference when organizers realized that the themes and activities were promoting wellness as a lifestyle. The conference director, Len Tritsch, estimated that the lives of 99 percent of Oregon school children had been touched in some way by the action plans developed by the teams in the first five years of the conference.

Recognizing the success of the conferences, the Office of Disease Prevention and Health Promotion (Department of Health and Human Services) and the U.S. Department of Transportation provided funding for out-of-state teams to attend. These teams were obligated to return to their states and attempt to provide a similar experience in health promotion. As a result of the funding, 25 states sent teams.

At this point, a National Network of School Conferences on School Worksite Wellness was established. The network attempts to maintain communication among the states and their expanding programs. Many of the programs have moved into small business health promotion. With strong leadership in a state, the potential for implementing health promotion activities at the grass roots level is unlimited.

State School Health Education Project

The Education Commission of the States (ECS) received a grant from the American Council of Life Insurance and the Health Insurance Association of America to develop a document on the health education of young people that would be a resource for the education and health professions.

ECS convened a meeting of representatives from the following agencies:
- state boards of education
- chief state school officers
- state legislators
- local school administrators

- U.S. Department of Education
- U.S. Department of Health and Human Services
- American School Health Association
- Association for the Advancement of Health Education
- American Public Health Association (School Health Education and Services Section)
- National Center for Health Education

This State School Health Education Task Force met several times with Mary Noak, project director, to study school health education and to develop a policy statement exemplifying state-level commitment to health education. The following ten recommendations were made (Noak, 1982):

1. State education agencies should encourage local school boards and administrators to include health education in the curriculum in elementary and secondary schools.
2. State education agencies should promote health education as a responsibility shared by the family, school and community.
3. State education policymakers should support the development and improvement of school health education programs by utilizing the direct and indirect means available to them in their official capacity.
4. State education agencies should provide technical assistance to local districts in planning and implementing school health education programs.
5. State education agencies should promote the development of comprehensive school health education programs.
6. State education agencies should encourage local school boards to undertake a participatory planning process in the development of school health education programs.
7. State and local education agencies should ensure the presence of trained and qualified teachers in school health education programs.

8. State and local education agencies should assist in developing a system of information exchange about health education.
9. State education agencies should encourage the evaluation of school health education programs and assist local districts in developing appropriate evaluation processes.
10. State education agencies should encourage federal agencies to channel categorical funds in a manner that will enhance comprehensive school health education program development.

These policy recommendations were expanded to include important considerations. The following statements and sections were included in the culminating publication, *Recommendations for School Health Education: A Handbook for State Policymakers* (1981):

• suggested policy statement on school health education for state boards of education
• the importance of school health education
• the current status of school health education
• problems in program development and implementation
• description of recommended content areas in comprehensive school health education

This document was distributed to governors, state legislators and educators for the improvement of school health education in their states.

The work of the project provides an excellent example of ways organizations and agencies outside of school health education can be supportive of a positive direction to strengthen the educational process and influence society. ECS, a nonprofit organization, has been in existence since 1966 and has influence on education within the states.

National Health Promotion and Disease Prevention Objectives

Soon after assuming office in 1977 as the Secretary of the Department of Health, Education and Welfare (now Health and Human Services), Joseph A. Califano, Jr., asked the Surgeon General to begin work on the first Surgeon General's Report on Health Promotion and Disease Prevention. The report was to emphasize the prevention of disease. "Its purpose," Califano stated, "is to encourage a second public health revolution in the history of the United States" (Public Health Service, 1979). (The first revolution was the struggle against infectious diseases.)

The document *Healthy People: The Surgeon General's Report on Health Promotion and Disease Prevention* was published in 1979. It is a landmark in the history of public health in the United States. The document focused on a healthier America. Risks to good health were examined and analyzed. Health goals to be achieved by 1990 were established for infants, children, adolescents and young adults, adults and older adults. The document identified actions for achieving the goals for these age groups through preventive health services, health protection and health promotion. The intention was to monitor the achievement of these goals nationally during the time period to 1990.

Some health agencies and organizations at the national, state and local levels began to assume responsibility for achieving these goals. The leadership of these groups attempted to integrate the national goals into the goals of their organizations. Progress was slow, not only in moving toward the goals but also in implementing activities targeted to the goals. The major objectives were to lower the death rate for four of the five age groups and to reduce the days of restricted activity for older adults. When the data were examined in 1987, three years before 1990, it was encouraging to see the progress. (Data for 1990 were not available at the time of this writing.)

Work on *Healthy People 2000: National Health Promotion and Disease Prevention Objectives* was initiated in 1987. The Healthy People Consortium consists of 271 national organizations and 54 state and territorial health departments. Testimony obtained from public hearings across the country served as resource material for the development of the health objectives. Once developed, the objectives were reviewed and commented on by more than ten thousand people. The objectives were then refined and revised to produce the final report.

This document reexamined the major health problems of the five age groups from the 1979 report and special populations (people with low income, minority groups and people with disabilities). The three major goals for the year 2000 were identified:

1. Increase the span of healthy life for Americans.
2. Reduce health disparities among Americans.
3. Achieve access to preventive services for all Americans.

These goals are to be achieved through health promotion, health protection and preventive services. Within each area, specific objectives are identified for action. Health promotion objectives deal with the following areas:

- physical activity and fitness
- nutrition
- tobacco
- alcohol and other drugs
- family planning
- mental health and mental disorders
- violent and abusive behavior
- educational and community-based programs

Health protection objectives fall within the following areas:
• unintentional injuries
• occupational safety and health
• environmental health
• food and drug safety
• oral health

Preventive services objectives deal with the following areas:
• maternal and infant health
• heart disease and stroke
• cancer
• diabetes and chronic disabling conditions
• HIV infection
• sexually transmitted diseases
• immunization and infectious diseases
• clinical preventive services

Health education program planners can find many objectives that will be relevant to their work setting in these three areas. Many objectives can be implemented through K-12 school curricula. The National Health Promotion and Disease Prevention Objectives can be achieved at the grass-roots level. Through shared responsibilities at the community level, the year 2000 will see a healthier population in the United States.

National School Health Education Coalition
The National School Health Education Coalition (NaSHEC) represents more than fifty national organizations with an interest in promoting quality and comprehensive school health education. Established in 1982, its goals include:
• cooperation and information sharing among member organizations

- supporting the establishment of state and local coalitions
- developing resource materials to support school health education
- acting as advocates for comprehensive school-based health education

NaSHEC includes organizations such as federal agencies, voluntary organizations, professional organizations and business agencies. The representatives meet regularly in Washington, D.C. The coalition provides an effective way of targeting issues in school health education and channeling the interests, materials and energies of the organizations toward support of comprehensive school health education.

The national organizations represented in NaSHEC have their counterparts in state and local settings. Thus, actions taken at the national level can reach the grass-roots level quickly if there is cooperation at this level. Coalition building at the state and local level is critical to comprehensive school health education.

NaSHEC also monitors legislation in Congress relevant to school health education. Newsletters with this information are circulated periodically, so if action is needed in the way of letters or phone calls to support or act against pending legislation, it can be accomplished quickly.

Met Life's Healthy Me Program

In 1985, Met Life launched a new national initiative designed to promote comprehensive school health education programs. Healthy Me, which took place over a five-year period from 1985 through 1989, was the latest in Met Life's long history of underwriting projects focused on helping children and youth make wise decisions about health. Committed to accomplishing this through schools to a large degree, Met Life discovered in a 1985 survey that only about one-third of the nation's public school children received comprehensive health instruction. The survey demonstrated a clear need to teach about health in ways that make a difference. Healthy Me sought to do this through identifying and rewarding exemplary programs that could serve as models for others.

This $5 million initiative was administered by the Health and Safety Education Division of Met Life and funded by the Metropolitan Life Foundation. Award recipients were chosen by a panel of ten health and education professionals around the country. In addition to the awards given to schools with outstanding comprehensive health education programs, funds were provided for community coalitions that actively promoted such programs, for classroom teachers who wanted to improve their health education skills, for wellness programs for teachers and other school personnel, and for information programs designed to raise awareness of effective school health education.

Awards to schools were the centerpiece of the initiative. One hundred fifty schools received Healthy Me awards of $5,000 for multitopic, multigrade programs, or $3,000 for multitopic programs designed for a single grade or special population. Schools that successfully incorporated HIV/AIDS education into their comprehensive program received an additional $2,000. A compendium of award-winning programs has been published (Metropolitan Life Foundation, 1990).

At the end of the five-year period, a three-part survey of public school students, teachers and parents of children attending public schools was designed and conducted by Louis Harris and Associates. The survey was designed to determine the knowledge, attitudes and behavior of school children on a range of topics, as well as teachers' and parents' perceptions of children's levels of knowledge. It covered specific areas regarding how much children know about nutrition, safety, health maintenance, smoking, substance abuse and HIV/AIDS; the state of their emotional health; and the extent of their physical exercise. The survey also was designed in part to assess the impact of comprehensive programs on the nation's school children. For that purpose, it included some of the Healthy Me award-winning schools. The results describe the current state of the nation's school health education, identifying where it is successful and where it falls short. The survey results also provide evidence that comprehensive programs are an effective approach. Complete results are contained in the publication *Health—You've Got to Be Taught* (Louis Harris and Associates, 1989).

Code Blue

In 1989, the National Association of State Boards of Education recognized the dangerous trends in adolescent health. They asked the American Medical Association to join them in the formation of a National Commission on the Role of the School and the Community in Improving Adolescent Health. The Division of Adolescent and School Health of the Center for Chronic Disease Prevention and Health Promotion, Centers for Disease Control and Prevention, supported the project financially through a cooperative agreement.

Many sectors of society with major concerns for adolescent health were involved through representatives to the commission. The focus was on adolescence, primarily ages ten through eighteen, a time when attitudes, knowledge and actions can affect present and future health and well-being.

The commission gathered data from many sources, including:
- an invitational conference on adolescent health held at the Carter Presidential Center in Atlanta
- field visits to the states of Vermont and Florida

- a national meeting of state officials in Michigan
- feedback on commission thinking from 300 individuals' knowledge of adolescent health and public policy
- conversation and written responses from adolescents

These data sources yielded a wealth of information to be organized for actions at the local, state, and national levels.

The commission prepared a document titled *Code Blue: Uniting for Healthier Youth*. The term *Code Blue* was used because it signals a life-threatening emergency in hospitals and sets in motion a number of actions to save an individual's life. The document should initiate action among agencies, organizations and others to focus on adolescence as a critical period of life. Strategies developed as the result of these actions have the potential to reverse the growing trend of adolescent health problems (National Commission on the Role of the School and the Community in Improving Adolescent Health, 1990).

The commission recommended four major actions:

1. Guarantee all adolescents access to health services regardless of ability to pay.
2. Make communities the front line in the battle for adolescent health.
3. Organize services around people, not people around services.
4. Urge schools to play a much stronger role in improving adolescent health.

The report explained each recommendation in detail, and then described specific actions to implement the recommendations. A significant aspect of the fourth recommendation was that schools should implement a comprehensive school health education program kindergarten through grade 12. Even though the document is about adolescents, starting health education at kindergarten will strengthen the foundation of developing attitudes, knowledge, and actions. *Code Blue* has been distributed nationally and provides an excellent call to action for community members.

School Health Education Today

Today, school health education is one component of a comprehensive school health program:

> ...the comprehensive school health program...includes the development, delivery, and evaluation of a planned instructional program and other activities for students pre-school through grade 12, for parents and school staff, and is designed to positively influence the health knowledge, attitudes, and skills of individuals. (Report of the 1990 Joint Committee on Health Education Terminology, 1991)

A more inclusive description was developed by the Division of Adolescent and School Health, National Center for Chronic Disease Prevention and Health Promotion, Centers for Disease Control and Prevention. This description is used by the division as they work with state and local education agencies:

> Health Education: A planned, sequential, K-12 curriculum that addresses the physical, mental, emotional, and social dimensions of health. The curriculum is designed to motivate and assist students to maintain and improve their health-related risk behaviors. It allows students to develop and demonstrate increasingly sophisticated health-related knowledge, attitudes, skills, and practices. The curriculum is

comprehensive and includes a variety of topics such
as personal health, family health, community health,
consumer health, environmental health, family life,
mental and emotional health, injury prevention and
safety, nutrition, prevention and control of disease,
and substance use and abuse. Health education is
taught by qualified teachers who have been trained to
teach the subject.

Recent data (Lovato, Allensworth and Chan, 1989) indicate
that 32 states (63 percent) require health education to be taught
sometime during kindergarten through grade 12, and 13 additional states (25 percent) require a combination of physical education and health education. If grade level requirements are reviewed,
19 states (37 percent) require that health education be taught
sometime during grades one through six, and three additional
states combine the health education requirement with physical
education. The combining of health with physical education is a
holdover from the early development of these two subject areas.
School systems and state legislatures have been slow to recognize
the differences and initiate change.

At the secondary level, 22 states (43 percent) require that
health education be taught sometime during grades seven and
eight, and four additional states still require health education
combined with physical education. Twenty-five states (49 percent) require a course in health education for high school graduation, and six additional states (12 percent) require the combination
for graduation. These statistics demonstrate that the goal of comprehensive school health education in all states and all schools
remains a challenge for the profession and for health educators.

References

Association for the Advancement of Health Education and the American College of Preventive Medicine. 1985. *Health education today: Investing in our children's future.* Washington, DC: American College of Preventive Medicine.

Cauffman, J. G. 1982. *A history of the coalition of national health education organizations: Its first ten years and future directions.* Muncie, IN: Eta Sigma Gamma.

Centers for Disease Control and Prevention, National Center for Chronic Disease Prevention and Health Promotion, Division of Adolescent and School Health. 1991. *Developing comprehensive school health programs to prevent important health problems and improve educational outcomes: A guide for state and local education agencies.* Atlanta, GA.

Committee on Health Education Terminology. 1973. Report of the Joint Committee on Health Education Terminology. *School Health Review* 6 (12): 25-30.

Committee on Terminology in School Health. 1963. Health education terminology. *The Journal of School Health* 35 (3): 119-122.

Committee on Terminology in School Health. 1951. Report of the Committee on Terminology in School Health Education. *The Journal of the American Association of Health and Physical Education* 51 (9): 14.

Committee Report of the Health Education Section of the APEA. 1934. Definition of terms in health education. *The Journal of Health and Physical Education* 25 (12): 16.

Davis, T. M., S. Koch and D. J. Ballard. 1991. The nature of Seaside-style health education conferences. *Journal of Health Education* 22 (2): 73-75, 123.

Department of Health, Education and Welfare, Health Services and Mental Health Administration. 1972. *The report of the President's Committee on Health Education.* Washington, DC.

Division of Adolescent and School Health. 1991. Developing comprehensive school health programs to prevent important health problems and improve educational outcomes. Paper. Atlanta, GA: Centers for Disease Control and Prevention.

Louis Harris and Associates. 1989. *Health—you've got to be taught: An evaluation of comprehensive health education in American public schools.* New York: Metropolitan Life Foundation.

Lovato, C. Y., D. Allensworth and F. A. Chan. 1989. *School health in America: An assessment of state policies to protect and improve the health of students.* 5th ed. Kent, OH: American School Health Association.

Metropolitan Life Foundation. 1990. *Healthy me initiative to promote excellence in school health education: A compendium of award winning programs, 1985-1989.* New York.

National Commission on the Role of the School and the Community in Improving Adolescent Health. 1990. *Code blue: Uniting for healthier youth.* Alexandria, VA: National Association of State Boards of Education.

National Task Force on the Preparation and Practice of Health Educators, Inc. 1983. *A guide for the development of competency-based curricula for entry-level health educators.* New York: National Center for Health Education Credentialing.

Noak, M. 1982. *State school policy support for school health education: A review and analysis.* Denver, CO: Education Commission of the States.

Public Health Service. 1979. *Healthy people: The surgeon general's report on health promotion and disease prevention.* Washington, DC: U.S. Department of Health and Human Services.

Report of the 1990 Joint Committee on Health Education Terminology. 1991. *Journal of Health Education* 22 (2): 97-108.

School Health Education Study. 1967. *Health education: A conceptual approach to curriculum design.* St. Paul, MN: 3M Education Press.

School Health Education Study. 1963. *Synthesis of research in selected areas of health instruction.* Washington, DC.

Shattuck, L. 1850. *Report of the Sanitary Commission of Massachusetts.* Boston: Dutton and Wentworth. (Facsimile ed.)

Sliepcevich, E. M. 1964. *School health education study: A summary report.* Washington, DC: School Health Education Study.

State School Health Education Project. 1981. *Recommendations for school health education: A handbook for state policymakers.* Denver, CO: Education Commission of the States.

U.S. Department of Health and Human Services, Public Health Service. 1991. *Healthy people 2000: National health promotion and disease prevention objectives.* DHHS Publication No. (PHS) 91-50212. Washington, DC.

Chapter 3

An Essential Strategy to Improve the Health and Education of Americans

Lloyd J. Kolbe, PhD

This chapter was presented as the Milton J. E. Senn Memorial Lecture at the 1992 American Academy of Pediatrics Annual Meeting. It outlines important challenges that currently confront the nation, describes why school health programs have become an essential strategy to improve both the health and education of our people, and portrays what the nation and its pediatricians must do if our schools are to meet the needs of Americans in the twenty-first century.

The demography and lifestyles of Americans changed during the twentieth century, and our health and education problems changed concomitantly. Today, one in four children lives with a single parent; one in five lives in poverty; one in five is of a minority race; and one in ten has a physical or mental disability (U.S. Department of Commerce, 1989, 1990; Commission on Minority Participation in Education and American Life, 1988; Hodgkinson, 1989). Each of these factors increases the likelihood of both health problems and educational failure.

The major health problems that confront our nation today are caused in large part by behaviors established during youth (e.g., tobacco, alcohol and drug use), and we pay increasingly to treat these health problems. In 1960 we paid 5 percent of our gross national product for health care; in 1991 we paid 12 percent; and by the year 2020 (given current trends) we will pay 23 to 32 percent (Advisory Council on Social Security, 1991). The increasing cost of health care is particularly detrimental to the one in five students who have no health insurance, and many health problems that afflict students erode both their health status and educational achievement.

Indeed, American students score no better today on standardized measures of educational achievement than their counterparts did twenty years ago (Mullis, Owen and Phillips, 1990). In science (Lapointe, Askew and Mead, 1992) and mathematics (Lapointe, Mead and Askew, 1992), American students score worse than their peers in most western industrialized nations. Furthermore, about 13 percent of White, 22 percent of African-American and 40 percent of Hispanic 19 to 20 year olds have not completed high school (National Center for Education Statistics, 1991). These measures of achievement bode ill for American youth, whose jobs will require more education, who will face more international competition, and who will support more retirees than their predecessors.

Given these challenges, school health programs could become one of the most efficient means the nation could employ to prevent the major health problems that confront us. By preventing health problems that afflict our young, and the adults they become, school health programs also could help improve educational outcomes, could help reduce the spiraling costs of health care, and thus could help improve economic productivity. Accordingly, during the past five years, about two dozen major reports have called for the nation to reconceive and regenerate its school health programs.

School health programs are essential to attain both national education goals and national health objectives by the year 2000. Between now and the year 2000, our nation will institute both education reform and health care reform. Thus, the actions we take (or fail to take) during the next few years to ensure that school health programs become part of education and health care reform will have a lasting impact.

What School Health Programs Could Become

From the late 1800s until the late 1900s, the school health program was conceived to have three components: health education, health services and health environments. During the 1980s, more sophisticated conceptions of the school health program were proposed. The Centers for Disease Control and Prevention (CDC) conceives the school health program to have eight interdependent components (Kolbe, 1986; Allensworth and Kolbe, 1987):

- health education
- health services
- biophysical and psychosocial environments
- counseling, psychological and social services
- integrated efforts of schools and communities to improve health
- food service
- physical education and physical activity
- health programs for faculty and staff

Such programs could enable the nation to efficiently implement and integrate primary, secondary and tertiary disease and injury prevention interventions for the 45 million youth who attend school every school day. In the lexicon of public health and medicine, this means that schools could prevent many health problems from occurring, detect health problems that do occur during their early stages when they are most treatable, and treat those problems that have not been or cannot be prevented, to preclude adverse effects on health and education. This chapter will focus on how two components of the school health program, school health education and school health services, could prevent and mitigate our most pressing public health problems.

Primary Prevention Through Comprehensive School Health Education

To understand how schools could prevent major health problems from occurring (i.e., through primary prevention), one must first understand the nature of those problems. Reviews of the leading causes of mortality and morbidity suggest that only six categories of behavior cause most of our major health problems:
- behaviors that cause unintentional and intentional injuries
- drug and alcohol use
- sexual behaviors that cause sexually transmitted disease (STD), including HIV infection, and unintended pregnancies
- tobacco use
- inadequate physical activity
- dietary patterns that cause disease

These behaviors usually are established during youth, persist into adulthood and are interrelated. They contribute simultaneously to poor health, education and social outcomes; and they are preventable (Kolbe, 1990; Kann, 1993).

One of the most efficient means of preventing these behaviors is comprehensive school health education, definitions of which have been offered by various groups during the past few decades

(Education Commission of the States, 1981; National Professional School Health Education Organizations, 1984; National Commission on the Role of the School and the Community in Improving Adolescent Health, 1990; Joint Committee on Health Education Terminology, 1991; U.S. Congress, 1991). CDC and many other agencies believe that planned and sequential, kindergarten through grade 12, comprehensive school health education programs, which purposefully integrate health education about important categorical topics (e.g., HIV, STD, unintended pregnancy, alcohol, drugs, tobacco), can be more effective and efficient than desultory school efforts to address single categorical topics without a broader school health education program framework.

Support for school health education grew during the late 1980s, principally through three initiatives. First, Congress provided roughly $500 million per year for the U.S. Department of Education to help schools provide drug abuse education. Second, Congress provided roughly $4 million per year for the Department of Education to support comprehensive school health education demonstration projects. And third, Congress provided roughly $40 million per year for CDC to help schools provide HIV education.

CDC Efforts to Improve School Health Programs

In 1988, CDC established a National Center for Chronic Disease Prevention and Health Promotion, within which it created a new Division of Adolescent and School Health (DASH). The mission of DASH is to identify major health risks and health problems among youth, monitor the prevalence of these health events over time, implement national programs to prevent these events, and evaluate the impact of those programs.

During the last few years, DASH has built the infrastructure necessary to enable the nation's 100,000 schools to prevent sexual and injecting drug use behaviors that spread HIV infection. This infrastructure, which has been described in more detail elsewhere (Moore et al., 1992), includes seven ongoing interactive elements:

- about sixty programmatic and scientific staff in DASH, about a third of whom comprise a program branch organized to provide technical and financial assistance to agencies, and about a third of whom comprise a research branch organized to assess and consequently improve those programs
- surveillance systems to identify and monitor major health events among youth and efforts to prevent those events
- fiscal and technical support for every state and 17 large city education agencies to implement programs
- fiscal and technical support for more than twenty national education and health agencies (e.g., the National Association of State Boards of Education and the American Medical Association) to support programs
- an information development and dissemination system, one function of which is to develop school health guidelines
- more than fifty school health training and demonstration centers across the nation
- an evaluation system to assess and improve the effectiveness of program efforts.

DASH also is implementing efforts to help prevent HIV infection and other important health problems among American college students and youth in high-risk situations, and among school-age youth globally.

From the very beginning, however, CDC built this infrastructure as a means not only to help prevent HIV infection but also to help prevent other important health risks and health problems as resources became available. Indeed, many believe that HIV education programs, and other such categorical programs, can be more effective if they purposefully are implemented as an integral part of the broader school health program.

In 1992, CDC started using the infrastructure established to help schools prevent HIV infection to also help schools prevent other important health problems in the District of Columbia and three states with the highest overall mortality rates: Arkansas, Florida and West Virginia. In 1993, Wisconsin was added to the list. West Virginia will serve as a national demonstration and training center and will provide funds for interested officials from other states to visit West Virginia and examine its efforts.

CDC will provide fiscal and technical support to each of these four states to accomplish two functions. First, CDC will provide support to establish a senior policy position in the office of the state school superintendent, and a similar position in the office of the state health commissioner, to work independently and jointly to improve all components of school health programs in that state. As a major part of this function, each state may help public and private health care providers and insurers to deliver health care services through schools by establishing the necessary organizational means, personnel, legal authorities and mechanisms for integrating and financing such services, especially for the most needy students.

Second, CDC will provide support for each of the four state departments of education to establish a comprehensive school health education position to integrate efforts to reduce risk behaviors in each of the six categories described earlier. As part of this function, CDC will provide support for these four states to reduce risk behaviors in each of the following categories: tobacco use, diets that cause disease, physical inactivity, and sexual behaviors that cause HIV infection and other STD. At this time, CDC is not providing categorical resources to reduce sexual behaviors that cause unintended pregnancy, behaviors that cause unintentional and intentional injuries, or drug and alcohol use (although cooperative agreements with these states are written to support such programs if resources become available).

To accomplish these two functions, CDC and the four demonstration states will work with four core federal agencies—the U.S. Department of Health and Human Services (DHHS) Office of Disease Prevention and Health Promotion, the DHHS Office of the Assistant Secretary for Planning and Evaluation, the DHHS Health Resources and Services Administration (HRSA), and the U.S. Department of Education Office of the Assistant Secretary for Elementary and Secondary Education—and with other relevant categorical agencies as warranted (e.g., the U.S. Department of Agriculture and the President's Council on Physical Fitness and Sports). In addition, these federal and state agencies hope to work with the Council of Chief State School Officers, the Association of State and Territorial Health Officers, and the American Public Welfare Association (which represent the nation's state school superintendents, state health commissioners and state social service directors respectively) to ensure the success of the four demonstration states and to examine the potential for replicating similar efforts in the other 47 states.

To help manage activities with the demonstration states, DASH has added a new special projects branch that includes staff with expertise in preventive health services, adolescent health, tobacco, diet and physical activity. In 1993, this branch will convene relevant national organizations to help CDC develop separate guidelines for school programs to prevent tobacco use, diets that cause disease, and physical inactivity, and guidelines for comprehensive school health education programs. These guidelines will address multiple components of the school health program, including the physical education program, the school food service program and policies governing tobacco use in the school environment. Staff in the special projects branch will help implement these school health guidelines in the demonstration states.

Also in 1993, CDC will invite the remaining 47 states to apply for support to perform the two functions summarized earlier. In 1993, CDC will provide support for one or two of these 47 states, and in subsequent years may provide support for other states that apply for and are approved for funding in 1993. In addition, in 1993, CDC will invite national education, health and social service organizations to apply for support to help improve the capacity of schools and other agencies that serve youth to prevent HIV infection and other important health problems among youth. CDC will provide such support for twenty to thirty national organizations.

In 1992 a bill, currently pending in Congress, was introduced to authorize $500 million to create healthy American schools. If Congress passes and funds this Healthy Students–Healthy Schools Act, it would enable CDC to provide fiscal and technical support for state and local education agencies to develop and maintain comprehensive school health education programs in our nation's schools.

National Health and Education Goals

Such school health education programs are essential to attain important National Health Objectives and National Education Goals. National Health Objective 8.4 states that "By the year 2000, [we should] increase to 75 percent the proportion of the Nation's elementary and secondary schools that provide planned and sequential kindergarten through twelfth grade quality [or comprehensive] school health education." Relatedly, other National Health Objectives call for schools to provide education about specific categorical health problems, "preferably as part of quality [i.e., comprehensive] school health education," including education about nutrition, tobacco, human sexuality, HIV, sexually transmitted disease, injury prevention, conflict resolution, and drugs and alcohol (U.S. Department of Health and Human Services, 1991).

Achieving the last three of these National Health Objectives (i.e., providing education to prevent injuries, violent conflicts and drug and alcohol use) will be vital to achieve National Education Goal 6, which states that "By the year 2000, every school in America will be free of drugs and violence and will offer a disciplined environment conducive to learning" (National Education Goals Panel, 1991).

In 1991, the U.S. Public Health Service (PHS) established a Life Science Education Initiative to achieve two goals: to foster scientific literacy (including biomedical scientific literacy) in the U.S. population, and to ensure that adequate numbers of well-trained biomedical personnel are available to meet future national needs (National Institutes for Health, 1992). As a key part of this initiative, CDC and other PHS agencies are acting to help schools improve and link life science education and health education, and to help American students understand the scientific basis for health promotion and disease prevention. Thus, this initiative could help achieve National Education Goal 4, which states that "By the year 2000, U.S. students will be the first in the world in science and mathematics achievement" (National Education Goals Panel, 1991).

Given the nature of health and education problems today, education about health is as important as education about science and mathematics. In effect, school health education could help immunize our young people against behavioral causes of illness and death, as school health services help immunize them against infectious causes. School health services also might provide secondary and tertiary disease and injury prevention.

Secondary and Tertiary Prevention Through School Health Services

Various preventive and acute health care services can be provided to youth largely through private medical practices, health maintenance organizations, hospitals, community health centers and schools. Schools could provide an efficient means to detect and address health problems (i.e., facilitate secondary and tertiary prevention) simply because they serve all children, rich and poor alike, every school day for thirteen developmentally critical years. If health services are to be provided through schools, however, health, education and social service agencies will need to establish the necessary organizational means, personnel, legal authorities and mechanisms for integrating and financing such services. Public and private health care providers and insurers will need to work closely with school administrators to determine means by which health care providers might systematically deliver health services through schools, especially for the most needy students.

During the course of the twentieth century, three means evolved to provide health services through schools: the traditional school nurse, nurse practitioners in schools, and school-based or school-linked clinics. Recent events have stirred more interest in the third means, school clinics. A U.S. Congress Office of Technology Assessment report entitled *Adolescent Health* described several options to support school-linked or community-based clinics for adolescents (U.S. Congress, 1991). The Advisory Council on Social Security recommended that the federal government enable states to establish health clinics in or near elementary schools and share with states the costs of providing health and dental services for poor children (Advisory Council on Social Security, 1991). State departments of health would operate the clinics either directly or through arrangements with health care providers.

In 1992, although funds were not provided, President Bush requested in his FY93 Budget $6 million for the Health Resources and Services Administration to enable 35 to 50 eligible agencies to provide school-linked or school-based health services to disadvantaged children three to twelve years old and to their families (Bureau of Health Care Delivery and Assistance, 1992). Eligible agencies would include funded community and migrant health centers, health care for the homeless programs, health care for the residents of public housing programs, and other federally qualified health centers.

Schools thus could provide preventive health services through one or some combination of three means—the traditional school nurse, nurse practitioners in schools, and school-linked or school-based clinics. For any of these means, the school nurse could serve as a linchpin for providing certain health services, as well as for helping to coordinate the broader school health program. Because these three means provide a progressively greater range of services, they require that school nurses and others acquire progressively greater training, credentials and legal authority (Pearson, 1992).

These three means also require progressively advanced mechanisms for integrating and financing necessary services. Indeed, because educational achievement suffers from fragmented efforts to serve children and families who have multiple education, health and social problems, the need to integrate, or co-locate, education, health and social services through schools has become more compelling. Numerous strategies and models have been designed to integrate preventive health and social services through schools, and the Department of Education and DHHS recently compiled a *Practical Guide to School-Linked Service Integration.*

In 1992 a bill, currently pending in Congress, was introduced to authorize $250 million per year to help coordinate and deliver comprehensive education, health and social services to youth in school-based, school-linked or community-based locations. Financing for school health services will need to be provided and integrated from a wide range of sources, including federal, state and local health, education, human service, agriculture, labor and juvenile justice programs (Farrow and Joe, 1992). One source of funds available to help state health departments improve school health programs is the Preventive Health and Health Services Block Grant (Public Law 102-531).

Two prominent sources of funds for school health services might be Medicaid and Chapter 1. Congress recently expanded the Medicaid program to phase in coverage for all poor children under 19 years of age by the year 2002. About 80 percent of Medicaid-eligible children currently receive Medicaid-reimbursed services in a given year (Health Care Financing Administration, 1993). Medicaid's Early Periodic Screening, Diagnosis and Treatment (EPSDT) Program is designed to provide comprehensive health services and case management for children enrolled in Medicaid. In 1992, the Health Care Financing Administration published *EPSDT: A Guide for Educational Programs* to acquaint school officials with state Medicaid agencies, the EPSDT program and benefits of participating.

Chapter 1 of Title I of the Elementary and Secondary Education Act is the chief federal program designed to meet special needs of educationally deprived children. In general, Chapter 1 funds can be used only for students who are educationally deprived. However, for schools in which at least 75 percent of the students are from poor families, funds may be used to benefit all students in the school. Currently, about 2,100 of 7,000 potentially eligible elementary schools have successfully applied to become such schoolwide Chapter 1 projects.

Differences in eligibility criteria between Medicaid and Chapter 1 programs create a barrier to integrating covered services for children in poor families and communities. To address this barrier, DHHS and the Department of Education have been examining whether states might be given the option to extend Medicaid EPSDT eligibility to all preschool and elementary school children in areas that receive schoolwide Chapter 1 funding, provided that the states deliver relevant school-linked health care services through case-managed, coordinated care mechanisms. Thus, a capitated, coordinated approach could be used to provide health services to all school-age and preschool-age children within such areas. California, Ohio, Pennsylvania, Texas and West Virginia are exploring the feasibility of using and integrating Chapter 1 and Medicaid in this way.

In addition, CDC is providing support for the Columbia University School of Public Health to identify major barriers that prevent schools from providing effective health services and to suggest actions to help schools address these problems.

National Health and Education Goals Revisited

Thus, schools could help ensure that all students, but especially the most needy, receive the health services they need to learn and stay in school. The first National Education Goal states that "By the year 2000, all children in America will start school ready to learn." The intent of this goal is to ensure that children receive the parental, social and health care support they need so that when they first enter preschool or kindergarten they are ready to learn.

To the extent that elementary schools include preschool programs, school health services could be a vital part of the overall strategy to achieve this objective. But, perhaps more important, school health services could help assure that after they first start school, all students in kindergarten through grade 12 continue to enter school every day healthy and thus ready to learn. Undoubtedly, such school services also could help achieve the second National Education Goal, that "By the year 2000, the high school graduation rate will increase to at least 90 percent."

In summary, the school health program could help in attaining more than one third of the 300 National Health Objectives, either directly (e.g.,"Establish tobacco-free environments and include tobacco use prevention in the curricula of all...schools....") or indirectly (e.g., "Reduce the initiation of cigarette smoking by children and youth...."). Analogously, school health programs could help attain all six of the National Education Goals, either directly (e.g., "Every school will be free of drugs and violence....") or indirectly (e.g., "American students will...[have] demonstrated competency in challenging subject matter....") (McGinnis and DeGraw, 1991; Novello, DeGraw and Kleinman, 1992).

What Does the Nation Need to Do to Improve School Health Programs?

What will the nation need to do to improve school health programs? There may be five strategic requirements. First, decision makers and the public, including school administrators, teachers and parents, must be informed about the current need for and nature of school health programs. Indeed, parents and concerned community members should be integrally involved in determining the nature of school health programs in their community. If decision makers and the public do not understand such programs, they are not likely to perceive them to be a priority for our schools and our young people.

Second, government education, health and social service agencies at the national, state and local levels will need to work together as partners to implement school health programs. Education agencies have the mandate to improve educational outcomes, the authority to establish education policies, and the organizational capacity to implement school programs. Health agencies have the mandate to improve health outcomes, access to fiscal resources for health, and a wide range of health expertise. Social service agencies have the mandate to support the disadvantaged, have access to social service resources, and have means and expertise to help improve health and education outcomes among the disadvantaged. Health, education and social service agencies need to establish administrative means to combine their respective resources.

Third, many important national nongovernmental organizations, and their constituents at the state and local levels, must be involved. Examples of these organizations include the Council of Chief State School Officers, Association of State and Territorial Health Officers, American Public Welfare Association, American Academy of Pediatrics, National Congress of Parents and Teachers, and the American Council for Education, which represents leadership in higher education.

Fourth, the nation's universities also need to be involved. Colleges of education, public health, medicine, nursing, social work, and allied health, among others, might establish interdisciplinary efforts in the following areas:
- help analyze the role of schools in improving health
- provide local, state and national leadership and technical assistance to improve school health programs

- modernize and provide preservice and inservice training for education, health and other professionals
- conduct research to assess and improve the impact of programs

Finally, many national, state and local philanthropies have accomplished much to improve school health programs. For instance, the Carnegie Corporation of New York has provided support for 27 states to facilitate educational reform in middle grades, including reform of school health programs (Council of Chief State School Officers, 1992), and the Robert Wood Johnson Foundation has provided support to establish demonstration school-based clinics throughout the United States (Lear et al., 1991). These philanthropies should be integrally involved in any national effort to improve school health programs.

National, state and local governmental agencies will need to plan and enact strategies to improve school health programs collaboratively with each other, and with relevant nongovernmental organizations, universities and philanthropies. Each of these agencies is dependent upon the others for its success. Accordingly, in 1993, and annually thereafter, CDC will convene representatives of these agencies to analyze and plan collaborative strategies for improving school health programs nationwide.

Much has been accomplished recently to establish the groundwork for improving school health programs. In the public sector, the DHHS Office of Disease Prevention and Health Promotion has spearheaded efforts to publish a *Directory of Federal Programs and Activities Related to Health Promotion Through the Schools* and to convene an Interagency Committee on School Health (comprised of about thirty federal agencies) and a National Coordinating Committee on School Health (comprised of about thirty national nongovernmental organizations). Both of these committees are cochaired by the DHHS Assistant Secretary for Health and the Department of Education Assistant Secretary for Elementary and Secondary Education. The U.S. General Accounting Office has launched a study of social services provided through schools and a study of clinical services provided through schools; and the DHHS Office of the Inspector General has initiated a study of school-based health services.

Additionally significant to school health programs, the U.S. Public Health Service recently established a Steering Committee on Adolescent Health, and the Congress authorized an Office of Adolescent Health in the Office of the Assistant Secretary for Health. To assess and monitor progress in improving the nation's school health programs, CDC recently initiated a study to describe the nature of various components of the school health program among a probability sample of the nation's 100,000 schools.

In the private sector, a National School Health Education Coalition and a National Health/Education Consortium have been established, and the American Cancer Society has launched a major effort to improve the nation's school health education programs (American Cancer Society, 1990, 1993). Much more remains to be done, however, and those entrusted with the health of our youth—the nation's pediatricians—have a critical role to play.

The Role of Pediatricians

If our nation's schools are to protect and improve the health of our young people, organizations that represent pediatricians will need to provide leadership at the national, state and local levels on two fronts simultaneously. First, pediatricians will need to work with educators, parents and other concerned community members to ensure that their schools provide effective health programs. Second, pediatricians will need to help determine the following:

- the type of health programs, especially health services, that schools should provide
- whether schools should provide such programs for all students or only the most needy
- the role of the pediatrician in the school health program
- ways to encourage, train and compensate pediatricians to work with schools

The American Academy of Pediatrics (AAP) traditionally has provided national leadership to improve school health programs. About 15 years ago, AAP called for better training of pediatricians to help improve school health programs (American Academy of Pediatrics, 1978), and the forthcoming AAP publication entitled *School Health: A Guide for Health Professionals* will be a vital instrument for improving school health programs in the future.

In September 1992, at the AAP Media Conference on "Crisis in the Classroom: The Undeniable Link between Health and School Readiness," AAP President Dr. Daniel Shea summarized what needs to be done:

> As a pediatrician, two thoughts emerge. First, I agree with educators that physicians and medical organizations must work in the public policy arena. [And second,] physicians need to enhance their working relationships with educators.... The bottom line is that health care professionals, schools and parents must work together to resolve this crisis.

References

Advisory Council on Social Security. 1991. *Commitment to change: Foundations for reform.* Washington, DC: U.S. Department of Health and Human Services.

Allensworth, D. D., and L. J. Kolbe. 1987. The comprehensive school health program: Exploring an expanded concept. *Journal of School Health* 57 (10): 409-473.

American Academy of Pediatrics. 1978. *The future of pediatric education.* Evanston, IN.

American Academy of Pediatrics. 1993. *School health: A guide for health professionals.* Elk Grove, IL.

American Cancer Society. 1990. *Report of the Planning Advisory Council.* Atlanta, GA.

American Cancer Society. 1993. Improving comprehensive school health education in the United States. *Journal of School Health.* 63 (1): 1-70.

Berryman, S., and T. Bailey. 1992. *The double helix of education and the economy.* New York: Columbia University Teacher's College, Institute on Education and the Economy.

Blum, R., K. Pfaffinger and W. Donald. 1982. A school-based comprehensive health clinic for adolescents. *Journal of School Health* 52 (8): 486-490.

Boyer, E. 1991. *Ready to learn: A mandate for the nation.* Lawrenceville, NY: Princeton University Press.

Bruhn, J., and P. Nader. 1982. The school as a setting for health education, health promotion and health care. *Family and Community Health* 4 (4): 57-69.

Bureau of Health Care Delivery and Assistance. 1992. *Proposed ready to learn school program—fact sheet.* Rockville, MD: Health Resources and Services Administration.

Carnegie Council on Adolescent Development. 1989. *Turning points: Preparing American youth for the 21st century.* Washington, DC.

Center for Collaboration for Children, California State University at Fullerton, and Human Services Policy Center, University of Washington. 1992. *Summary: Interprofessional Training Conference, July 24-25.* Greenwich, CT: Annie E. Casey Foundation.

Cherlin, A., ed. 1988. *The changing American family and public policy.* Washington, DC: Urban Institute Press.

Center for the Future of Children, The David and Lucile Packard Foundation. 1992. *The future of children: School linked services,* Vol. 2, No. 1. Los Altos, CA.

Commission on Minority Participation in Education and American Life. 1988. *One third of a nation.* Washington, DC: American Council on Education and Education Commission of the States.

Congressional Record. U.S. Senate. July 28, 1992. *Comprehensive services for youth act.* 102d Cong., 2d sess. S10512-S10532.

Council of Chief State School Officers. 1991. *Beyond the health room.* Washington, DC.

Council of Chief State School Officers. 1992. *Turning points: States in action.* An Interim Report of the Middle Grade School State Policy Initiative. Washington, DC.

Council of Chief State School Officers. In press. *Student success through collaboration: A policy statement.* Washington, DC.

Coye, M. 1992. Health care for California's children. *California Pediatrician* 8 (2): 25-28.

DeFriese, G., C. Crossland, C. Pearson and C. Sullivan, eds. 1990. Comprehensive school health programs: Current status and future prospects. *Journal of School Health* 60 (4): 127-190.

Dryfoos, J. G. 1988. School-based health clinics: Three years of experience. *Family Planning Perspectives* 20 (4): 193-200.

Dryfoos, J. G. 1990. *Adolescents at risk: Prevalence and prevention.* New York: Oxford University Press.

Education Commission of the States. 1981. *Recommendations for school health education: A handbook for state policymakers.* Denver, CO.

Education and Human Services Consortium. 1991. *What it takes: Structuring interagency partnerships to connect children and families with comprehensive services.* Washington, DC.

Farrow, F., and T. Joe. 1992. Financing school-linked, integrated services. In *The future of children: School linked services.* Vol. 2, No. 1. Los Altos, CA: Center for the Future of Children, The David and Lucile Packard Foundation.

Federal Interagency Ad Hoc Committee on Health Promotion Through the Schools, U.S. Department of Health and Human Services. 1992. *Healthy schools: A directory of federal programs and activities related to health promotion through the schools.* Washington, DC: Office of Disease Prevention and Health Promotion, Public Health Service, U.S. Department of Health and Human Services.

Fox, H. B., L. B. Wicks and D. J. Lipson. 1992. *Improving access to comprehensive health care through school-based programs.* Washington, DC: Fox Health Policy Consultants.

Fuchs, V. 1974. *Who shall live: Health, economics and social choice.* New York: Basic Books.

Hamburg, D. 1992. *Today's children: Creating a future for a generation in crisis.* New York: Random House.

Health Care Financing Administration. 1993. Medicaid statistics: Program and financial statistics fiscal year 1991. Washington, DC: Medicaid Bureau, Health Care Financing Administration, U.S. Department of Health and Human Services.

Hechinger, F. 1992. *Fateful choices: Healthy youth for the 21st century.* New York: Hill and Wang.

Hodgkinson, H. 1989. *The same client: The demographics of education and service delivery systems.* Washington, DC: Institute for Educational Leadership.

Igoe, J. B., and E. Campos. 1991. Report of a national survey of school nurse supervisors. *School Nurse* 7 (4): 8-20.

Interagency Task Force on Family Resource and Youth Services Centers, Kentucky Family Resource and Youth Services Centers. 1991. *Interagency task force: State implementation plan.* Frankfort, KY: The Secretary for Human Resources, Commonwealth of Kentucky.

Jehl, J., and M. Kirst. September 1992. Spinning a family support web among agencies, schools. *The School Administrator* 49 (8): 8-15.

Johns, E. 1973. Health education in schools. *World Medical Journal* 20 (Sept./ Oct.): 87-90.

Johnson, W., and A. Packer. 1991. *Workforce 2000: Work and workers for the 21st century.* Indianapolis: Hudson Institute.

Joint Committee on Health Education Terminology. 1991. Report of the 1990 Joint Committee on Health Education Terminology. *Journal of Health Education* 22:97-106.

Kann, L., ed. 1993. Measuring adolescent health behaviors: The Youth Risk Behavior Surveillance System (YRBSS) and recent research reports on reaching high-risk adolescents. Atlanta, GA: *Public Health Reports.*

Klein, J., S. Starnes, M. Kotelchuck, J. Earp, G. DeFriese and F. Loda. 1992. *Comprehensive adolescent health services in the United States.* Carrboro, NC: Center for Early Adolescence, University of North Carolina at Chapel Hill.

Kolbe, L. J. 1986. Increasing the impact of school health promotion programs: Emerging research perspectives. *Health Education* 16:47-52.

Kolbe, L. J. 1990. An epidemiological surveillance system to monitor youth behaviors that most affect health. *Health Education* 22:252-255.

Kolbe, L. J., L. Green, J. Foreyt, L. Darnell, K. Goodrick, H. Williams, D. Ward, A. Korton, I. Karacan, R. Widmeyer and G. Stainbrook. 1986. Appropriate functions of health education in schools: Improving health and cognitive performance. In *Child health behavior: A behavioral pediatrics perspective,* ed. N. Krasnegor, J. Arasteh and M. Cataldo, 171-216. New York: John Wiley & Sons.

Kolbe, L. J., D. Tolsma, H. Dhillon, D. O'Byrne and J. Jones. 1992. School health education: Challenge for national and international agencies. *Hygie* 11:72-76.

Lapointe, A., J. Askew and N. Mead. 1992. *Learning science: The international assessment of educational progress.* Princeton, NJ: Educational Testing Service.

Lapointe, A., N. Mead and J. Askew. 1992. *Learning mathematics: The international assessment of educational progress.* Princeton, NJ: Educational Testing Service.

Lavin, A., G. Shapiro and K. Weill. 1992. *Creating an agenda for school-based health promotion: A review of selected reports.* Boston, MA: Harvard School of Public Health.

Lear, J., H. Gleicher, A. Germaine and P. Porter. 1991. Reorganizing health care for adolescents: The experience of the School-Based Adolescent Health Care Program. *Journal of Adolescent Health* 12 (6): 450-458.

Mason, J. 1989. Forging working partnerships for school health education. *Journal of School Health* 59:18-20.

McGinnis, J., and C. DeGraw. 1991. Healthy schools 2000: Creating partnerships for the decade. *Journal of School Health* 61 (7): 292-328.

Means, R. 1975. *Historical perspectives on school health.* Thorofare, NJ: Slack.

Medicaid Bureau. 1992. *EPSDT: A guide for educational programs.* Washington, DC: Health Care Financing Administration.

Moore, J., L. Daily, J. Collins, L. Kann, M. Dalmat, B. Truman and L. J. Kolbe. 1992. Progress in efforts to prevent the spread of HIV infection among youth. *Public Health Reports* 106:678-686.

Morrill, W., and M. Gerry. 1990. *Integrating the delivery of services to school-aged children at risk: Toward a description of American experience and experimentation.* Falls Church, VA: Mathtech, Inc., National Center for Service Integration.

Mullis, I., E. Owen and G. Phillips. 1990. *America's challenge: Accelerating academic achievement.* A summary of findings from 20 years of the National Assessment of Educational Progress. Princeton, NJ: Educational Testing Service.

Nader, P. 1990. The concept of "comprehensiveness" in the design and implementation of school health programs. *Journal of School Health* 60 (4): 133-138.

National Academy of Sciences. 1989. *AIDS: Sexual behavior and intravenous drug use.* Washington, DC: National Academy Press.

National Academy of Sciences. 1990. *AIDS: The second decade.* Washington, DC: National Academy Press.

National Association of School Nurses. 1990. *Guidelines for a model school nursing services program.* Scarborough, MA.

National Center for Educational Statistics. 1991. *Dropout rate in the United States 1990.* Washington, DC: U.S. Department of Education.

National Commission on Children. 1991. *Beyond rhetoric: A new American agenda for children and families.* Washington, DC.

National Commission on the Role of the School and the Community in Improving Adolescent Health. 1990. *Code blue: Uniting for healthier youth.* Alexandria, VA: National Association of State Boards of Education.

National Education Goals Panel. 1991. *The national education goals report: Building a nation of learners.* Washington, DC: U.S. Department of Education.

National Health/Education Consortium. 1990. *Crossing the boundaries between health and education.* Washington, DC: Institute for Educational Leadership.

National Health/Education Consortium. 1991. *Bridging the gap: A health care primer for health and education professionals.* Washington, DC: Institute for Educational Leadership.

National Health/Education Consortium. 1992. *Creating sound minds and bodies: Health and education working together.* Washington, DC: Institute for Educational Leadership.

National Institutes for Health. 1992. *Meeting the challenge: U.S. Public Health Service strategic plan for life sciences education and public science literacy—Part I.* Bethesda, MD: U.S. Public Health Service.

National Institutes for Health. In press. *Meeting the challenge: U.S. Public Health Service strategic plan for life sciences education and public science literacy—Part II.* Bethesda, MD: U.S. Public Health Service.

National Professional School Health Education Organizations. 1984. Comprehensive school health education. *Journal of School Health* 54 (8): 312-315.

National Research Council. 1987. *Risking the future: Adolescent sexuality, pregnancy, and childbearing.* Washington, DC: National Academy Press.

National School Boards Association. 1991. *School health: Helping children learn.* Alexandria, VA: National School Boards Association.

National School Health Education Coalition. 1992. *Comprehensive school health education and coalition building resource guide.* Washington, DC.

Natriello, G., E. McDill and A. Pallas. 1990. *Schooling disadvantaged children: Racing against catastrophe.* New York: Teachers College Press.

Novello, A., C. DeGraw and D. Kleinman. 1992. Healthy children ready to learn: An essential collaboration between health and education. *Public Health Reports* 107 (1): 3-15.

Office of the Assistant Secretary for Planning and Evaluation. In press. *Practical guide to school-linked service integration.* Washington, DC: U.S. Department of Health and Human Services.

Parron, D., F. Solomon and C. Jenkins. 1982. *Behavior, health risks, and social disadvantage.* Washington, DC: National Academy Press.

Pearson, L. 1992. 1991-92 update: How each state stands on legislative issues affecting advanced nursing practice. *Nurse Practitioner* 17 (1): 14-23.

Presidential Commission on the Human Immunodeficiency Virus Epidemic. 1988. *Report of the Presidential Commission on the Human Immunodeficiency Virus Epidemic.* Washington, DC.

Proctor, S., S. Lordi and D. Zaiger. In press. *School nursing practice: Roles and standards.* Scarborough, MA: National Association of School Nurses.

Public Law 102-531. Preventive Health and Health Services Block Grant. Section 1901 to 1907 of Title XIX of Public Health Services Act.

Robert Wood Johnson Foundation. 1985. *Special report: National School Health Services Program.* Princeton, NJ.

Schultz, G. 1988. National success and international stability in a time of change. In *Thinking about America, the United States in the 1990s,* ed. A. Anderson and D. Bark, 515-526. Stanford, CA: Hoover Institution Press.

Shea, D. 1992. *Crisis in the classroom: The undeniable link between health and school readiness.* Speech given at the 1992 AAP Media Conference, 15 September 1992. Elk Grove, IL: American Academy of Pediatrics.

Smith, G., and M. Egger. 1992. Socioeconomic differences in mortality in Britain and the United States. *American Journal of Public Health* 82:1079-1081.

Stone, E. 1990. Access: Keystones for school health promotion. *Journal of School Health* 60 (7): 298-300.

St. Peter, R., P. Newacheck and N. Halfon. 1992. Access to care for poor children. *Journal of the American Medical Association* 267:2760-2764.

Task Force on Standards of School Nursing Practice. 1983. *Standards of school nursing practice.* Kansas City, MO: American Nurses' Association.

U.S. Congress. 1990. *Omnibus Budget Reconciliation Act of 1990.* (Public Law No. 101.508). Washington, DC.

U.S. Congress. House. 1992. *Preventative Health Amendments of 1992, Conference Report.* Report 102-1019. Washington, DC.

U.S. Congress. House. Select Committee on Children, Youth and Families 1992. *A decade of denial: Teens and AIDS in America.* Washington, DC.

U.S. Congress. Office of Technology Assessment. 1991. *Adolescent health.* Washington, DC.

U.S. Congress. Office of Technology Assessment. 1992. *Does health insurance make a difference? Background paper.* Washington, DC.

U.S. Congress. Senate. 1990. *Senate Appropriations Committee FY90 Report.* Washington, DC.

U.S. Congress. Senate. Committee on Labor and Human Resources. 1992. Hearing on the *Healthy Students–Healthy Schools Act* (S. 2191). Washington, DC.

U.S. Congress. Senate. Subcommittee on Oversight of Government Management of the Committee on Governmental Affairs. 1992. *Healthy schools, healthy children, healthy futures: The role of the federal government in promoting health through the schools.* 102d Cong., 1st sess. S-2191. Washington, DC.

U.S. Department of Commerce, Bureau of the Census. 1989. Money income and poverty status in the United States. *Current Population Reports, series P-60, no. 168.* Washington, DC: U.S. Department of Commerce.

U.S. Department of Commerce, Bureau of the Census. 1990. Table C—marital status and living arrangements: March 1989. *Current Population Reports, series P-20, no. 445.* Washington, DC: U.S. Department of Commerce.

U.S. Department of Education. 1991. *America 2000: An education strategy.* Washington, DC.

U.S. Department of Health and Human Services, Public Health Service. 1991. *Healthy people 2000: National health promotion and disease prevention objectives.* DHHS Publication No. (PHS) 91-50212. Washington, DC.

Woodfill, M., and M. Beyrer. 1991. *The role of the nurse in the school setting: A historical perspective.* Kent, OH: American School Health Association.

World Health Organization; United Nations Educational, Scientific, and Cultural Organization; and United Nations Children's Emergency Fund. 1992. Comprehensive school health education: Suggested guidelines for action. *Hygie* 11:8-15.

Programmatic
Issues

Chapter 4

Planning for a Comprehensive School Health Program

William M. Kane, PhD, CHES

S tructuring schools to provide opportunities for children to reach their fullest health potential requires collaboration among parents, families, communities and school leaders. The foundation for planning an effective school health program consists of family and community values and aspirations; community, school and family resources; epidemiologic data; and educational and behavioral research. (See Figure 1.)

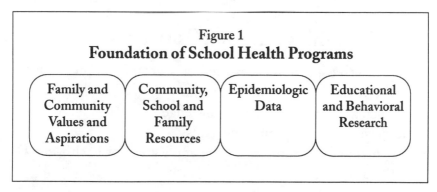

Figure 1
Foundation of School Health Programs

| Family and Community Values and Aspirations | Community, School and Family Resources | Epidemiologic Data | Educational and Behavioral Research |

The schools' role in fostering the healthy development of children and youth goes beyond the teacher providing a health education class. Although health education is a critical component in a child's healthy development, schools must undertake other efforts to support the healthy development of children. Diane Allensworth and Lloyd Kolbe (1987) identified several areas in which schools should establish efforts to promote the health of children, youth and staff. Their framework identifies the following eight components of schools that can be organized and combined to create a comprehensive program:

- school health education (instruction)
- healthy school environment
- school health services
- physical education and fitness
- school nutrition and food services
- school-based counseling and personal support
- schoolsite health promotion
- school, family and community health promotion partnerships

These components can provide guidance as school leaders strive to provide leadership in organizing the resources of the community and school to promote the healthy development of children and youth.

School Health Education (Instruction)

School health education or instruction is a combination of educational activities with the following aims:

- to increase students' health knowledge
- to develop health-promoting skills
- to provide opportunities for the application of health knowledge and skills

- to reinforce and foster the continued practice of healthy behaviors

Health education is the classroom curricular component of the overall plan to foster healthy development of children and youth. The end goal of school health education is to give children and youth the knowledge, skills, opportunities and support to develop to their fullest potential. School health education should be based on a planned and sequential curriculum that interacts with other components of the comprehensive health education program to enable young people to achieve optimal health.

The curriculum is planned in that it should be based on the current documentable threats to the health of young people. School leaders can look to national, state and local morbidity and mortality statistics for some of this data. Behavioral risk factor data that identify behaviors that put youth at increased risk of future health problems is available from the Centers for Disease Control and Prevention and state departments of health.

The aspirations of families and communities, as well as the hopes of the students themselves, are also important foundations upon which to base health curricula. Successful school health education programs involve a wide range of individuals, including:

- students and their families
- community members
- representatives of business, health and social service professions
- clergy
- community activists

All of these people should be represented in the process of planning a curriculum that is appropriate and sensitive to the cultural needs and values of the community and school. A health education curriculum based on a collectively shared vision of the importance of the health of children is the first step toward helping all children develop to their optimal health potential.

Curriculum Content

Although school districts often have different names for the content areas of their particular curriculum, the range of topics included in most school health curricula can be grouped into the following ten areas:
* prevention of alcohol and other drug use
* nutrition and healthy eating
* family life education
* mental and emotional health
* environmental health
* injury prevention and safety
* personal health and fitness
* disease prevention and control
* community health
* selecting health options (consumer health)

Not all ten content areas are covered at each grade level. Decisions regarding scope and focus of the curriculum at each grade level are based on what is appropriate to interests, needs and physical and mental development of students. The health education curriculum and content should be sequential, each year building on and reinforcing the knowledge learned and the skills developed at earlier grade levels.

Health Skills

Health education curricula include both content and process. The process, or *skills development,* is a major focus of the curriculum and classroom activities. These health-related skills are defined a bit differently by each school district, but fall into the following general categories:

- assessing personal health and risks
- gathering and assessing health information
- rewarding healthy behavior
- communicating with others
- making decisions
- negotiating for health
- managing stress
- setting and achieving goals

School leaders will want to develop a curriculum that provides learning opportunities for students to acquire health awareness and the knowledge, skills and opportunities to practice healthy behavior, and encourages and reinforces the development of healthy lifestyles. A curriculum of this type relies heavily on experiential learning.

Unlike curricula in many areas, a health curriculum is in a constant state of change, reflecting developments in culture, society, technology and behavioral sciences. An annual review should be conducted to determine the continuing relevance of the curriculum to the priorities and needs of the local community and the growing body of health and medical science.

Instructional Time

Planning for instructional time is another important issue for school leaders to consider in developing the school health education program. Most authorities recommend that elementary and middle school students experience the equivalent of two to three hours of health education each week. Integration of health education learning experiences into other subject-oriented learning experiences can be successfully accomplished.

However, experience shows that many schools that report using the integrated approach are not successful in helping students gain the knowledge, develop the skills and find the opportunities to practice healthy behaviors. This lack of success many be due not to the integrated approach, but to the level of commitment, time and priority the teachers and school place on quality health instruction. Many leaders recommend that elementary schools establish specific times for health instruction, as well as integrating health education with other subjects in the curriculum.

Health education should continue beyond elementary school. Early adolescence is a critical time; young people are exploring various behaviors, making choices and establishing lifetime health behaviors. Health education in middle school grades should include sixty to seventy hours of direct instruction and learning experiences each year. At the high school level, students should be encouraged to include at least two semesters of health instruction in their schedule.

Teacher Skills and Preparation

The skills and preparation of the classroom teacher are critical to the success of school health education. Teachers should be professionally prepared, either through preservice or inservice education, to implement health curriculum, to foster health-related learning, to help students develop health and life skills, and to work with the school, families and community to provide opportunities to practice this healthy behavior.

Teachers should keep in mind that the health needs and interests of their students will be personal and will differ from student to student, from class to class and from community to community. The optimal school health education program will allow the skilled teacher to modify learning opportunities accordingly.

Teachers should be fully prepared in the following areas:
- handling controversial health issues and content
- experiential learning
- peer education, cooperative learning and cross-tutoring
- questioning strategies to foster development of critical thinking
- health counseling
- family relations and counseling
- advocacy
- life-skills training
- rewarding healthy behavior
- modeling healthy behavior

Administrative Leadership

Administrative leadership in providing policy, funding and support for training and materials to implement successful health education programs is also important. School leaders have a responsibility to work with their communities, initiating action and providing leadership in policy and funding areas.

Instructional Materials

Instructional and educational materials for health instruction include a wide range of textbooks, prepackaged curricula and supplementary texts, videos and other materials that can be used in conjunction with local and state-developed curricula or commercial curricula.

Healthy School Environment

A safe and healthful environment is important for education. Schools should not be places where students and teachers fear for their personal safety. Harassment from gang members and drug pushers and resolution of conflict by violent actions has no place in the school.

Commitment to regular safety inspections and emergency drills, provision of safe and orderly transportation, adherence to environmental regulations and standards, and clean, safe and well-maintained school grounds and buildings communicate a message to all by establishing health norms and expectations. The physical surroundings in which students and teachers are expected to work should promote healthy behaviors.

Likewise, students' personal achievements and social growth are fostered by the psychological environment of the school. Not surprisingly, research has found that a favorite teacher is frequently a positive role model in a child's life. Teachers not only help students develop academic skills, but also provide positive models for students' personal identification and development. The emotional and physical health and the social, problem-solving and conflict-management skills demonstrated by teachers influence young people.

The health norms and social expectations created by the school support healthy development of students. Benard (1991) has identified the level of caring and support within the school as a powerful predictor of positive outcomes for youth. Researchers have concluded that schools that are successful in helping young people overcome problem behaviors project clear expectations and regulations, emphasize academics, have high levels of student participation, foster high self-esteem and promote social and scholastic success. Schools that establish high expectations for all students and provide the support necessary to achieve these expectations have high rates of academic success. Benard's review of the research on the school's role in developing resilient youth concludes that the caregiving environment of the school can serve as a protective shield in reducing levels of alcohol and other drug use.

School Health Services

The provision of health services by schools emerged near the end of the nineteenth century in response to compulsory education laws. The focus of these services was to prevent and control infectious diseases and exclude children who represented a health threat to others.

Much has changed over the past one hundred years. The 1990 Joint Commission on Health Education Terminology definition of school health services identified both the school health services personnel and their responsibilities. (See Appendix B for the full text of the report.) School health service personnel include the following individuals who appraise, protect and promote the health of students and school personnel:

- physicians
- nurses
- dentists
- health educators
- allied health personnel
- social workers
- teachers

The definition goes on to describe school health services as those activities designed to:

- ensure access to and appropriate use of primary health care services
- prevent and control communicable disease
- provide emergency care for injury or sudden illness
- promote and provide optimum sanitary conditions in a safe school facility and environment
- provide concurrent learning opportunities conducive to the maintenance and promotion of individual and community health

For example, health services provided by the school and community to all students in one Massachusetts school district include:

- immunizations
- vision and hearing screening
- fluoride dental rinse program
- dental screening, sealants and cavity repair
- physical evaluation
- speech therapy
- postural screening
- pediculosis (body lice) screening
- health assessment and individual education plans
- child abuse assessment
- prekindergarten and kindergarten screening
- management of asthmatics
- mental health counseling and referral
- family outreach/parent support groups
- inservice education for staff
- supplemental health education in classrooms

School nurses have traditionally been the focal point for health services in the schools. School nurses are also a key resource for the other components of the overall school health program, as they provide health education and act as consultants on community and family health. Unfortunately, there are only about 30,000 school nurses throughout the United States to serve 42 million students. The National School Nurses Association recommends a ratio of one nurse for every 750 students. To achieve this ratio, we would need more than twenty thousand additional school nurses. In the absence of adequate funding for school nurses, many schools rely on a school secretary to administer first-aid and minor medications.

Rapidly escalating health care costs have combined with today's unstable employment market to leave many adults and their children without medical insurance and with limited access to primary health care. As a result, many schools and communities are exploring alternative methods of providing health services for young people.

More than one hundred health clinics based in schools have emerged over the past decade. These clinics provide a full range of primary health care services and act as a point of referral for students requiring more extensive diagnostic work, treatment and rehabilitation. Unfortunately, many of these clinics have become embroiled in controversy surrounding the provision of sexuality counseling and birth control devices. By the end of high school, 60.8 percent of males and 48 percent of females report they have had sexual intercourse (U.S. Department of Health and Human Services, 1991). About 60,000 babies are born each year to adolescent girls under fifteen years of age. Family planning counseling and provision of services are appropriate roles for school-based clinics.

Some schools (and communities) are experimenting with health insurance coverage for students. Actually, the concept of accident insurance for students has been around for decades. Today's student health insurance has been expanded to cover regular checkups, immunizations, hospitalizations, outpatient care, prescriptions, eyeglasses and drug and alcohol treatment and rehabilitation. These insurance plans are being financed through community fundraising, public health agencies and private insurance carriers.

In every school, the physical and mental health needs of some students will exceed the immediate resources of the school and its personnel. Paying for health care is an expensive and complex societal issue. However, good health is essential for learning and for achieving one's fullest potential. School leaders need to work closely with families, community leaders and health and social service providers to establish a systematic health care system for students.

Physical Education and Fitness

It is widely held that participation in physical education activities promotes health development. More than 97 percent of this country's elementary school children and 80 percent of its secondary school students have access to organized physical education. Students in elementary schools take physical education an average of 3.1 times weekly, with 36.4 percent taking classes daily. At the high school level, students take physical education an average of 3.9 times weekly, with 36.3 percent taking classes daily (Office of Disease Prevention and Health Promotion, 1984).

The popular literature attributes a large range of benefits to physical exercise, including:
- improved cardiovascular and physiological functioning
- reduction of stress
- reduction of weight and body fat
- improved skeletal and muscle structure
- increased sense of self-worth
- improved academic performance

Indeed, research findings seem to support many of these popular beliefs. Yet despite the growing body of knowledge regarding the effects of physical fitness and exercise on health, and the long existence of physical education programs in America's schools, all is not well. The National Children and Youth Fitness Study released in 1984 cited the following problems:
- Body fat of today's youth is significantly greater than in the 1960s.

- Only 50 percent of today's youth participate in appropriate physical activity.
- Only 50 percent of the students in twelfth grade participate in physical education classes.
- Physical education teachers devote most classroom time to competitive sports and other activities that have questionable health effects and that cannot readily be performed once one reaches adulthood.

Recognizing the importance of exercise, the U.S. Department of Health and Human Services *Healthy People 2000* (1991) recommends that by the year 2000 "schools increase by at least 50 percent [from 36 percent to 54 percent] the proportion of children and adolescents in 1st through 12th grade who participate in daily school physical education" (Objective 1.8).

The proportion of students participating in daily physical education is one measure of the quality of school-based physical education. Another measure of quality identified by *Healthy People 2000* is students' exposure to information about how and why to partake in activities, and encouragement to develop skills that allow for out-of-school and lifetime activities. Lifetime physical activities are defined as those activities in which individuals can participate throughout their lives. They include tennis, badminton, golf, hiking, individual exercise, swimming and bicycling. They do not include football, soccer, baseball, basketball or most of the competitive team activities that commonly dominate the high school curriculum.

Healthy People 2000 recommends that by the year 2000 we "increase to at least 50 percent [baseline 27 percent in 1984] the proportion of school physical education class time that students spend being physically active, preferably engaged in lifetime physical activities" (Objective 1.9). Studies indicate that only 27 percent of the current physical education classroom time is spent in actual physical activity, while 26 percent is spent in instruction, 22 percent in administrative tasks and 25 percent waiting.

Physical education is another area of the school health program that requires coordination between schools, families and communities. The typical student in fifth through twelfth grades reports that more than 80 percent of his or her physical activity takes place outside of physical education classes. The majority of this time is spent in activities sponsored by community organizations, including religious groups, parks and recreation programs, local teams and private organizations.

Healthy People 2000 calls for more class time to be spent engaged in lifetime activities and more emphasis given to developing knowledge, attitudes, cognitive skills and physical skills students need to remain physically active throughout life. To achieve these objectives and provide physical education experiences that promote healthy development, teachers responsible for physical education programs need preservice or inservice training. District or school level physical education specialists can become responsible for the inservice education of nonspecialized teachers responsible for physical education classes. In addition, a team including the physical education specialist should assume responsibility for overall curriculum scope, sequence and implementation.

School Nutrition and Food Services

The history of school nutrition in the United States is a study in politics. It wasn't just by chance that the establishment of school lunch programs coincided with the nation's overproduction of food. School lunches became a convenient "dumping ground" for surplus food commodities, providing low-cost food for America's children. However, surplus farm products (milk, eggs, meat, cheese) were not always the healthiest foods.

At the same time, nutrition education emerged as an important function of the U.S. Department of Agriculture, the same organization that had encouraged overproduction of food and established the school lunch assistance programs. In the late 1970s, the U.S. Department of Health and Human Services, after long and difficult negotiations with the Department of Agriculture, made a series of recommendations in *Dietary Guidelines for Americans*. The 1990 edition of these recommendations urged Americans to make the following changes in their eating habits:

- reduce intake of fat to less than 30 percent and saturated fats to less than 10 percent of the total dietary intake
- increase consumption of fruits and vegetables
- reduce intake of sugar
- increase consumption of whole-grain products
- reduce consumption of salt
- reduce total calorie intake

These guidelines established new criteria for measuring the nutritional value of school lunch programs. Although many schools today incorporate the principles of the *Dietary Guidelines*, such nutritional planning should be universal.

Healthy People 2000 recommends we "increase to at least 90 percent the proportion of school lunch and breakfast services...that are consistent with the nutritional principles in the *Dietary Guidelines for Americans*" (Objective 2.17). To accomplish this objective, school meals must provide choices that include low-fat foods, vegetables, fruits and whole-grain products. Doing so will also provide opportunities for students to practice the health knowledge and food selection skills introduced in school-based health education instruction.

To support this learning experience, *Healthy People 2000* recommends that schools offer "point-of-choice" nutrition information in the school cafeteria. Point-of-choice nutrition information includes information on nutrient value and calories of the foods being served. Such information enables students to choose healthy food. *Healthy People 2000* further recommends that school fundraising activities that involve food sales, on-site vending machine offerings and food service offerings at concession stands during recreational and other events should also reflect the principles of the *Dietary Guidelines for Americans*.

For many children, especially poor children, school breakfast, lunch and snack programs constitute a significant portion of their daily nutritional intake. In these cases, school food service personnel, and particularly cafeteria managers, are the gatekeepers to childrens' food supply. The school's nutritional program provides an excellent opportunity to establish health norms and model healthy nutritional behaviors. Schools that provide healthy food choices and discourage availability of unhealthy foods send a clear message to developing youth. Schools can also involve students in the planning of menus and preparation of food as a hands-on learning experience.

Nutritional policies consistent with scientific health findings and in the best interest of students demonstrate a school's commitment to the development of healthy youth. Such policies, with opportunities for students to practice nutritional knowledge and food selection skills in the lunch line, are consistent with the overall concept of a healthy school.

In some communities, school food service personnel spend time in the classroom working with teachers delivering nutrition instruction to students and preparing educational materials that enable students' families to support the classroom instruction. For students with special nutritional needs, close cooperation between school health services personnel and food services personnel is a critical factor in these students' achievement of optimal health.

School-Based Counseling and Personal Support

The school counseling program was originally implemented in the 1960s to provide vocational guidance for students. Today, school counselors and psychologists work in partnership with teachers, parents and community personnel to respond to special needs and provide personal support for individual students, teachers and staff. In addition, in many schools, counseling staff have initiated programs that promote schoolwide mental, emotional and social well-being.

The American School Counselor Association (ASCA) identifies the major aims of school-based counseling as follows:
- help students increase communication skills
- improve the quality of interaction between adults and youth
- encourage the learning process
- sensitize administrators and teachers to the necessity of matching the curriculum to the developmental needs of the students

The school counselor works to meet these goals by "structuring developmental guidance to promote psychological aspects of human development; individual and small group counseling; consultation with and inservice training for staff, parents and community groups; and performing needs assessment to guide interventions" (Klingman, 1984).

A recent study found that school counselors routinely interact with students on the following issues:
- divorce
- substance abuse by students or their parents

- teen sexuality and pregnancy
- depression
- suicide
- sexual and physical abuse
- problems with family members or friends
- concerns about career and future
- questions about the meaning of life

Counselors also often become involved in providing assistance to teachers and other school staff and their families. The activities of school counselors frequently bring them in contact with families of students and with community health and social service workers. Counselors often become advocates for students' interests.

Like teachers, counselors must be sensitive to the unique cultural backgrounds of students and their families. An understanding of the family and cultural values that guide students' priorities and decisions is critical for all who are responsible for helping young people grow up healthy. Schools should make special efforts to implement inservice education programs to ensure that counselors have background in and understanding of the communities and cultures in which students live.

Counselors can provide broad-based intervention programs to promote the health of students. They can initiate individual and small group programs aimed at preventing the onset of mental and emotional health problems, as well as interventions designed to reduce the consequences of stress or rehabilitate those who are experiencing difficulty in coping with stress (Klingman, 1984). These interventions include:

- problem-solving training
- assertiveness training
- life skills training
- peer-led problem-solving groups

- programs to build self-esteem and address loss of control, peer pressure and adolescent rebellion

Many schools employ school psychologists. The role of the psychologist varies from school to school, but much of the school psychologist's time is spent on pyschoeducational evaluation and educational programming for students with special needs. In addition, the school psychologist provides:
- group appraisal of students
- coordination with other pupil personnel workers
- coordination with child- and youth-serving community agencies
- counseling and psychotherapy
- preventive mental health consultation
- participation on curriculum committees
- inservice education
- data collection and research

School counselors and psychologists are important members of the school team who contribute to the healthy development of students. Both counselor and psychologist play an important role in linking schools with families and community health and social service workers and agencies. These resulting partnerships are crucial to creating an environment that supports young people in growing up healthy.

Schoolsite Health Promotion

Health promotion is a combination of educational, organizational and environmental activities designed to stimulate students and staff to establish healthy lifestyles and become better consumers of health services. Like all components in a comprehensive school health program, school-based health promotion is intertwined with and closely linked to the other components.

School leaders should view health promotion as a systems approach that enables the school to bring together the various health-related components to foster a culture that supports healthy development and the practice of healthy lifestyles. Health promotion establishes a social climate with the following characteristics:

- Teachers and family members are encouraged to model healthy behaviors.
- Opportunities are provided for students, faculty and staff, and parents and community members to practice health-promoting behaviors.
- Reinforcement is built in through recognizing and rewarding those who practice healthy behaviors.
- Health services are linked to health instruction.
- Assessment, counseling and, when necessary, referral of students experiencing health-related problems is provided.
- School policies and administrative procedures consistently support the healthy development of youth, teachers and staff.

The documented effects of health promotion programs on staff include increase in energy levels, increased productivity, improved morale, decreased absenteeism and decreased teacher burnout.

Teachers and school staff who model the health knowledge, skills and behaviors learned by students in the classroom encourage students to adopt healthy behaviors. School policies and practices that provide a health-promoting environment free from violence and pressures to engage in self-destructive health behaviors provide an opportunity for students to adopt healthy behaviors.

Providing for the safety of students is only the first step in establishing a health-promoting environment in the school. Schools can provide other health promoting opportunities as well. These include:

- opportunities in the school cafeteria to select food which is low in fat, high in nutrients and prepared in a healthy manner
- a smoke-free environment in which to learn
- opportunities for all students to engage in physical activities that promote cardiovascular fitness, flexibility, strength, coordination, and that can be practiced over the life span

Social values and cultural beliefs and traditions are important determinants of health behavior. The school must reach beyond the schoolyard gate and work with families and communities to understand the cultural aspects of health. Then it can help communities and families develop culturally specific programs that provide health-promoting activities to reinforce those of the school.

The health and social norms of the home and community support or detract from a school's ability to foster the development of healthy youth. Communities that value healthful behavior can send a clear message supporting young people's adoption of healthy behaviors. The following activities can be part of that message:

- modeling healthy behavior
- providing environmental support (such as enforcement of laws against the sale of alcohol to minors)
- having health care providers inquire about and offer counseling regarding healthy behaviors
- providing opportunities for young and old alike to practice health-promoting behavior

The school's role in establishing the health-promotion component includes:

- appointment of a leader
- formation of a school and community health council

- work with the community and families to conceive and articulate a vision for the healthy development of children
- analysis of the current school, community and family environment for health promotion and support of the healthy development of students
- development and implementation of new policies, programs and strategies that fully utilize the resources of the school, community and families to help children grow up healthy

As with all programs, education and training will enhance the success of the school health promotion program. In more than one-half of the states, department of education and department of health leaders offer five-day statewide summer wellness conferences for school teams comprised of administrators, teachers, staff and community leaders.

These teams learn how to incorporate the concept of "wellness as a lifestyle" into their personal and professional lives. When these teams return to their home communities, they have knowledge, skills and commitment to establish health promotion efforts in their schools and communities.

School, Family and Community Health Promotion Partnerships

Smoking, alcohol and other drug use, sexual activity at an early age, violence and abuse, delinquency and school dropout are not school problems. These threats to the future health of youth are interrelated. They share common roots in the community, families and school.

Partnerships to unite schools, families and communities are being established across America to help solve these community-wide problems. These effective collaborative partnerships focus on health promotion and disease prevention. They are the corner-stone of prevention and the foundation upon which children develop to their fullest potential. School officials have a leadership role to play in these collaborative efforts.

Schools and communities cannot ignore the role poverty plays in limiting children's access to health and education and, subsequently, opportunities for success in their adult lives. Appropriate health education for poor children and children of diverse ethnic backgrounds should be devised in consultation with those who represent their culture.

Partnerships formed to support healthy development of children must involve parents from all cultures, business and community leaders representing the diversity of the community, and parents and members of poor communities. To ignore this area will result in social and educational failure for millions of young people. For many, this failure will be the precursor of an adult life of poor health, crime, unemployment, welfare dependency and premature death. This is an unacceptable vision for our children. Coalitions and partnerships driven by mutual aspirations sharing a common vision of healthy young people can effectively help schools meet the needs of youth.

Code Blue: Uniting for Healthier Youth, a report of the National Commission on the Role of the School and the Community in Improving Adolescent Health (1990), issued a call for national action to improve the health of youth. The commission was jointly convened by the National Association of State Boards of Education and the American Medical Association. The report identified all sectors of society as important actors, including:

- individual Americans
- federal and state governments
- local communities
- health and social services communities

- businesses and corporations
- media, entertainment and advertising industries
- churches, youth-serving agencies and other community organizations
- the education community

Recommendations for collaborative action were directed to each of these sectors. Among those recommendations aimed at the education community were the following:

- Education and health are inextricably intertwined. Achieving the educational mission requires attending to the health needs of students.
- Recognize the necessity of working not only with students, but with their families, whatever the composition of such families might be.
- Promote the concept of collaboration within the school and welcome other health professional and service delivery organizations to the school as full partners in working with students.
- Permit sharing of information with collaborating agencies on a need-to-know basis that maintains confidentiality.
- Allow schools to serve as locations for student health care if the local community determines that school sites are the most effective location for providing collaborative services.
- Make school buildings available as sites for recreation, services and other community activities outside school hours.
- Provide all students opportunities to engage in community service.

The commission concluded its recommendations to the educational community by urging education leaders to ensure that teachers are trained in collaborative approaches and given sufficient time to work with other professionals, community members and families.

Collaboration with families requires that schools engage families in the education of their children. This can be done by giving families meaningful roles in school governance, communicating with families about the school program and student progress, and offering families opportunities to support the learning process at home and at school (Carnegie Council on Adolescent Development, 1989). For example, homework assignments that draw on their family's history and experiences or views regarding current health affairs help engage youth and their families with the school.

School Leaders' Steps to Health Program Planning

The following step-by-step approach, outlined in detail in *Step by Step to Comprehensive School Health* (Kane, 1993), walks school leaders through the development of a comprehensive program to support the healthy development of children and youth. The steps include:

- needs assessment
- organization of support and working groups
- goal development
- program status assessment
- resource analysis
- development and implementation of a strategic plan
- evaluation
- a process for monitoring and managing change

The Ad Hoc Advisory Committee
Prior to the planning process, school leaders will need to establish an ad hoc advisory committee. This committee acts as a "cabinet" to assist and advise school leaders in their efforts to initiate planning for the school's comprehensive school health program.

The ad hoc advisory committee advises school leaders during the initial stages of planning; it is discontinued once a Committee for Healthy Students is established. Members of the ad hoc committee should be selected based on the following criteria:
- the school's need for health expertise
- their access to ongoing community initiatives
- their vision of health and education challenges
- their knowledge of and access to school and community organizations
- their visibility and established leadership qualities

The nature of this committee's responsibilities suggests it should have five to eight members. Ideally, membership should include:
- a school board member
- a local or state epidemiologist
- community leaders (church, social, organizational, political)
- teachers and other school leaders

The functions of the committee are as follows:
- Reviews and clarifies the need for a vision of a comprehensive school program that supports healthy development of children.
- Identifies strategies and opportunities for schools, families and communities to come together to develop that vision.
- Advises school leaders on assessing community aspirations.
- Assists school leaders with the epidemiological assessment of the health status of children in the community.
- Advises school leaders regarding the establishment and membership of the Committee for Healthy Students.

Needs assessment includes assessing the aspirations of the community and a thorough review of epidemiologic data regarding the health status and behaviors of children and youth.

Assessment of Community Aspirations

The community's aspirations and perceptions of health needs can be identified by gathering information from:

- students
- parents and family members
- church leaders
- community leaders
- health and social services professionals
- teachers and other school personnel
- supportive community members

Community aspirations and values, when described, should provide a philosophical foundation for establishing the school's comprehensive school health program. Consulting with community members regarding their concerns not only provides valuable input that can guide program development, but is also an important first step in establishing community ownership of the program.

Because each community is different, school leaders will have to determine the most effective methods of working with their community to collect information. Issues related to reading levels, written and spoken language proficiency, cultural differences, and access to decision making need to be considered in this process. School leaders should collect information from all segments of the community to ensure a clear understanding of the community's concerns.

Epidemiologic Data

Identifying, assembling and interpreting epidemiologic data can best be carried out by public health personnel who have a background in and understanding of epidemiology. Including a public health epidemiologist on the ad hoc committee helps ensure that the school's programs consider the latest health and risk-factor data pertinent to school-age children and youth.

There are three types of epidemiologic data school leaders should consider when establishing health program priorities—mortality, morbidity, and risky or unhealthy behaviors.

Mortality (death) data, although a crude measure of health status, will provide school leaders with information regarding the causes of death among children and youth. The leading cause of mortality (death) and morbidity (sickness or injury) among children and youth has been historically mislabeled as "accidents." Use of the term *accident*, which implies a random and uncontrollable event, is widely discouraged by public health leaders. The term suggests that such injuries are not preventable, when in fact, many are. Most automobile crashes, for example, are neither random nor uncontrollable. More than half of all automobile-related deaths involve drivers who have been drinking. High speeds and careless driving account for the large majority of the remainder. School leaders will want to consider injury prevention a high priority in their planning efforts.

Behavioral risk-factor data, a third type of epidemiologic data, quantifies the presence of risky or health-protective behaviors in a population. Many experts consider the presence or absence of health-compromising behaviors or risk factors a more relevant measure of the health status of children and youth than mortality or morbidity.

Identifying behavioral risk factors among school-age youth is an important step in developing educational and preventive interventions. Typical risk factor information will include the incidence, prevalence and age at onset of:

- tobacco use
- alcohol and other drug use
- sexual intercourse

- unprotected sexual intercourse
- nonuse of safety belts
- engagement in violence
- levels of nonexercise
- unhealthy eating patterns

Specific questions that school leaders should ask include:
- What are the leading causes of mortality (deaths) among school-age youth in this community?
- What are the leading causes of morbidity (sickness and injury) among school-age youth in this community?
- What are the unhealthy or risky behaviors of our children and youth that will result in future morbidity and mortality?
- At what age do our youth develop these unhealthy or risky behaviors?

Data sources for mortality, morbidity and risky behaviors include local, state and federal agencies.

A report outlining the community's aspirations for children and youth and the epidemiological factors that influence health should be developed by school leaders. This information will become the boiler plate for the development of the school's comprehensive plan to support the healthy development of children and youth.

Community Awareness Meeting

Once school leaders have completed and digested the community needs assessment and the epidemiologic assessment of the health status of children and youth, an open community forum should be held. This meeting should be planned well in advance. It provides an opportunity for school leaders and community members to discuss the health of children and youth and ways for schools, families and the community to work together to promote healthy development. The awareness meeting can strengthen the commitment of the community to support development of school-based programs to foster healthy development of children and youth.

The Committee for Healthy Students

A Committee for Healthy Students, responsible for securing broad-based community support and input for the comprehensive school health program, should be established following the community awareness meeting. The committee membership needs to be broad enough to represent the various organizations and agencies with an interest in the healthy development of youth. Every attempt should be made to include individuals who can represent an organization's unique perspective, but can forgo the organization's individual agenda in favor of the broad agenda of establishing a systematic and comprehensive school health program.

A Shared Vision Statement

An important early step to the success of your community's efforts to provide a school program that promotes the development of healthy youth is to develop a vision for the program. Students, parents, community leaders and school personnel should all contribute to the development of this vision statement. Once developed, the vision statement needs to have high visibility in the community and in all activities related to the school's program.

There are three types of information that the Committee for Healthy Students needs to consider in the process of developing a vision statement:
- the community's aspirations and perceptions of the health needs of its children and youth
- epidemiological data about the health status and risk behaviors of children and youth

- information regarding proven methods for helping children and youth develop in healthy ways

Working Groups

School leaders will want to establish working groups charged with developing the school program to promote the health of children and youth. One efficient approach is to establish a working group responsible for each of the eight areas that contribute to the healthy development of students, as identified by Allensworth and Kolbe (1987).

Each working group will take responsibility for shaping one component of the school program so that it fosters healthy development of children and youth. Each working group will also be responsible for ensuring that its component fits with other components to constitute a comprehensive program.

Responsibilities of the working groups include:
- identifying and prioritizing new program needs
- developing program goals and objectives
- conducting resource assessment
- developing and presenting reports to the Committee for Healthy Students

The Strategic Plan

Reports from each of the working groups should be received and reviewed by the Committee for Healthy Students. This committee is responsible for developing a strategic plan that brings the eight components of the school together into a comprehensive health plan. The plan should include overall goals to be achieved over a five-year period and specific activities, tasks and outcomes for the coming two years. This plan provides a comprehensive approach for the school's efforts to foster the healthy development of children and youth. The strategic plan should include:

- long-range goals
- short-range objectives
- activities
- materials and resources needed
- staff responsible for implementation
- timeline for implementation of activities
- a framework for evaluating activities and outcomes

Presentation to the Board of Education
The strategic plan is presented to the school board of education along with the request for additional resources. The school district's board of education has the ultimate responsibility and power to make programmatic and funding decisions to support programs for healthy development of children and youth. The school board establishes the priorities and identifies the funding necessary to implement a program. The Committee for Healthy Students has the responsibility of advising the board of education.

The presentation to the board of education should include:
- the community's aspirations for its children and youth
- the needs of the community's children and youth
- the vision for healthy children and youth
- the goals and objectives of the comprehensive school health program
- the proposed plans for meeting the health needs of students
- the request for resources needed to carry out the plan

Annual Reviews
The Committee for Healthy Students should meet annually with working groups to review the status of all past-year activities and to reestablish the strategic plan for the upcoming year. Working groups for the eight areas should be responsible for reviewing and making adjustments to the following items:

- vision statement
- identified needs
- priorities assigned to each need
- activities and programs implemented in the previous year

In addition, each working group is responsible for identifying priorities, outlining activities and programs, and identifying resources available and resources needed for the coming year. The reports of each working group are annually presented to the Committee for Healthy Students for action. Every two years, the Committee for Healthy Students needs to reestablish the five-year plan for the comprehensive school health program.

Evaluation

Evaluating the health program once it is established is important for several reasons. Thoughtfully designed evaluation strategies will provide data about daily activities, management, strategies, learning experiences and community involvement (process evaluation); data about the health knowledge, skills and behaviors of children and youth (impact evaluation); and data about longitudinal changes in health status indicators (outcome evaluation).

Process evaluation should be ongoing. The data collected should be continually reviewed and used to improve existing programs. Process evaluation data is most useful to those directly involved in delivery of educational programs, services, counseling, and those involved in the day-to-day operations of the school.

Impact evaluation collects data that measures the program's effectiveness in producing gains in knowledge and achievement in the health behaviors targeted by the program. School leaders should conduct an annual review of impact evaluation data. This review should guide planning for the upcoming years.

Outcome evaluation attempts to measure changes in health

status over periods of time—usually years. Improved health status outcomes are an intended goal of health education and health promotion programs. They are an indicator of the success of school and community efforts to foster healthy development of children and youth. These changes can only be measured by careful, longitudinal analysis of health status data. Although longitudinal data is very abstract, school leaders need to understand the importance of small changes in health status indicators. For example, a community that can prevent ten unintended teenage pregnancies has actually saved hundreds of thousands of dollars and provided ten young women the opportunity to continue with their schooling and develop to their fullest potential.

Process, impact and outcome evaluation strategies need to be built into the health education program plan from the beginning.

Implementation of the Plan

The Committee for Healthy Students and the working groups provide excellent and appropriate opportunities to involve community members in identifying aspirations and developing the vision, goals, objectives and plan for the comprehensive school health program. However, school leaders know that committees are not viable mechanisms for implementing plans that establish systematic programs.

Implementation of activities and programs to support the healthy growth and development of children and youth are the responsibility of teachers and other school personnel. A clear blueprint that identifies each program goal and the objectives and activities related to that goal must be established.

A numbering system that allows for easy reference should be used to identify each activity. Figure 2 shows a sample blueprint. In this example, Goal 3, Objective 1, Activity 1 is written as 3.1.1.

Figure 2
Sample Blueprint

Goal 3: Involve all students in daily fitness activities which promote healthy physical development.

Objective 3.1: Provide all teachers in grades 1-6 with necessary knowledge and skills to provide daily fitness activities for children and youth.

Activity 3.1.1: Review the literature to determine knowledge and skills needed by teachers to implement appropriate fitness programs for school-age children and youth.
   Individual(s) Responsible: Assistant Superintendent will contract with consultant
   Materials and Resources Needed:
   • Literature reviews of school-based fitness programs
   • Evaluation studies of fitness programs
   • Expert consultant(s)

Activity 3.1.2: Develop inservice training modules designed to enable all teachers to provide daily fitness activities for children and youth. Develop process and impact evaluation instruments.
   Individual(s) Responsible: District Coordinator for Physical Education
   Materials and Resources Needed:
   • Examples of other training modules
   • Example evaluation instruments
   • Materials to provide learning experiences
      (videos, guides, equipment)

Activity 3.1.3: Secure faculty to conduct inservice training of teachers.
   Individual(s) Responsible: District Curriculum Coordinator
   Materials and Resources Needed:
   • Listing of fitness experts in local community, university, state

Activity 3.1.4: Secure facilities and schedule inservice training sessions.
   Individual(s) Responsible: Secretary for District Curriculum Coordinator
   Materials and Resources Needed:

Figure 2 (continued)
- Schedule of events and sites planned for the school year
- Listing of possible facilities and contact person and telephone number to reserve those rooms

Activity 3.1.5: Develop and circulate announcements of inservice education for all teachers.
> *Individual(s) Responsible:* District Curriculum Coordinator
> *Materials and Resources Needed:*
> - Completed announcement
> - Listing of all teachers and addresses

Activity 3.1.6: Conduct first inservice education session for teachers.
> *Individual(s) Responsible:* Consultants
> *Materials and Resources Needed:*
> - Equipment: overhead projector; VCR
> - Facilities: exercise mats

Activity 3.1.7: Review evaluation data. Modify the inservice based on the evaluation results.

The blueprint includes the following items:
- goals
- specific objectives
- activities
- individual(s) responsible
- materials and resources

Figure 3 shows a sample implementation timeline for the blueprint.

The Goals of Comprehensive School Health

Properly designed school-based health education programs help children and youth acquire the necessary awareness, knowledge

Figure 3
Sample Timeline

Activity	Individual(s) responsible	Sept	Oct	Nov	Dec	Jan	Feb	Mar	Apr	May	June
3.1.1	Assistant Superintendent/ Consultant	X	X								
3.1.2	District Coordinator for Physical Education			X	X						
3.1.3	District Curriculum Coordinator					X—X					
3.1.4	Secretary for District Curriculum Coordinator					X					
3.1.5	District Curriculum Coordinator							X			
3.1.6	Consultants								X		
3.1.7	Consultants									X	X

and health-related skills, and provide opportunities within the classroom and school for students to practice healthy behaviors. Quality school programs also recognize that the family and community play an important role in students' learning and provide wider opportunities to practice and reinforce healthy behaviors. School health education programs committed to working with families and communities to provide health education, health and social services, and an environment that promotes and rewards healthy behaviors will be an important step in supporting the healthy development of children and youth. This is the goal of comprehensive school health efforts.

References

Allensworth, D. D., and L. J. Kolbe. 1987. The comprehensive school health program: Exploring an expanded concept. *Journal of School Health* 57 (10): 409-412.

American School Health Association, Association for the Advancement of Health Education and Society for Public Health Education. 1989. *National adolescent student health survey.* Oakland, CA: Third Party Press.

Benard, B. 1991. Fostering resiliency in kids: Protective factors in the family, school and community. *Western Regional Center for Drug-Free Schools and Communities.* Portland, OR: NWREL.

Carnegie Council on Adolescent Development, Task Force on Education of Young Adolescents. 1989. *Turning points: Preparing American youth for the 21st century.* Washington, DC.

Kane, W. M. 1993. *Step by step to comprehensive school health: The program planning guide.* Santa Cruz, CA: ETR Associates.

Klingman, A. 1984. Health-related school guidance: Practical application in primary prevention. *Personnel and Guidance Journal* 62:576-579.

National Commission on the Role of the School and the Community in Improving Adolescent Health. 1990. *Code blue: Uniting for healthier youth.* Alexandria, VA: National Association of State Boards of Education.

Office of Disease Prevention and Health Promotion. 1984. *Key findings: National children and youth fitness study II.* Washington, DC.

U.S. Department of Agriculture and U.S. Department of Health and Human Services. 1990. *Nutrition and your health: Dietary guidelines for Americans.* 3d ed. Home and Garden Bulletin No. 232. Washington, DC.

U.S. Department of Health and Human Services, Public Health Service. 1991. *Healthy people 2000: National health promotion and disease prevention objectives.* DHHS Publication No. (PHS) 95-50212. Washington, DC.

Chapter 5

Instructional Planning for Health Education

Evelyn E. Ames, PhD, CHES

The classroom can be an exciting, stimulating and thought-provoking environment in which to promote health behaviors and attitudes and impart accurate knowledge for the purpose of promoting healthy lifestyles and preventing disease. Teaching personal and social health competencies and health-enhancing skills to young people cannot be left to chance or to the teachable moment.

Childhood is the prime time of human development. This is no less true for development of good health than it is for social, educational, emotional, and moral development. It may be easier to prevent the initiation of some behaviors, such as smoking and alcohol and drug abuse, than to intervene once they have become established. Likewise, it may be easier to establish healthful habits, such as those related to basic hygiene and those related to dietary and physical activity patterns, during childhood than later in life. Childhood is the opportune period for such healthy development. (U.S. Department of Health and Human Services, 1992a)

Studies document that significant and preventable health problems and risk-taking behaviors that pose serious health risks for young people can be addressed through effectively planned and implemented comprehensive school health education (Louis Harris and Associates, 1988; American School Health Association, 1989). Health-related behaviors and lifestyles established during young people's formative years have a direct effect on their lives as adults.

A comprehensive K-12 school health instruction program is the logical and effective way to ensure that children's health needs and interests are met at the appropriate developmental stages of growth. A sequenced program that reflects the process of health education and is based upon the growth and developmental characteristics of children and youth can reduce or eliminate the frustration caused by trying to deal with the multiple health concerns facing young people in a "one-shot" approach (what health educators call the "disease-of-the-month syndrome"). Proponents of the comprehensive approach point to research that indicates that "children who have repeated exposures to key topics at different stages in their education form attitudes that help them avoid bad health habits when they are older" (Pine, 1985).

The philosophy, goals and curriculum objectives of a school district's health education program give direction to the development of lesson objectives; the selection of teaching strategies, resources and materials; and the development of student outcome assessment procedures. Those planning the instructional curriculum need to know the definitions of the field and process, the philosophy, and the content of health education. They also need to understand the following:

- the school district's philosophy and goals
- what health curricula are available or mandated
- what resources and teaching aids are available
- who the students are (i.e., their needs, the community values, their developmental characteristics)
- how students influence the planning of instruction
- what good teaching entails or what students' perception of good teaching is
- topics taught in other subject areas that relate to health education

Understanding all of these factors requires considerable time, effort and thought. It requires leadership from individuals with expertise in health education who have a detailed understanding of the health needs and interests of young people. These leaders must be familiar with both the field and process of health education.

The field of health education is defined as "that multidisciplinary practice, which is concerned with designing, implementing, and evaluating educational programs that enable individuals, families, groups, organizations, and communities to play active roles in achieving, protecting, and sustaining health." The process of health education is defined as "that continuum of learning which enables people, as individuals and as members of social structures, to voluntarily make decisions, modify behaviors, and change social conditions in ways which are health enhancing" (Association for the Advancement of Health Education, 1991).

Establishing the Basis for Content Selection

All dimensions of the individual—physical, mental, emotional, social and spiritual—are integrated into health topics and issues of a K-12 comprehensive program. Selection of content is oriented to the skills, knowledge and attitudes that contribute to the development of healthy lifestyles and promote a sense of well-being. Relevant and necessary content focuses on preventable health problems of children and youth such as intentional and unintentional injuries, substance use, sexually transmitted disease, low self-esteem and physical inactivity.

Determining Content

Individuals appointed to determine content (subject matter) of the school health curriculum should first expand their horizons as to what the content of health education could be. The next step is to narrow the identified content so that it adheres to the school district's philosophy and goals and fits within the curriculum time frame. Professionals in the field of health education suggest that comprehensive school health instruction includes, but is not limited to, ten major content areas: community health, consumer health, environmental health, family life, mental and emotional health, injury prevention and safety, nutrition, personal health, prevention and control of disease, and substance use and abuse (Association for the Advancement of Health Education, 1991).

Some teachers may opt to change these headings to reflect more closely their school district's health education curriculum. For example, elementary teachers involved in developing a health education scope and sequence for kindergarten through grade five for the Bellingham Public School District in Washington chose to make the following changes:
• broaden family life to family life/social skills

- narrow mental and emotional health to emotional health
- combine prevention and control of disease and personal health to form personal care/disease prevention and control
- list growth and development as a separate content area

In regard to the family life heading, teachers said they focused on social skills when teaching family relationships and felt the combined heading more adequately reflected what they taught in their classrooms (Ames and Sherwood, 1992).

Instructional planners need to know what subject matter falls within the rubric of school health instruction. Descriptions of subject matter within the ten major content areas are found in various state health education frameworks and health education texts. For example, descriptors of the minimum knowledge for the area of substance use and abuse in one state's framework are "personal goals, individual responsibility, substances beneficial to mankind, classifications of substances and their effects on the body, implications of use of substances, how habits are formed and influence health, use and misuse of tobacco, alcohol and other drugs, treatment and rehabilitation programs, respect for self and others" (Ames et al., 1992). But planners should keep in mind that "there should be no hard and fast rule for organizing topics into health areas; in any curriculum, placement of a topic under a particular health area is arbitrary. Discussion, for instance, of non-prescription drugs could be included when studying drugs, disease control, consumer health, or safety" (Trucano, 1984).

Student Interests

Another basis for selecting content is to look at the interests of young people. Two well-known studies, *Teach Us What We Want to Know* (Byler, Lewis and Totman, 1969) and *Students Speak* (Trucano, 1984), revealed what students said were their health interests. For each grade level, students indicated what health topics interested them, what their perceptions of the value of health education were, and how they wanted to be taught.

In the Trucano study, students expressed interest in learning about "fears and worries" at all grade levels. There was a high interest in learning about drugs at all grade levels; and almost all grade levels mentioned divorce. Students also wanted to be involved in the learning process and to be taught by competent teachers.

A later study of adolescents by Louis Harris and Associates (1988) provided data that showed which health topics from a list of eleven were very important to students. Of the adolescents surveyed, 75 percent rated not taking or experimenting with drugs as very important, 68 percent rated not smoking cigarettes very important, and 60 percent rated not being overweight very important.

Student Health Needs

Content selection is also based upon what students know and believe about health (their knowledge and attitudes) and what health behaviors they practice or do not practice. There are many sources of data about students' health knowledge, behaviors and attitudes, including the following:
- government agencies such as the Centers for Disease Control and Prevention (CDC), in particular the National Center for Chronic Disease Prevention and Health Promotion and its Division of Adolescent and School Health
- state departments of education and health
- school districts
- community agencies and organizations
- private foundations

The CDC's 1990 *Youth Risk Behavior Survey* contains a wealth of information about adolescents' health behaviors relating to intentional and unintentional injuries, tobacco use, alcohol and other drug use, sexual behaviors and dietary behaviors. (See box.)

Youth Risk Behavior Survey

Motor vehicle crashes account for 31 percent of the causes of death among 1 to 24 year olds.

Nearly half of all deaths from motor vehicle crashes among students in grades nine through twelve involve alcohol.

Homicide accounts for 13 percent of the deaths among this age group.

Suicide rates for adolescents ages 15 to 19 have quadrupled from 1950 to 1988.

Approximately 86 percent of all sexually transmitted diseases occur among persons ages 15 to 29.

Only 37 percent of students in grades nine through twelve report being vigorously active, with physical activity being significantly less common among females and African-American students (U.S. Department of Health and Human Services, 1992b).

The 1987 *National Children and Youth Fitness Study II* identified physical activity needs of young children. The study found the health-related fitness of young children to be significantly associated with the physical activity behaviors of the children themselves and their parents. Today, young children weigh more and have more body fat than they did twenty years ago. They eat more while they watch television; they also eat more of the foods they see advertised on television. The average child in grades one through four spends two hours, two minutes watching television on school days and three hours, twenty-six minutes watching television on the weekends (U.S. Department of Health and Human Services, 1987).

Community and Societal Needs

Instructional planners must also examine community and societal needs. Information about community needs can be obtained by contacting local health-related organizations, health care providers, public health departments, youth and social service organizations, and religious groups. For societal needs, an excellent place to start is a review of the *Healthy People 2000* Summary Report. This government document provides a database targeting important health issues. Approximately 33 percent of the year 2000 objectives focus on school-age children and youth. Attainment of these objectives relies substantially on improvements in comprehensive school health education.

Other national sources are the Children's Defense Fund, which provides useful data about health problems of American youth, and two frequently cited documents, *Code Blue: Uniting for Healthier Youth* (National Commission on the Role of the School and the Community in Improving Adolescent Health, 1990) and *Turning Points* (Carnegie Council on Adolescent Development, 1989), which target adolescents. The Children's Defense Fund's 1990 report indicates that every 47 seconds an American child is abused or neglected; every 67 seconds an American teenager has a baby; and every seven minutes an American child is arrested for a drug offense.

Special Concerns

Instructional planners need to reflect upon the special concerns that affect health instruction and be cognizant that planning for health education may differ from planning for other subject areas. Parental, community and religious values can be antagonistic or supportive forces that drive the curriculum. Legislative mandates influence not only health content but at which grade level certain topics are to be taught. For example, most states have legislated

HIV/AIDS prevention education to be taught at specific grade levels.

Therefore, the selection of health content is guided not only by the health needs and interests of young people, but by a school district's philosophy and goals, state legislative mandates, parental and community values, and research about young people's behaviors and health status.

Narrowing the Scope of Health Education

Needless to say, not all major content areas and identified health topics and issues can be taught every year or at every grade level. The scope of health content needs to be narrowed before proceeding in the sequencing of selected content. The process of narrowing the scope (i.e., the range of health topics that could or should be taught at each grade level) can be facilitated through the use of agreed-upon criteria (Ames et al., 1992). Pertinent questions to ask when narrowing the scope include:

- Are topics and skills consistent with the philosophy and goals that have been established?
- How important is the health topic in relation to the health needs of the target population?
- Is the topic relevant to the specific characteristics and needs of the identified population?
- What is the relative importance and urgency of the health topic to society?
- Is the topic of a high level of interest to the learners?
- Can one distinguish between unnecessary repetition and desirable reinforcement?

A curriculum committee with representation of teachers from each grade level (including those from combined grades), school support staff, parents and community health care providers can provide answers to these questions.

Sequencing Health Content

Sequencing means that health topics are arranged at various grade levels in such a way as to meet the developmental needs and interests of young people. The many topics and issues the health education curriculum planning committee identifies as necessary and relevant need to be sequenced and placed at appropriate grade levels. This arrangement of topics and issues at particular grade levels must meet the developmental growth patterns, health needs and interests of students, and impart the related desired health knowledge, attitudes and practices, as well as meet the needs of the school district, parents and community.

Keep in mind that health topics are placed at various grade levels not only to introduce new issues but also to review and reinforce what students have previously been taught. Curriculum and lesson objectives are developed to encourage students to build on their prior knowledge. Sequencing encourages the consideration of different aspects of a health topic and the application of acquired knowledge to new situations. Some health topics will be of interest to students at all grade levels, but different aspects of these topics will be studied at different age levels (Ames et al., 1992).

Sequencing is determined by the developmental growth patterns of children and youth as well as societal needs, family needs, individual needs and current events. Instructional planners, therefore, must be knowledgeable about the physiological and psychosocial developmental characteristics of children and youth.

For example, early adolescents undergo vast and rapid physical changes. Young adolescent females are reaching menarche and subsequent fertility at earlier ages than ever before. Young females are maturing physiologically, from the standpoint of being able to become pregnant, at age 12, 13 or 14, but have yet to reach the equivalent maturity in their psycho-social development, especially when it comes to decision-making skills. And what about young males? They have not changed much in respect to the onset of puberty during the past several decades. The implications of this are very interesting. Who are the young females dating? What is happening to same-age males in respect to dating patterns? What decision-making skills should these young people be practicing?

Understanding these changes and differences is essential to effective sequencing of sexuality education subject matter. Those planning health instruction must wisely select health content, lesson objectives and student outcomes, teaching strategies, resources and evaluation procedures that effectively address the changing developmental needs of youth.

The following example illustrates the relationship of developmental characteristics to desired health knowledge, attitudes or behaviors. Young people ages 12 to 15 are described as being "ambivalent between independence and need for adults; self-identity strong at times to a point of rebellion." If one of the goals of a school district's health education program is to educate students to practice behaviors that promote and maintain mental health, then the desired health knowledge, attitudes or behaviors corresponding to these developmental characteristics would be that the student "strengthens self-concept and self-understanding; explores effect of selected situations; assesses own feelings about selected risk behavior" (Ames et al., 1992).

This example illustrates the need for instructional planners to review growth and developmental characteristics of each age group and relate these to the health knowledge, attitudes and behaviors desired for young people. As a further illustration of this relationship, it is known that young people ages 9 to 12 are "concerned with differences in growth patterns; may be embarrassed about their own and others' physical development." If a second health education goal of the school district is to educate the students about patterns of healthy growth and development, then the desired health knowledge, attitudes and behaviors would focus on students understanding the normalcy of differences in growth patterns and cycles (Ames et al., 1992).

Planning Lessons and Selecting Methodology

Planning lessons is like serving a full-course meal. Certain ingredients are requisite for the completion of a successful learning activity in health education. The lesson is a plan a teacher follows to facilitate the process of learning so particular student outcomes are accomplished.

> Lesson plans are step-by-step procedures the teacher will follow to assist students in meeting the lesson objective(s). Lessons can last fifteen minutes or continue over several days. Lessons include lesson objectives (what is to be learned), generally an introductory activity (to develop interest and/or to explain what will be expected of the students), the actual learning experience (what the students will be doing to achieve the objective), resources needed, and (if a lesson is evaluated by itself rather than as part of a unit) what evaluation will be used. (Ames et al., 1992)

Planning instructional lessons requires determining how many minutes and hours (especially at the elementary grade level) or days (more likely at the secondary level) teachers have to teach health. It requires selecting curriculum objectives that address the school district's curriculum goals for health education. These are grade-specific objectives written for instructional planning that provide direction for deciding what learning activities and materials are to be used in a particular lesson or course of instruction. It also requires choosing a variety of teaching strategies to enable teachers to meet different student learning styles and elicit student enthusiasm.

Lesson objectives need to be written for the selected teaching strategies. Lesson objectives define what students will be able to do, know or feel after completing a particular lesson. Planning lessons also requires a school district to obtain materials that will assist teachers in accomplishing their lessons and in preparing evaluation procedures by which student outcomes can be assessed.

The basis for selecting teaching strategies is related to the following:
- the characteristics of the students
- the comfort level of the teacher in using a particular method
- the availability of teaching materials and resources
- the adaptability of the strategy to the teaching center
- the time it takes to complete the strategy
- the hands-on involvement of students

Whatever the basis, ultimately the strategy should accomplish the lesson objective.

It is a challenging task to find appropriate and usable resources for teaching health lessons. A considerable number of resources are available from nonprofit and for-profit businesses and organizations, as well as governmental agencies. All resources need to be evaluated for their usefulness. When choosing resources, be sure the content is accurate, current and complete, and free from racial, ethnic, sex, age, disability and cultural bias. Resources need to be age-appropriate and interesting to young people, have instructional merit, and meet the district's philosophical point of view. They should address stated curriculum objectives and goals, be realistic in cost, and pose little or no difficulty in use by teachers and students (Ames et al., 1992).

Special Concerns When Planning Health Instruction

The subject matter of health education encompasses many things that are a part of everyday life; the issues it addresses focus on immediate and future personal health needs and interests. These issues are personal and arise out of values; therefore, parents, young people, community members, religious leaders and school administrators have strong feelings and opinions about what should or should not be taught to children and youth. Whether the teacher presents one viewpoint or allows for many, teaching about human sexuality, substance use and abuse, self-image, risk-taking behaviors, nutrition, health care practitioners, values, emotional well-being, family relationships and a host of other health-related topics has the potential to create controversy.

Students who want to search out facts, evaluate the information and learn how to make the "right" decisions will be heavily influenced by the values they bring with them from their own homes. This means that students will not all make the same decisions. Creating a classroom environment that allows various viewpoints to be expressed is basic to a democracy. Education that teaches critical thinking and good decision making is requisite for such a democratic classroom.

An awareness and understanding of the people and organizations who can influence health education is crucial. The school board, school district and building administrators, teachers, health education coordinators, school support staff, students and parents influence the curriculum. Other key players include community members, religious leaders, health care providers and agencies, public health officials, state lawmakers, and departments of education. Both teachers and administrators must be aware of issues that could polarize the community. Therefore, it is wise to adopt policies and procedures for governing the treatment of sensitive and controversial health issues in the classroom.

As previously mentioned, planning for health instruction may differ from planning instruction for other curricular areas. For one thing, health education, as yet, is not an entrenched subject within the total school curriculum as are math, science and English. This results in fewer comprehensive curricula and resources being avail able in the district's curriculum library. For another, fewer teachers are professionally prepared in health education when compared to the number prepared in other teaching areas. Health education is less likely to be part of university and college teacher preparation core requirements. Following graduation, when teachers are as-signed to teach health, they require more inservice training about curricula, content and pedagogical skills needed to teach health. "No matter how inclusive, enriched, and updated the curriculum is, it has little value if the delivery or the instructional method to teach the concepts, skills, and information is not effective. Teach-ing students involves more than just reaching them" (Klavas, 1991).

For a curriculum to be carried out as planned, inservice training of teachers is crucial. Such training gives teachers a clear under-standing of the expectations related to the health education cur-riculum and helps them buy into the program. (See Chapter 28 for more information on inservice training.) Those who do teacher inservice training should be cognizant of factors that can contrib-ute to successful programs. A two-year project in which 56 elementary teachers received inservice training and mentoring in comprehensive school health education identified several key factors that contributed to a highly successful inservicing and mentoring program (Ames and Sherwood, 1992). These factors include:

- Project staff respect and value teachers.
- Speakers are credible and enthusiastic.
- Workshops meet teacher needs based on needs assessments and site visits.
- A safe climate for open discussion is created.
- The training atmosphere is upbeat, with music and humor incorporated daily.
- Strategies encourage team bonding.
- Background information substantiates health teaching.
- Practical lesson ideas are presented.
- Grade-appropriate strategies are emphasized.
- Time is allotted for processing and debriefing information.
- Activities are highly interactive and student-centered.
- There is time in class for participants to make and take materials for classroom use and to plan school year activities.
- The inservice schedule accommodates teachers' needs.
- Incentives and teaching materials are provided.
- Basic creature comforts are met and good food is provided.
- Facility for instruction is spacious and accommodating, with convenient parking provided.

Inservice programs organized to update and prepare teachers to teach health education frequently target categorical curricula and methodology pertaining to the specific curricula. Inservice seldom focuses on comprehensive school health instruction. Usually omitted is education about students' health needs and interests; their developmental characteristics and the corresponding desired health knowledge, attitudes and practices; and an operational definition of comprehensive school health instruction.

Health education is often integrated or infused into other teaching areas such as science and social studies. Curriculum coordinators may mistakenly believe this to be an effective means of educating youth about health. Rather than establishing separate health classes at the middle and secondary levels, health education is "inserted" into other classes for a few days or weeks. A common saying is that when health instruction becomes everybody's business, it generally becomes nobody's business!

The problem with this "one-way street" philosophy is that it leads nowhere. There should be two-way streets, or better yet, several streets (i.e., curricular areas) converging to tackle societal and student health issues. Teachers of three, four or five curricular areas (e.g., math, science, social studies, health and English) could work together to focus on a specific health issue, such as environmental pollution, for one or two weeks. A team approach to health instruction could bring life to learning. "Where possible, curriculum delivery systems with similar learner outcomes should be integrated and coordinated to form a better instructional program" (Wisconsin Department of Public Instruction, 1992). Making connections among curricular areas should be given high priority as schools move toward the twenty-first century. These connections require a concerted effort by teachers and administrators.

Preparing Teachers to Teach Health Education

Implementation of comprehensive school health instruction is hampered by inadequately prepared teachers. Poorly prepared teachers and a lack of interest by staff assigned to teach health have been documented by national studies to be critical contributing factors as to why quality school health education programs have not become a reality for more than 25 years (Coalition of National Health Education Organizations, 1990).

Teachers' awareness of the importance of a healthy classroom and how this contributes to the well-being of students must be increased. What teachers say and do can have a lasting impact on students. Creating a healthy classroom constitutes a vital ingredient in the recipe for being an effective and successful teacher. Understanding the learning process and professional preparation are important as well.

Understanding the Learning Process

Master teachers know that individuals learn in different ways. Therefore, a variety of teaching strategies and learning experiences must be chosen to meet the needs of those who learn best through reading or hearing or seeing or doing, or through a mix of these learning modes. The more teachers involve students in the learning process and the more actively students' five senses are involved, the more learning will take place.

Master teachers know that students differ in their learning styles, i.e., the way they concentrate on, process and retain new and difficult information. Learning style is defined as a combination of many variables, including physical, environmental, emotional, psychological and sociological stimuli. Some students process information analytically, in a step-by-step sequential pattern that builds toward a conceptual understanding. Other students, global learners, learn by understanding the concept first and then by concentrating on the details.

> Many analytics tend to prefer learning in a quiet, well-illuminated, informal setting; they often have a strong emotional need to complete the tasks they are

working on, and they rarely eat, drink, smoke, chew, or bite on objects *while* learning. Conversely, globals appear to work with what teachers describe as distractors; they concentrate better with sound (music or background talking), soft lighting, an informal seating arrangement, and some form of intake. In addition, globals take frequent breaks while studying and often prefer to work on several tasks simultaneously. (Dunn, 1989)

Master teachers know that there is a period of readiness for learning. Involving young people in planning learning activities and in carrying out projects will assist teachers in determining their students' readiness to learn. Master teachers also know that when children feel success, they are motivated to learn. Children continue to be productive if they experience such feelings. Therefore, it is necessary for teachers to set short-term, realistic goals that make success an obvious element. Students can also help set classroom goals. The more students apply the learning to their own interests, values and needs, the more interesting the learning and the more permanent the application will be (Ames et al., 1992).

Professional Preparation

Until such time as universities and colleges and education accrediting bodies deem it relevant to require course work in instructional methods in health education as part of the core requirements for all elementary education majors, health education will be poorly taught in the elementary grades. The route to improvement in secondary health instruction is preservice professional preparation in an academic major in health education. The program major should meet the accrediting standards of AAHE/NCATE (Association for the Advancement of Health Education/National Council on Accreditation of Teacher Education). Additionally, all teacher education majors, both elementary and secondary, should be educated in ways to enhance their own lifestyle behaviors. Healthy role modeling by teachers does have an impact on students. (See Chapter 27 for more information on preservice education.)

Whether teacher preparation is preservice or inservice, a guiding light is provided by what students have to say about teachers who teach health. When asked what they thought teachers should do and know when teaching health (Trucano, 1984), students said teachers should:

- "Be prepared—know what they are talking about."
- "Teach the things involving our life now and in the future."
- "Talk to us and tell us things of health so we can understand instead of just reading it out of the book."
- "Be knowledgeable; have a clue; be competent."
- "Go more into the subject. Talk about every little thing a body does and how it works and how it stops working, and then use a model and point to every part of the body."
- "I would like teachers to be well educated for the area they teach."

Special Concerns for Elementary Teachers

A typical comment of the elementary teacher is, "I don't teach health! I don't have time to teach another subject. The curriculum is already too crowded." In reality, however, elementary teachers *do* teach health—they just don't recognize that they do! Visit an elementary classroom on any given day and look at the bulletin boards. Ask to see student activities that focus on self-esteem, relationships, injury prevention, nutrition, and growth and development. Health education is happening, but often the elementary teacher is not aware of it until it is pointed out. Elementary teachers participating in a project to enhance and update their pedagogical skills and strategies and increase their comfort level for teaching health were astonished to find that health education is central to much of what they do on a daily basis. Elementary teachers are truly concerned with the health and well-being of their students.

Elementary school health instruction can be strengthened by showing teachers how to connect lesson objectives and subject matter content among various disciplines. The Wisconsin curriculum supplement *Healthy Kids* suggests the coordination and management of people, time and resources to achieve curriculum goals and student objectives that are mutually beneficial and interrelated. The focus is on establishing "models of specific content area integration at the elementary level which can be simultaneously achieved through a coordinated, integrated approach toward classroom instruction" (Wisconsin Department of Public Instruction, 1992). Health instruction at the elementary grade level also can be strengthened by helping teachers feel more comfortable about teaching health and be more knowledgeable about their own health behaviors.

Requirements for Instructional Planning

Planning comprehensive school health instruction requires an understanding and knowledge of the health needs, interests and developmental characteristics (growth and development patterns) of young people. Health needs and interests define the health content of the curriculum; developmental characteristics define the age-appropriateness of content and materials and the methodology used to educate young people about health. Those planning the instructional program must know the field of health education and its content and philosophy, what good teaching entails, what curricula and resources are available, why a variety of teaching strategies need to be selected, why individuality must be remembered when evaluating student outcomes, and how developmental characteristics direct the selection of content, objectives and learning experiences.

References

Ames, E., L. Trucano, J. Wan and M. Harris. 1992. *Designing school health curricula: Planning for good health.* Dubuque: William C. Brown.

Ames, E., and L. Sherwood. 1992. Project health 1990-1992. Comprehensive school health education: Inservicing and mentoring elementary education teachers. Unpublished data. Bellingham, WA: Western Washington University.

Association for the Advancement of Health Education. 1991. Report of the 1990 joint committee on health education terminology. *Journal of Health Education* 22 (2): 97-108.

Byler, R. V., G. M. Lewis and R. J. Totman. 1969. *Teach us what we want to know.* New York: Mental Heath Materials Center.

Carnegie Council on Adolescent Development. 1989. *Turning points: Preparing American youth for the 21st century.* Report of the Task Force on Education of Young Adolescents. Washington, DC.

Children's Defense Fund. 1990. *Children 1990: A report card, briefing book and action primer.* Washington, DC.

Coalition of National Health Education Organizations. 1990. *Incentives for strengthening elementary school health education.* Position paper by the delegates to the Coalition of National Health Education Organizations. Chapel Hill, North Carolina, January.

Dunn, R. 1989. Introduction to learning styles and brain behavior: Part 1 of 2, suggestions for practitioners. *Inter-Ed* 15 (47): 6-8.

Klavas, A. 1991. Teaching health education through students' individual learning styles. *Proceedings of six regional workshops: Strengthening health education for the 1990s.* Reston, VA: Association for the Advancement of Health Education.

Louis Harris and Associates. 1988. *Health—you've got to be taught: An evaluation of comprehensive health education in American public schools.* New York: Metropolitan Life Foundation.

National Commission on the Role of the School and the Community in

Improving Adolescent Health. 1990. *Code blue: Uniting for healthier youth.* Alexandria, VA: National Association of State Boards of Education.

Pine, P. 1985. *Critical issues report: Promoting health education in schools—problems and solutions.* Arlington, VA: American Association of School Administrators.

Trucano, L. 1984. *Students speak: A survey of health interests and concerns.* Seattle, WA: Comprehensive Health Education Foundation.

U.S. Department of Health and Human Services. 1987. Summary of findings from National Children and Youth Fitness Study II. *Journal of Physical Education, Recreation and Dance* 58 (9): 50-96.

U.S. Department of Health and Human Services, Public Health Service. 1991. *Healthy people 2000: National health promotion and disease prevention objectives.* DHHS Publication No. (PHS) 91-50212 Washington, DC.

U.S. Department of Health and Human Services, Public Health Service. 1992a. *Healthy people 2000: Summary report.* Boston: Jones and Bartlett.

U.S. Department of Health and Human Services, Public Health Service. 1992b. *1990 youth risk behavior survey.* MMWR Series. Atlanta, GA: Centers for Disease Control and Prevention, National Center for Chronic Disease Prevention and Health Promotion.

Wisconsin Department of Public Instruction. 1992. *Healthy kids: A team approach to integrating developmental guidance and health education.* Madison, WI: Bureau for Program Development.

Chapter 6

The Importance of a Healthy School Environment

Alan C. Henderson, DrPH, CHES

Traditionally, the school environment has been viewed as a basic ingredient for education. Much attention has been given to the planning, construction and maintenance of the physical plant of the school. However, traditional views of the school environment can be broadened by looking at the school as a web of interdependent and interacting components. These components include the physical plant, emotional tone and social climate. All of these factors are important for achieving educational goals as well as conserving scarce human and material resources at the school.

The broadened concept of the school environment as key to the formation and reinforcement of healthy behavior places greater demands on school personnel. Yet by putting this idea into practice, school personnel may be healthier and happier in their work and may be able to offer opportunities for their students to obtain more from their education.

The Importance of the School Environment

Millions of students, teachers, administrators and staff spend their working days at schools throughout the United States. Thousands of public and private schools are found in all parts of the nation—urban, suburban and rural. Schools are highly diverse organizational units, from private schools, one-school rural districts, elementary or secondary school districts to huge, urban, unified districts containing hundreds of thousands of students. While school is one of our most common shared experiences, each school contains a unique blend of physical, social and emotional elements that create its character and help to shape the teaching/learning process and educational outcomes.

Much attention is paid to teaching and learning in schools and how these things are assessed and improved. Local, state and national attention is given to observations, analyses and recommendations for changing and improving our schools. Educational reform and restructuring proposals have dominated the nation's attention in the 1980s and into the 1990s, with the intent of helping our schools to better prepare children and youth for responsible adulthood in our society. Rarely have these proposals looked upon the school as a worksite, both for students and for those responsible for the education, health and safety of students.

Education at all levels is a labor-intensive endeavor. The quality of the teaching/learning process is determined by the skills and knowledge of those responsible for education. The outcomes of education are dependent upon the willingness and ability of learners to participate in the educational process. The location and physical facilities of the school, its learning resources, support services, staff and administrators are the underpinnings of teaching and learning; they influence the outcomes of the process.

The school's physical facilities, once constructed and equipped, are difficult to change without substantial capital improvements. As population patterns change, some schools lose their student populations as other schools become overwhelmed with students. Unfortunately, schools can't easily be moved once built. Through time and use, essential equipment becomes dated or worn. The necessary replacements may entail significant financial investment to modify the school's physical plant.

Teaching resources are particularly subject to change as evolving technology and knowledge become translated into new teaching resources. Decisions to adopt one or more new instructional programs are involved and are often quite costly. Related equipment, such as computers, may be required to fully adopt new resources.

These conditions and decisions are familiar challenges to educators; they are part of the nature of K-12 education. What may be less understood is the effect of the social and emotional as well as the physical school environment on students and school personnel. Educational progress of students is affected by their health status; it affects their ability and willingness to learn. Educational effectiveness of school personnel is affected by their health status; it affects their ability to carry out their responsibilities. The health status of both groups can be maintained, protected and improved by conscientious efforts to recognize and support opportunities for health promotion at the school.

A major reason for addressing the school environment as a means for school improvement is the evolving concept of health as applied to the school. Most of us are familiar with particular health concerns affecting children and youth, including the following:

- communicable and noncommunicable disease
- intentional and unintentional injury
- hearing, vision and ambulatory limitations

- premature sexual behavior and pregnancies
- sexually transmitted disease, including HIV and AIDS
- alcohol and other drug dependencies
- behavioral problems

Each of these concerns is well described in popular and scientific media. What has been missing has been the development and implementation of concepts that can help educators link these issues and concerns together.

In the last several years, an evolution of thought has begun to crystallize and shape approaches to these numerous health concerns. The perspective presented here is that health for all in our schools and educational processes are inseparable. Students cannot properly learn if they have health difficulties. Similarly, teachers and other school personnel cannot be effective if they, too, have obstacles to health.

Palpable but often intangible factors such as the emotional or social climate can support or undermine educational objectives. Schools are total experiences for students and staff alike—what occurs in and out of the classroom forms a seamless background that helps shape the well-being of all.

Schools' Basic Responsibilities for Health

Aside from recent developments in our understanding of environmental influences on learning, there is no question that schools have basic responsibilities for protecting and promoting the health and safety of all who go to school, including teachers, administrators and staff. Schools consist of not only the physical plant and grounds that make them identifiable as schools, but also the facilities, equipment, books, curricular materials, consumable supplies and the people occupying the physical plant. The responsibility to protect health begins at the onset when new schools are planned and continues until the school no longer is used for education.

As a legal and ethical matter, school officials are responsible for looking after the health and safety of their students. The schools act *in loco parentis*, meaning the schools take the place of the parents in a special way. Schools are obligated to return children to their parents or guardians at the end of the school day with the same health status they had when they left home to go to school. Schools are responsible for children and youth on the way to and from school as well as during the school day. This responsibility requires that teachers and administrators take positive action in two ways.

First, school personnel must take reasonable steps to protect students from potential harm stemming from hazards created by the physical environment of the school building and its surroundings, as well as hazards created by students' actions or those of others. Children and youth frequently act impulsively or fail to think through the risks they may encounter. Because school personnel should understand these qualities of young people, they are accountable for dealing with and removing harmful situations, whether physical, personal or interpersonal.

Second, school personnel must discipline students who misbehave, holding them accountable for their behavior. Discipline may take the form of requiring students to serve detention after school or, when statutory laws have been broken, legal steps involving law enforcement.

Both aspects of the school's duty to act require that teachers and administrators, as well as any other designated school officials, supervise the conduct of students. Active supervision and an adequate number of supervising school personnel help to reduce or eliminate risks to the greatest extent possible. Much case law in the courts has demonstrated the adverse consequences when teachers and administrators fail to provide supervision when called for, supervise inadequately by ignoring or neglecting supervising duties, or fail to provide enough supervisors.

The importance of the school's ethical and legal obligation to protect its students warrants annual review, discussion and revision of school policies and procedures by all school personnel to try to identify the best means for doing so. Administrators and teachers new to the school, as well as student teachers, should receive an orientation to their supervisorial and legal duties. They should also become familiar with the policies and procedures established by the school and school district. Specific problem areas need to be identified and action plans developed to address them, with a firm date for resolution identified. New problems arising during the school year should be the subject of staff meetings as needed and should be resolved at the earliest possible date.

Adapting the Physical Environment

Another basic area of responsibility for health protection at the school is the adaptation or modification of the school's physical environment and daily schedule to meet the needs of those who attend the school each day. As the physical plant and equipment ages and as characteristics of the surrounding community and students change, the need for altering the school becomes apparent. If schools are to continue to meet needs, then classrooms, offices, gyms, fields and equipment must be adapted to fulfill changing educational missions.

First consideration should be given to identifying and correcting physical hazards in the schools. These changes involve many physical aspects of the school, including:
- worn or dangerous building materials (e.g., gym floors or non-fire-retardant draperies)

- broken or inadequate ventilation systems
- holes in playing fields
- broken toilets
- leaking faucets and water coolers
- asbestos ceiling and/or floor tiles
- rickety stair railings and slippery, worn steps
- inoperable communications systems
- poorly maintained fire hoses and fire extinguishers

The life cycle of many of these parts of school buildings can be estimated and replacement budgeted. However, in recent years, the infrastructure of the school has often taken a back seat to other demands, such as new instructional programs to meet compelling educational needs, until such time as the physical plant's hazards to its occupants result in unavoidable and unfortunate personal or property damage. Many health and safety hazards are silent until other changes in the environment cause these threats to become manifest.

In the last several years, changes in law and in educational philosophy have demanded and encouraged the mainstreaming of students with handicaps into the school. Equal employment opportunity statutes have made it possible for those with handicaps to acquire teaching and administrative credentials to work in schools. As a consequence, school facilities have had to be modified or designed to accommodate these students and workers.

Meeting Basic Responsibilities in Schools at Risk
Many of our schools, and inner-city urban schools in particular, are experiencing an unrelenting deterioration of their capacity to deliver education. Problems include:
- poverty
- widespread alcohol and other drug use

- violence
- unemployment
- youth gangs
- deteriorating housing and closed businesses
- low educational attainment by parents
- premature pregnancies
- inadequate tax support for education and social and health services

These and other social and health indicators combine to create formidable barriers to meeting the educational needs of children and youth. Despite our increasing capabilities for education overall, changes in significant parts of our society have diminished the capacity of far too many schools to provide the basic necessities that make education possible.

Deteriorating schools, like all others, are total environments. There are reciprocal and interactive connections between the school's services, instruction and environment and the surrounding community. Substantial social problems in the community are reflected in the schools. School personnel can play an important role in counteracting the deleterious effects of impoverished communities on education. Despite the constraints of the environment, educational progress can be made.

The first priority of the school must be to provide a safe and healthy environment to protect students during the school day and on their way to and from school. Conditions in the inner-city environment make it increasingly difficult to meet this basic requirement. Schools have taken extraordinary steps to achieve this priority, with limited success. Yet educators recognize that without this foundation schools are greatly inhibited from developing an atmosphere supportive of learning.

School leaders need to make sure that unwanted outside influences are kept away or removed from the school. These disruptive influences, such as drug dealing and gang activity, undermine campus authority. School authorities have the legal responsibility and right to make sure that these unwanted groups are kept from school grounds. In some instances, these provisions extend to areas near the campus.

Disruptions at school wreak havoc with education and must be dealt with in a swift and effective manner to remove the individual or individuals precipitating the problem. School officials must also take steps to establish an environment that respects teaching and learning and the rights of youth to participate in the process without distraction.

To reinforce these measures, school officials need to develop contacts with community agencies interested in and responsible for services that will support a safe atmosphere for the school. They must also involve parent and community groups. Parents need to be given information about the progress being made at the school. Parents and other community members can offer feedback and help to reinforce the policies and procedures developed to create a safe haven at school.

Once the basic provisions for safety have been established and a stable environment has been created, school leaders can begin to expand health-promoting activities. All affected parties must be involved in this process under the consistent leadership of school administrators. Consistency and commitment must be translated into the daily schedules and activities of the school and into the attitudes and behavior of teachers, staff and students. This time-consuming process will have periods of progress and setback. Yet without a commitment to these procedures, schools at risk will not be able to provide the benefits of education to youth in these troubled environments.

Good Health as a Vital School Component

Once basic responsibilities for health and safety are met, schools can focus attention on the more substantive qualities of education. Underlying school improvement is the recognition that the health of all those learning and working at school is vital to the educational process. Health was identified as one of the seven cardinal principles of education more than a hundred years ago, with the recognition that being healthy makes it possible for learning to occur. This principle also applies to teachers and staff. Health is a foundation factor in education, as in most other aspects of life, because it is instrumental to all activities.

Health of Today's Children and Youth

Overall health of children and youth has improved over the years. According to the federal publication *Healthy People 2000* (U.S. Department of Health and Human Services, 1991), death rates for children decreased by 21 percent from 1977 to 1987. Death rates also declined for adolescents and young adults during this same period.

For children and adolescents, unintentional injuries are now the major cause of death. Most of these deaths are due to motor vehicle crashes. Even these rates have been declining, although a disturbing upward trend has occurred for adolescents and young adults in recent years. For children, mandatory safety seats and the use of automobile safety belts have helped to reduce this rate. However, the rate of child and youth homicide has increased, with death by homicide becoming the leading cause of death among African-American males 15 to 19 years old.

Infectious and respiratory illnesses remain problems for children and youth. Influenza and other respiratory diseases account for most school days missed. Recent estimates of the prevalence of chronic health conditions for those under 18 years of age suggest that 31 percent, or almost 20 million children nationwide, have one or more chronic conditions. Of those with such conditions, 70 percent have one, 21 percent have two and 9 percent have three or more. Most children affected by these conditions report that their activities are not limited by the presence of the conditions most of the time.

The most commonly reported of these conditions are respiratory allergies and repeated ear infections. Other common chronic conditions include asthma, eczema and skin allergies, frequent or severe headaches, and speech defects. Less common conditions include diabetes, sickle cell disease and cerebral palsy. Chronic conditions are more prevalent among boys than girls and among White children than African-American. The cumulative impact of these conditions on school attendance in 1988 resulted in 41 million absences.

An additional concern is that diet and exercise patterns for our children and youth are changing. Youth are becoming a less physically fit and fatter group. Between 1965 and 1985, skinfold thicknesses (a measure of body fat) of children have increased. As measured by the U.S. Public Health Service, 15 percent of youth ages 12 to 19 were overweight in the 1976 to 1980 period.

Levels of fitness among youth in recent years have decreased, and the proportion of those leading sedentary lives has increased. Attempts to establish habitual physical exercise among elementary school children have indicated it is one of the most difficult of health habits to influence. As overweight, unfit children age into adulthood, they face increased risks of developing heart disease, cancer and stroke, the current leading causes of death among adults.

From these and other data, it appears that children in our society are moving in two directions. One group is moving toward a healthier, better educated and higher socioeconomic status. This is reflected in the data indicating a decline in death rates among children and youth and improvement in overall indexes of health status and longevity.

These young people are in position to excel in society. They have high achievement test scores, suffer from less disease and fewer disabling conditions, are more physically fit and will have the opportunity to maintain or improve their socioeconomic status as they assume adult roles. The improvement of status for this group of youth has contributed to improved health statistics for the nation's children and youth as a whole.

In contrast, however, a second group of children faces an alarming decline in health status due to the circumstances of their birth and living conditions. Statistics from public hospitals in major American cities indicate that 15 percent of babies are born alcohol- or drug-addicted. Low birth weight (less than 2,500 grams) occurs in about 7 percent of all births. Factors associated with low birth weight include pregnancy before age 18, lack of prenatal care, maternal smoking and use of alcohol and other drugs.

Effects of Poverty

According to the Maternal and Child Health Bureau of the U.S. Public Health Service, in 1989 there were 12.6 million children under age 18 living in poverty—almost 40 percent of the nation's poor. This represents an increase of 1 million since 1980. Slightly more than 20 percent of children have no form of health insurance coverage for health and medical services.

African-American or Hispanic children are three times more likely to live in poverty than White children. Poverty contributes to many difficulties for children and youth, including:

- learning disorders
- poor educational attainment and increased dropout rates
- inadequate nutrition
- more involvement with the criminal justice system
- psychological and emotional difficulties
- chronic physical conditions

Many children living in poverty live in two-parent families in which both parents work outside the home. However, these parents cannot earn sufficient wages to get their families out of poverty. This situation is complicated by parents' growing incapacity to achieve better jobs.

In California, for example, educational attainment of parents living in poverty has dropped over the past twenty years. Two results follow. First, parents are limited in finding better-paying jobs. Second, parental educational attainment is a predictor of educational attainment of their children. Thus, children living in poverty may remain there as they become adults with low education levels.

Children living in poverty are less likely to see a physician than those living above the poverty line. When these children do see a physician, it is more often in a hospital than any other place. Children living in poverty spend nearly 60 percent more days in the hospital than those from higher-income families.

Children without health insurance receive about half the care of those with health insurance, and this lack of care occurs when children are most vulnerable. It affects children's schooling as well as their development. If the nation is to see substantial improvement in the health status of its children and youth, serious attention must be paid to the circumstances of daily living for children in poverty.

Other Changes

Other changes in society have affected and will continue to affect school-age populations well into the next century. Working patterns for parents have changed. Today, 54 percent of mothers of children ages six to fourteen are working outside the home either full- or part-time. Thirty-seven percent of mothers of children under age six are working outside the home. Teenagers are working as well: 45 percent work sixteen hours or more per week.

Family structure has also changed. In 1990, 15.9 million children, almost 25 percent of those under age 18, lived in families with only one parent. This percentage had more than doubled since 1970. Experts estimate that approximately 60 percent of all children will live with a single parent at some time prior to age 18. However, when remarriages are considered, 75 percent of children do live in two-parent households for at least some part of their youth.

A recent study indicates that children living with only one parent are less likely to finish school, particularly boys who live with their mothers. Nearly 40 percent of children live in single-parent households with less than $10,000 annual income. African-American children are nearly three times as likely as White children to live with a single parent. In California, for example, one child in four is born to a single mother, and more than half of all African-American children are born to single mothers.

The increased presence of other cultures, languages and ethnicities has also had and will continue to have an impact on education. For example, by the year 2000, 42 percent of California's schoolchildren will be White, 36 percent Hispanic, 13 percent Asian, and 9 percent African American. Currently, one out of four California schoolchildren speaks a language other than English at home.

Other major metropolitan areas in the country are also experiencing this demographic shift. These changes have required schools to adapt school schedules, curricula and relationships with parents and other family members.

Health Care Needs of Teachers and Staff

Changes in the school-age population provoke much discussion and planning by state and local education agencies. However, looking only at students and their needs misses a substantial component of schools—administrators, teachers and other staff. Schools are among the largest employers in the nation. According to 1988 statistics, more than 4.3 million people work in public school districts and schools throughout the nation. Add the slightly more than 539,000 private elementary and secondary school employees, and the total is almost 5 million school employees overall.

As significant employers, schools are faced with the same concerns that businesses and industries have in regard to providing a comprehensive package of benefits. Sick-care costs and health insurance rates continue to increase at a dramatic rate. The United States spends approximately 12 percent of its gross national product on health care services. This cost has translated into an ever-increasing burden for those providing health insurance to their employees; for employees, who must directly bear increased rates; and for those who continue to drop out of insurance coverage either due to lack of employer-provided benefits or low wages that make health insurance unaffordable.

School districts and schools have responded by reviewing their capability to provide comprehensive health insurance benefits. Many districts have increased the number of part-time employees to save benefit costs. Other districts have passed along increased health care coverage costs to employees.

Districts and schools have also taken steps to create "Preferred

Provider Organizations" (PPOs) with local health care providers. This arrangement makes it possible for schools to negotiate a discounted rate for health care services with one or more providers to gain adequate coverage. In many instances, however, this represents only a one-time savings over a prior period or year, because costs increase at the same rate of acceleration as the Consumer Price Index in subsequent years, unless steps are taken to reduce utilization.

Another major strategy is for districts and schools to become self-insured, meaning that the district or school provides benefits to employees directly without using a third party such as an insurance company. Districts and schools must create an effective administrative and fiscal organization to manage this arrangement lest employee use of benefits exceed the funding the school has appropriated to cover them.

Business and industry have used other means to help control sick-care costs and health insurance. Many have adopted policies known to promote health, such as banning smoking in the workplace. Cigarette smoking contributes significantly to sick-care costs and lower productivity, due to illnesses from smoking itself and those such as colds and flu that are exacerbated by smoking.

Many of the behavioral factors affecting health can be positively influenced by the development of health promotion and disease prevention programs at the school worksite. These programs take positive and affirmative action to assist employees to take some control over their health by reducing risks for disease and to improve productivity and job satisfaction. Employers in business and industry as well as schools have increasingly recognized that organized programs of health enhancement—from stress management to weight reduction to smoking cessation—provide a return on investment for the costs of such programs aside from savings that may accrue from reduced sick-care costs.

Adults have the opportunity to protect and improve their health status through practicing behaviors consistent with good health. Most of the leading causes of death and disability can be avoided through modification of lifestyle. Cumulative evidence during the last half of this century has amply demonstrated that health and lifestyle are linked. For example, there has been a 40 percent reduction in coronary heart disease deaths and a 50 percent decline in stroke deaths since 1970. This change was largely achieved through reduced rates of cigarette smoking, lower average blood cholesterol levels, and increased control over high blood pressure. Deaths from motor vehicle crashes declined almost 30 percent from 1970 to 1990, primarily due to lower rates of alcohol use, increased safety belt use and changes in speed limits.

While these developments are encouraging, American patterns of adult living continue to produce results that, unless changed, will prevent further substantial progress and will contribute to the escalation of health care costs, lost productivity, absenteeism and premature years of life lost. Only one in five adults exercises lightly to moderately five or more times in a given week. Only one in ten exercises seven or more times weekly. Less than one in ten exercises vigorously enough to produce cardiorespiratory fitness.

One in four does not participate in physical activity at all. Almost one in three suffers from hypertension. One in four is overweight. Twenty-six percent of adults smoke. One in ten is addicted to alcohol, and almost one in twelve has difficulty with alcohol.

These statistics indicate that there is a significant amount of avoidable disease, disability and death among school personnel—avoidable because the behaviors contributing to these statistics are acquired over time as part of lifestyle. The personal, family and social effects of these conditions further justify efforts to intervene to avoid lost productivity, unnecessary absenteeism, employee turnover and premature death.

When health factors of children, youth and school personnel are combined, it can be seen that the health of all those learning and working at school has a substantial impact on what happens there. Health merits incorporation into planning and design of school buildings and grounds; curricula; student and staff services; and personnel recruiting, retention and retirement, including employee benefits.

The School as a Total Environment

Schools are influential, total environments for students and staff alike. The layout, quality and condition of the physical plant of the school have an effect on all who study and work there. Many studies have demonstrated the influence physical environment has on performance of tasks. Most of the nation's attention is focused on the curricular aspects of schools, i.e., reading, writing and arithmetic. Indeed, the largest proportion of school personnel are hired to teach. Yet schools contain far more complex and important influences. Just as the physical environment affects feelings about the school, the manner in which the school day is conducted also plays a significant role. The physical environment, the social environment, and the psychological results produced by the physical and social environment interact to have a profound effect on all who come in contact with the school.

For students, school policies and procedures—the rules—and the way they are carried out offer important guidelines for learning how to get along in society. Odds are that school rules will be different from those at home and require the student to adapt to the school's environment. As stated and unstated rules are applied through years of schooling, students quickly learn to pay attention to those that have priority and to ignore or avoid rules that they understand to be irrelevant or unenforceable. Students learn the required curriculum in the context of the rules, social structure and organization of the school.

Students make a contribution to this school structure based on their family, ethnic, linguistic and cultural backgrounds and their prior experiences in society and other schools. In a similar fashion, the backgrounds of school personnel and their roles and responsibilities in the school make a significant contribution to the environment of the school. Because teachers and other professional staff have different disciplinary academic backgrounds and teaching responsibilities, especially at the secondary level, their diversity has an important effect on the flow of the school day and the expectations, values and behavior of others.

As students interact with each other and school personnel in the context of the social and physical organization of the school, the character of the school is formed. Once formed, it changes through the progress of society and the changing qualities of students and personnel alike. It can also be altered through a more deliberate process—altering organization, social structure, curricular patterns, services, etc., and introducing technical and social innovations in the school. Changes may be as simple as repainting classrooms, offices and hallways. They may range from designing staff development programs to identify and work on problems in the way the school functions on a daily basis, to substantive redesign and re-equipment of the physical plant and grounds. Recent examples of deliberate alterations include the proliferation of magnet schools offering specific programs, computerized educational technology intended to augment instruction, and health promotion programs for school personnel.

One characteristic of most schools is the separation between students and teachers. Teachers are responsible for carrying out policies and procedures as well as teaching. Students often see their role in the school as very different from that of their teachers.

The view that the interests of teachers and students are separate will influence the social and emotional climate of the school. The gaps created by such a mindset can hinder communications and make it more difficult to address significant problems that affect students and staff.

Evidence from schools and districts with high dropout rates and lack of achievement, as measured by standardized test scores, indicates that adverse school environments contribute to students' lack of progress. Conversely, schools in inner-city environments that promote school achievement through policies and procedures, teacher/student interactions and the physical plant give evidence that schools have powerful tools to help with learning, often despite students' home and community conditions. Optimum conditions for learning exist when there is consonance between home, school and community and when school staff and students share common backgrounds.

Planned Health Promotion Programs for Staff

Personnel responsible for education need to feel they are important to the educational process and that their efforts are valued by school officials, students and parents. School leaders must implicitly and explicitly value the importance and the contributions of teachers, aides, counselors, support staff and students. Attention to both the achievement of specific, measurable goals and objectives and the interpersonal qualities of school life are important to the teaching/learning process. School leaders' clear specification of expectations of students and staff in a supportive environment helps reconcile humanistic and achievement orientations.

Morale, productivity and capability of teachers and other staff are essential to reaching the quantitative goals and objectives set for educators. School leaders can recognize and conserve the skilled labor force essential to education by providing a supportive environment and initiating health promotion programs. Such programs are designed to counter the often fatiguing process of guiding children and youth as they develop cognitively, psychologically and socially. By offering such programs and paying attention to the needs of school staff, leadership implicitly acknowledges the value and worth of school staff.

Schools have the personnel to protect and promote health. Schools retain health service, guidance and counseling professionals, as well as nutritionists for school meal programs. Within the instructional program many teachers have instructional expertise important to health, e.g., biology, home economics and physical education. By organizing collaborative efforts between teachers of these subjects, schools can offer important preparation to protect and promote the health of school staff as well as students.

Among the expected results of a schoolsite health promotion program is improvement in staff morale. Morale is strongly associated with commitment to the goals and objectives of an organization and is reflected in measurable terms such as absenteeism and productivity. Health promotion programs also have had demonstrated success in changing adverse health outcomes generated by behaviors deleterious to health, such as smoking, sedentary living, overweight and poor diet. These changes have had the effect of reducing health care costs. Health problems are minimized by a more healthful approach to managing the rigors of working in the school and an emphasis on the importance of individual staff members and their contributions.

Because of the interactive nature of the school environment, successes of health promotion programs with staff can affect students. Enthusiastic teachers and staff produce a climate of optimism around the goals and objectives of the school. Student expectations of their teachers and other school staff may be significantly altered as a result. Students then rethink and reorient themselves to their education in positive ways. Thus, promoting the health of school staff has multiple beneficial effects.

Beyond Teaching: The Social Environment

The social experiences gained at school include the formal processes governed by policy and procedure, teaching/learning and extracurricular activities, and the informal exchanges between students, staff, faculty and administrators. Social experiences are important to behavioral development as children mature. Children and youth, as well as adults, learn important cognitive and behavioral skills in a social context, either purposefully in a teaching/learning environment or through situations that call upon past experience or introduce new experiences, either directly or indirectly, through others. Social experiences include interactions between persons within the school and between school and family and school and community. These social experiences help shape the health attitudes, values and practices of youth as they mature into adults.

Children must be able to successfully adapt to the demands of new environments as they grow and develop. The demand for the ability to adapt increases as children get older. Therefore, young people must learn how to use social experiences to benefit themselves. They need to acquire cognitive and behavioral skills important to success, and social skills essential to coping with the social environment. These skills and others are learned in and out of the classroom, in school, at home and in the community. Children are faced with many conflicting messages. The must learn how to make critical analyses of situations, solve problems, make decisions and live with the consequences of their actions.

Children begin to learn how to adapt at home and then apply

their skills to school and community environments as they experience them. The early imprint of values, attitudes, world view and modes of adaptation at home directly influences how children cope with the environment of the school.

Conflicting demands and expectations between these settings and with different people in these settings (e.g., parent and teacher) often produce stressful situations for students. There are many areas of potential and real conflict between home, school and community regarding students' health behavior. Standards of personal hygiene, nutrition, alcohol and other drug use, family life and human sexuality, use of health products, services and information may vary widely—a reflection of the complex nature of health as it is woven into lifestyles and world views.

Schools need to recognize the sources of social support for children and youth in the school environment. If support is lacking at home, children may have little incentive to strive for school success. Conversely, if support at home is strong, the probability of school success is higher. These divergent scenarios illustrate the need to match school conditions with those of families and communities, particularly social and economic conditions.

Schools must also recognize that the quality of the interactions between teachers and between teachers and administrators affects the social environment, as do demands on teachers and teacher morale. Chronic teacher turnover, lack of enthusiasm in the classroom, excessive absenteeism and lowered expectations of students indicate a poor social environment for learning. These conditions are transmitted to students in varied ways. They establish and reinforce the message that school is a difficult and unrewarding place. Consider the following questions:
- How much time and attention do teachers give students?
- How enthusiastic are teachers in presenting their lessons?
- What level of performance do teachers expect from students?

- How are students treated individually and as a group?
- Do teachers model the behavior of responsible adults?
- Do teachers follow through on their duties in the school outside the classroom?
- Are student problems recognized and handled promptly, either directly or through referral?
- Do teachers and administrators interact with students at school outside of required assignments?

We know that students can learn in spite of what is done to them in the classroom, but the cumulative effects of a negative social environment are antithetical to student achievement and deliver strong negative messages about the value of schooling. Poor conditions for learning in the classroom and school environment are reflected in lower achievement and higher dropout rates.

Reversing adverse trends in the social experiences of students and staff at school is difficult. Organizations, including schools, develop modes of functioning both in terms of the amount done and the way things are done. The principle of physics that objects in motion tend to stay in motion applies to school environments as well. To make changes in the social environment and the outcome of teaching/learning transactions, other aspects of the school must be changed.

Individuals in key positions, such as school administrators, must become champions for change toward a more supportive and healthful environment. Many schools have turned to building partnerships with community agencies to help make them more productive. The "I Have A Dream" Foundation was set up by a businessman in New York who visited the elementary school from which he graduated. He made a promise to the sixth graders he visited that if they would finish school, he would guarantee their college expenses. Another example of making substantial changes that directly speak to youth is the guarantee of jobs to all graduates of inner-city high schools by the city of Boston. These types of programs can have a positive effect on the social environment of the school, helping school officials, teachers, staff and students, as well as their families, reorder and redefine their expectations toward broader possibilities.

To alter the social experiences of students and staff in the school environment, changes must fit within existing conditions and patterns of the school. Examples of projects that successfully met their objectives but failed to be integrated into the regular life of the school are abundant. Applying fiscal and human resources to make changes is almost always possible, but lasting change occurs only with deliberate leadership and planning by those who can effect and those who are affected by changes, including families and community interests that have a stake in the success of the school.

The Importance of Role Models

Modeling is learning that occurs by witnessing another person perform a behavior. Modeling is sometimes called "imitative learning" or "observational learning." It is marked by the fact that it occurs without obvious direct reinforcement. The opportunity to witness the actions of others and the consequences of those actions enables us to acquire needed knowledge, attitudes, values and skills beyond the limits of our own direct experiences.

Our contemporary environment provides both students and school personnel with a volume of information and social experiences. Our internal systems for acquiring, sorting, evaluating and incorporating useful intelligence to manage our daily lives and our futures are first formed by early socialization experiences at home. These systems are developed, augmented, refined and extended through experiences in the community and at school. Beliefs, internal standards, perceptions of the environment, prior experiences, rewards and punishments help us to formulate systems for managing experiences and acquiring knowledge and skills. Capabilities acquired in school help us develop behaviors important to successful social functioning.

Influences on this process of development begin with the family. The family provides the fundamental socialization to enable youth to function in society. The family instills values, beliefs, outlooks and hierarchies of permissible and nonpermissible behaviors. Included in this family socialization are important attitudes and practices about health—nutrition, personal hygiene, coping with illnesses, protective behaviors (e.g., wearing safety belts and immunization against disease), to name just a few.

These attitudes are either repudiated or reinforced by the community. School supplies the technical knowledge and skills essential for full participation in society, from mathematics and English to health. But because social experiences are seamless, formal and informal learning in and out of school blend together.

To minimize confusion and ambiguity, youth need and expect consistency between the messages they receive and the behavior of the messengers. School learning experiences designed to improve nutritional habits are unlikely to be incorporated as a value or behavior if school meals and snacks negate the educational message. Attempts to promote vigorous physical activity are unlikely to succeed if the school or teacher delivering the message offers little support for regular physical activity. Young people can easily detect that one or more teachers smoke or that the teachers' lounge is, in fact, a smoking lounge. This can carry far more weight than in-class messages about the dangers of smoking.

Does this mean that those who come into contact with students each day—teachers, administrators and staff (to say nothing of parents and peers)—must be exemplary in the health behavior they display? It is easy to say that this is, indeed, what adults must do to demonstrate consistency: Do as I say, as well as I do. However, the complex nature of modeling behavior makes this directive problematic.

There is no question that noting the behaviors of others that have been consistently rewarded is valuable learning. Youth who are able to see behaviors and their consequences learn valuable lessons without having to use time-consuming and potentially costly trial-and-error methods to arrive at the same end. But people come from different backgrounds with different experiences and expectations, and behaviors and their consequences are not always seen. Therefore, the power of a role model for any given individual will vary. If there are differences between the potential role model and the youth, such as gender or ethnicity, these differences may mediate the potential effects of the role model.

Teachers and other school officials need to keep in mind that their positions of power and importance in the classroom and school give them a great deal of potential influence. Students quickly learn, through personal and vicarious experience, that school officials exert broad influence in the school. This recognition is not limited to official school duties, but is generalized to other aspects of life, as the many requests for advice directed by students to teachers attest. Included among these generalized influences are the more overt aspects of adult authority figures— general appearance, speech, style, age, symbols of success or status, established or apparent expertise, and health behavior.

Young people are particularly vulnerable to influences that they would imitate. As children, youth take their cues from older and authoritative adults at home and in school. These figures are perceived as reliable guides to proper behavior. However, with the onset of adolescence, as they begin the process of shedding a child's identity and acquiring an adult role, youth do not look at adult authority figures in quite the same way. Media influence and the kinds of feedback children experience when they try to mimic adult behaviors may accelerate this process.

Adolescence stimulates youth to develop their own identities and modes of functioning, without the assistance of traditional authority figures. They often turn to their own or somewhat older peers as guides. Peers have been identified as important role models in adolescence, as well as in other periods of development. Unfortunately, peers are often in the same situation as their contemporaries as they try to sort out how to think, feel and perform—a process filled with trial and error for all involved.

Young people, as well as adults, are attracted to individuals who have an aura of confidence and authority or who have apparent success in desirable areas. Teachers and other school officials often have great potential to influence youth because of the quality of their interactions with young people in and out of the classroom or because they possess qualities with which young people closely identify. These qualities could be the relative youth or youthful appearance of a teacher, the teacher's gender or ethnicity, or her or his involvement with extracurricular activities in school or outside of school.

School officials are more likely to be influential role models if they share the background and characteristics of the student body of the school. They also may be attractive to youth if they display interest in and concern about young people and conduct themselves in ways that indicate that they are fair minded and reliable. None of these qualities necessarily relate to what teachers teach, but they do affect the way school figures conduct themselves in and out of the classroom and how they handle their interactions with students and others in the school. Adult role models can give reassurance to adolescents during a turbulent period of life.

Health Messages and the School Environment

Students recognize the similarities and differences between the messages adult authority figures present in and out of the classroom and the way they conduct themselves in the social environment of the school. Those who teach about health topics, whether health educators or not, are the most vulnerable to student comparisons of what is said and what is practiced. This is particularly true when health messages conflict with or contradict behaviors practiced in the school, home and community environment.

Rather than demand strict consistency between what is said and done in classroom settings, which puts an inordinate amount of pressure on individual students and teachers, attention should be focused on the environment of the school, home and community. Positive role models have the most effect when the environment supports their cognitive and behavioral messages. This gives the would-be follower the opportunity to witness the professed behavior in more than one environment, performed by more than one role model. Nothing could be more difficult than to be a lone voice for health in an adversarial, deteriorating physical and social environment.

Role-modeling messages must be supported by others in the school environment to be effective. Naturally, the messages supporting health urge individuals to take control over areas where they can act in healthful ways. But much of society makes it difficult for youth as well as adults to see the benefits of such behavior when the social environment clashes with messages given in the classroom.

For example, students have every right to question health messages about smoking when they see that cigarettes are widely and legally available, that cigarette makers sponsor any number of athletic and cultural events, that the federal government supports tobacco farming, and that smoking is allowed in virtually every environment, including the home and school. The fact that the teacher with the antismoking message does not smoke plays only a small part in students' understanding of the use of tobacco in society.

When actions are taken to match the school environment with antitobacco messages, the modeled behavior and messages are substantiated. Students receive feedback that health messages against the use of tobacco are to be taken seriously as more social environments become smoke free, including the school.

Health messages are up close and personal. Health messages are immediately evaluated by students as they reflect on their own current behaviors as well as the behaviors of others who are significant to them. Disparities between messages and behaviors often lead to questioning the credibility of the individuals who are health advocates rather than thoughtfully evaluating the social environment and the factors that contribute to or compromise health. This tendency is natural in a society that extols the importance of the individual and the right to self-determination. Tales of personal successes against obstacles found in society, whether economic, social or educational, are used to illustrate that the grit and determination of the individual will overcome all barriers. Missing in this scenario, however, is consideration of the physical and social environments that help to shape opportunities for self-determination.

As educators, we know that success stories help to stimulate and motivate individuals to exert efforts for their own success. At the same time, we know that there are key ingredients for successful lives in society. Among these key ingredients is success in school, which often translates into opportunities for success in life. There is a relation between supportive home environments, school successes and successful adult roles. To the extent that disjunctions or conflicts between home, school and community exist, opportunities will decrease and the individual's potential for growth and development will be subordinate to social circumstances.

Any school environment designed to help young people protect and promote their health will reflect society's many inconsistencies and contradictions about health practices. After all, it takes many years of living for most of our significant health problems—heart disease, cancer and stroke—to occur, and school employees face the same choices and consequences of health behavior as their students. But because these employees have responsibility for millions of impressionable youth, they need a supportive environment to protect and promote their health.

The Larger Mission

We have an even larger mission for developing healthier environments, because students cannot learn well if they are not healthy. They cannot learn if their lives are at constant risk for intentional and unintentional injury. Health status is directly linked to school achievement. A total school environment dedicated to promoting health can have multiple beneficial effects for learners, teachers and other staff, effects that can be measured by such diverse markers as educational achievement and medical care insurance claims. Investment in personnel, services and facilities to promote the optimal well-being of students and staff has the potential to pay vast dividends over time as school personnel and graduates lead healthy lives.

References

Allensworth, D. D. 1987. Building community support for quality school health programs. *Journal of School Health* 18 (5): 32-38.

Allensworth, D. D., and W. Patton. 1990. Promoting school health through coalition building. *Eta Sigma Gamma Monograph Series* 7 (2): 1-89.

American School Health Association, Association for the Advancement of Health Education and Society for Public Health Education. 1989. *National adolescent student health survey*. Oakland, CA: Third Party Press.

Anspaugh, D. J., and G. O. Ezell. 1990. *Teaching today's health*. 3d ed. Columbus, OH: Merrill.

Bandura, A. 1977. *Social learning theory*. Englewood Cliffs, NJ: Prentice-Hall.

Blair, S., L. Tritsch and S. Kutsch. 1987. Worksite health promotion for school faculty and staff. *Journal of School Health* 57 (10): 469-473.

Bradshaw, R. 1991. Stress management for teachers: A practical approach. *The Clearing House* 65:45-47.

California: The state of our children. 1992. *Saving the dream*. Los Angeles, CA: Children Now.

Cleary, M. J. 1991. Restructured schools: Challenges and opportunities for school health education. *Journal of School Health* 61 (4): 172-175.

Cornacchia, H. J., K. L. Olsen and C. J. Nickerson. 1988. *Health in the elementary schools*. 7th ed. St. Louis, MO: Times Mirror/Mosby.

Council of Chief State School Officers. 1989. *What are the characteristics and components of effective comprehensive school health programs?* Washington, DC.

Creswell, W. H., Jr., and I. M. Newman. 1989. *School health practice*. 9th ed. St. Louis, MO: Times Mirror/Mosby.

Davis, J. H. 1983. A study of the high school principal's role in health education. *Journal of School Health* 53 (10): 610-612.

Delgado-Gaitan, C. 1991. Involving parents in the schools: A process of empowerment. *American Journal of Education* 100 (1): 20-46.

Deputat, Z., and M. S. Pavlovich. 1988. School health programs: A comprehensive plan for implementation. *Health Education,* Obersteuffer Symposium on Administrative Aspects of School Health Education, October-November.

Floyd, J. D., and J. D. Lawson. 1992. Look before you leap: Guidelines and caveats for schoolsite health promotion. *Journal of Health Education* 23 (2): 74-84.

Gingiss, P. L. 1992. Enhancing program implementation and maintenance through a multiphase approach to peer-based staff development. *Journal of School Health* 62 (5): 161-166.

Golaszewski, T. J., M. M. Milstein, R. D. Duquette and W. M. London. 1984. Organizational and health manifestations of teacher stress: A preliminary report on the Buffalo teacher stress intervention project. *Journal of School Health* 54 (11): 458-463.

Health Insurance Association of America/American Council of Life Insurance. 1985. *Wellness at the school worksite: A manual.* Washington, DC.

Joki, R. A. 1988. Health education: Program development and implementation. *Health Education,* Oberteuffer Symposium on Administrative Aspects of School Health Education, October-November.

Kirst, M. 1989. *Conditions of children in California,* Policy Analysis for California Education (PACE). Palo Alto: SRI International.

Lavin, A. T., G. R. Shapiro and K. S. Weill. 1992. Creating an agenda for school-based health promotion: A review of selected reports *Journal of School Health* 62 (6): 212-228.

Mitchell, J. T., and D. J. Willover. 1992. Organizational culture in a good high school. *Journal of Educational Administration* 30 (1): 6-16.

Natale, J. A. 1992. Shopping for health benefits. *The American School Board Journal* 179 (1): 17-23.

National Center for Educational Statistics. 1991. *The condition of education: Elementary and secondary education* Washington, DC.

National Commission on the Role of the School and the Community in Improving Adolescent Health. 1990. *Code blue: Uniting for healthier youth.* Alexandria, VA: National Association of State Boards of Education..

Nelson, B. B., Jr. 1988. Principal's commitment: A key to success. *Health Education,* Oberteuffer Symposium on Administrative Aspects of School Health Education, October-November.

Nelson, S. 1986. *How healthy is your school? Guidelines for evaluating school health promotion.* New York: National Center for Health Education.

Nettles, S. M. 1991. Community involvement and disadvantaged students: A review. *Review of Educational Research* 61 (3): 379-406.

Newacheck, P. W., and W. R. Taylor. 1992. Childhood chronic illness: Prevalence, severity, and impact. *American Journal of Public Health* 82 (3): 364-371.

Newman, F. M., R. A. Ruter and M. S. Smith. 1989. Organizational factors that affect school sense of efficacy, community and expectations. *Sociology of Education* 62:221-238.

Perry, C. L. 1984. Health promotion at school: Expanding the potential for prevention. *School Psychology Review* 13 (2): 15-37.

Pollock, M. B. 1987. *Planning and implementing health education in schools.* Palo Alto, CA: Mayfield.

Pruitt, B. E., D. J. Ballard and L. G. Davis. 1990. The school health promotion profile: Measuring a school's health. *Health Education* 21 (5): 20-24.

Recommendations for school health education. 1981. Denver, CO: Education Commission of the States.

Report of the 1990 Joint Committee on Health Education Terminology. 1991. *Journal of Health Education* 22 (2): 97-108.

Report of the Task Force on Education of Young Adolescents. 1989. *Turning points: Preparing American youth for the 21st century.* Washington, DC: Carnegie Council on Adolescent Development.

Rose-Culley, M., J. M. Eddy and B. Cinelli. 1989. A study of school health promotion programs: Implications for planning. *Health Values* 13 (6): 21-30.

Smith, W. M., and R. L. Andrews. 1989. *Instructional leadership: How principals make a difference.* Alexandria, VA: Association for Supervision and Curriculum Development.

Trickett, E. J., and D. Birman. 1989. Taking ecology seriously: A community development approach to individually based preventive interventions in schools. In *Primary prevention and promotion in the schools,* ed. L. A. Bond and B. E. Compas, 361-390. Beverly Hills, CA: Sage Publications.

U.S. Department of Health and Human Services, Public Health Service. 1991. *Healthy people 2000: National health promotion and disease prevention objectives.* DHHS Publication No. (PHS) 91-50212. Washington, DC.

Wentzel, K. R. 1992. Social competence at school: Relation between social responsibility and academic achievement. *Review of Educational Research* 61 (1): 1-24.

Chapter 7

School Health Services: Issues and Challenges

Diane D. Allensworth, RN, PhD, CHES

> Learning does not take place in isolation. Societies therefore must ensure that all learners receive nutrition, health care and general physical and emotional support they need in order to participate actively in and benefit from their environment. (World Conference on Education for All, 1990)

Two concepts undergird the comprehensive school health program: healthy children learn better, and children provided the opportunity to adopt health-enhancing behaviors in childhood will become healthier adults. The school health services program, one component of the comprehensive school health program, is designed to ensure a safe, healthy environment conducive to learning and to provide professional care for those who become ill or injured while at school. The primary purpose of the health services program is the optimal maintenance, promotion, protection and improvement of student, staff and community health through counseling, instruction, appraisal, screening, referral and follow-up services (Snyder, 1991).

Rationale

It has been said that children are one-third of our population and all of our future. A cursory review of the health of children and youth in our nation does not portend a healthy future. The National Commission to Prevent Infant Mortality states that our nation's mothers and children are in trouble. The United States ranks behind 31 other nations in the number of children born with low birth weight, twenty-second in the number of infants who die in their first year of life and twentieth in the number of children who die before their fifth birthdays (National Commission to Prevent Infant Mortality, 1992). While there were improvements in several health measures during the 1980s for children and youth, including a reduction in infant mortality and overall childhood death rates, there was no change in the teenage pregnancy rate and the percent of low-birth-weight infants. Furthermore, the death rates due to homicide and suicide actually increased (U.S. Department of Health and Human Services, 1991a).

The leading causes of death for children and youth ages 5 to 19 are unintentional injury, cancer, homicide, suicide and congenital anomalies. In all age categories, unintentional injuries lead in cause of mortality; for children ages 5 to 14 cancer is the second leading cause of death, but for those ages 15 to 19, homicide is the second leading cause of death (U.S. Department of Health and Human Services, 1991a). (See Figure 1.)

Because the leading causes of death in adults (heart disease, cancer and accidents) are related to nutritional, fitness and safety habits established while young, it is important to understand the extent of health-debilitating behaviors common among today's students.

Figure 1
Leading Causes of Death for Ages 5-19
(death rate per 100,000)

Ages 5-9

Unintentional Injury	11.7
Malignant Neoplasms	3.3
Congenital Anomalies	1.6
Homicide	1.0
Disease of the Heart	0.8

Ages 10-14

Unintentional Injury	12.7
Malignant Neoplasms	3.1
Homicide	1.7
Suicide	1.4
Congenital Anomalies	1.3

Ages 15-19

Unintentional Injury	46.7
Homicide	12.7
Suicide	11.3
Malignant Neoplasms	4.1
Congenital Anomalies	2.2

Adapted from U.S. Department of Health and Human Services, Public Health Service. 1991. *Child Health USA '91.* DHHS Publication No. HRS-M-CH91-1. Washington, DC.

- One in four fourth graders (26 percent) and four in ten sixth graders report that many of their peers have tried beer, wine or distilled spirits (U.S. Department of Health and Human Services, 1991b).
- More than one in three secondary school students (36 percent) had consumed five or more drinks on at least one occasion in the past month (CDC, 1991a).

- Almost one in four adolescents ages 12 to 17 have tried an illegal drug (Irwin et al., 1991).
- One in three high school seniors (33 percent) reported having five or more drinks on one occasion within the past two weeks (Inter-Agency Commission, WCEPA, 1990).
- Only 40 percent of students ages 10 to 18 engaged in appropriate physical activity on a year-round basis (Ross and Gilbert, 1985).
- One in two adolescents will become sexually active by the time they graduate from high school (Inter-Agency Commission, WCEPA, 1990).
- One in four sexually active teenagers will become infected with a sexually transmitted disease before graduating from high school (Gans and Blyth, 1990).
- Nineteen percent of high school students report daily use of cigarettes. One in two eighth grade students report having tried cigarettes; almost two in three tenth grade students (63 percent) have tried smoking (ASHA, AAHE and SOPHE, 1989).
- Two in twenty students in grades 9 through 12 reported that they had carried a weapon at least once during the past month. Of those students carrying weapons, 36 percent reported doing so six or more times (CDC, 1991c).
- Almost three in ten students in grades 9 through 12 (27.3 percent) reported that they had thought seriously about attempting suicide in the 12 months preceding the survey (CDC, 1991b).

These behaviors contribute to a disease classification which has been called the "social morbidities," the threats to the well-being of children and youth that are primarily the result of the social environment and behavior: suicide, homicide, sexually transmitted disease including HIV infection, unintended pregnancy and substance abuse (Gans and Blyth, 1990).

A number of reasons have been proposed to explain both the status of students' health and their behaviors: the number of children in poverty, inadequate health insurance coverage, family composition and working mothers (U.S. Department of Health and Human Services, 1991a; Fox, Wicks and Libson, 1992). While one in five children live in poverty, this age group represents nearly 40 percent of the nation's poor. In 1989, a family of four was considered to be living in poverty if its annual income was below $12,675. Eleven percent of children living in poverty were publicly insured, primarily through Medicaid, but 33 percent of these children had no health coverage (U.S. Department of health and Human Services, 1991a).

Children from low income families are less healthy than children whose families are more affluent. Further, their relative ill health is compounded by difficulty in obtaining medical care. Compared to their more affluent peers, they are significantly less likely than other children to receive physical examination, vision testing, immunizations and dental care (Williams and Miller, 1991).

During the past two decades the percentage of children not living with both parents has increased from 12 percent to 25 percent. Currently, approximately 25 percent of all children live with only one parent, usually the mother (U.S. Department of Health and Human Services, 1991a). It is estimated that half of the children born today will spend a part of their childhood in a single parent home (Children's Defense Fund, 1990). In 1970, 29 percent of mothers with preschool children and 43 percent of mothers with school children were working. Today the numbers have risen to 58 percent and 75 percent (U.S. Department of Health and Human Services, 1991a).

To help children who are struggling to survive the challenges of poverty, teen pregnancy, substance abuse and chronic disease, the Education and Human Services Consortium suggests structuring interagency partnerships to connect children and families with comprehensive services (Melaville and Blank, 1991). Because schools offer the critical point of access, they become an ideal location for health and human services to be provided along with educational programming.

There has been a renewed interest in school-based health promotion, according to the Harvard School Health Education Project, which conducted a national policy analysis of 25 different reports published between 1989 and 1991 (Lavin, Shapiro and Weill, 1992). (See Appendix D.) The common themes emerging from these reports included the following points:

- Education and health are interrelated.
- The biggest threats to health are "social morbidities."
- A more comprehensive, integrated approach is needed.
- Health promotion and education efforts should be centered in and around schools.
- Prevention efforts are cost-effective; the social and economic costs of inaction are too high and still escalating.

Phil Porter, an associate professor in the Department of Pediatrics, Harvard, has articulated a variety of advantages of locating health services programs in schools: (1) care is easily accessible and immediately available; (2) students will miss less school traveling to health care; (3) schools have well-developed health record-keeping and tracking systems; and (4) all children and youth have an opportunity to participate in the health care system early in their lives and form good habits for their health and well-being (Policy Studies Associates, 1992).

Traditionally, the school health services program has tried to serve as the bridge between education and health and between services in the school and services provided by the community. The school health services program, like the comprehensive school health program, employs multiple interventions to promote the health of students, staff and families. The variety and scope of the interventions may vary but in general they can be characterized as belonging to one of three delivery models: basic health care, expanded health care and comprehensive primary health care (Schlitt, 1991). (See Figure 2.)

Organization of School Health Services

Thirty-three states have educational codes or legislation establishing a legal basis for school health services (Lovato, Allensworth and Chan, 1989). While state mandates for health services vary, those states that do mandate health services usually require only minimum basic services. However, the continuum of care that may be provided within the school health program—from basic screening and first-aid to comprehensive primary health care—may be found within state statutes (National Health/Education Consortium, 1990). The extent of health services provided in any local school is dependent upon state guidelines and the model chosen by that school district. While three distinct models will be described here, schools organize their programs to meet their health needs and financial constraints. Therefore, in any given school, elements of one or more of the models may be in existence.

Traditional Basic Care

Lawton Chiles, the governor of Florida, had the following to say:

> We absolutely cannot afford to wait until the school
> bell rings to attend to our children's health and de-

Figure 2
School Health Services

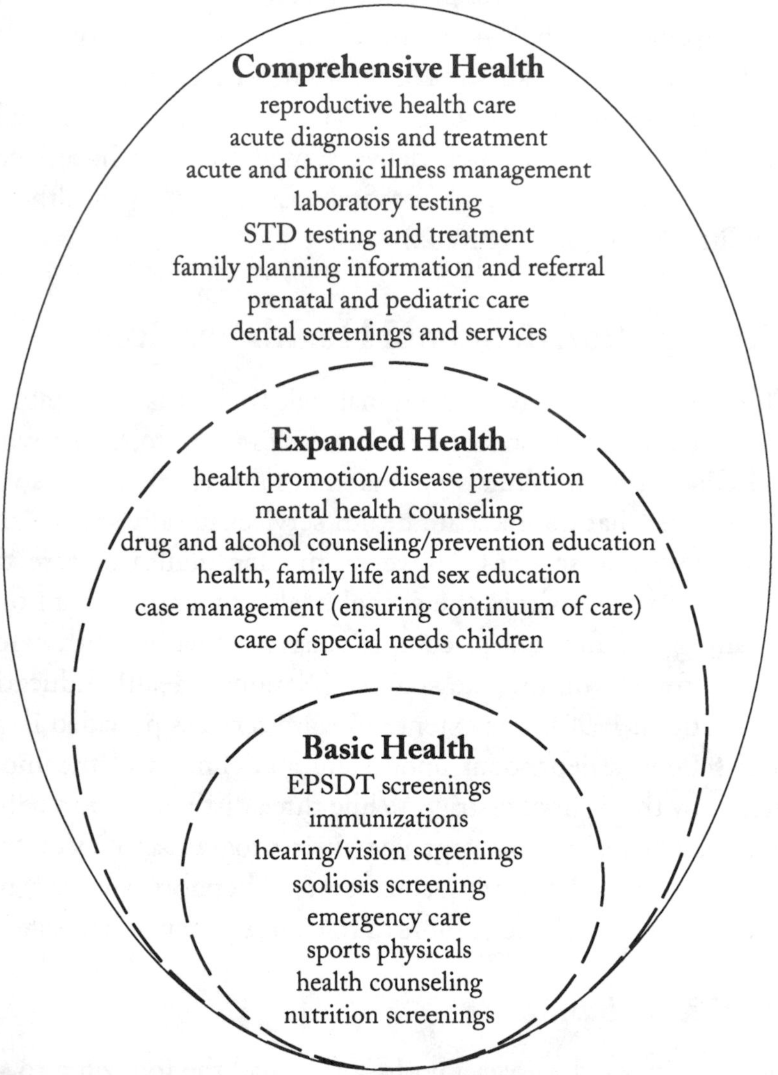

Comprehensive Health
reproductive health care
acute diagnosis and treatment
acute and chronic illness management
laboratory testing
STD testing and treatment
family planning information and referral
prenatal and pediatric care
dental screenings and services

Expanded Health
health promotion/disease prevention
mental health counseling
drug and alcohol counseling/prevention education
health, family life and sex education
case management (ensuring continuum of care)
care of special needs children

Basic Health
EPSDT screenings
immunizations
hearing/vision screenings
scoliosis screening
emergency care
sports physicals
health counseling
nutrition screenings

Adapted with permission from the Southern Center on Pregnancy Prevention. J. J. Schlitt. 1991. *Bringing Health to School: Policy Implications for Southern States.* Washington, D.C.: Southern Center on Adolescent Pregnancy Prevention.

velopmental needs. We need to start thinking of immunizations and well-child care, health screening, proper
food and prevention of health problems as being just as
important as books and pencils and chalkboards and
teachers. (National Health/EducationConsortium, 1990)

The predominant model across the nation is one of basic
screening provided by the school nurse. This model is an out-
growth of the initial school health program founded at the turn of
the century in which physicians were appointed as public school
health officers to reduce contagion and absenteeism. By 1910,
337 cities in the United States required medical inspections (Snyder,
1991). Although the number of school physicians employed in
1910 outpaced school nurses by three to one, over the years school
nurses have become the predominate providers of services. The
school nurse, with assistance from health aides, usually staffs this
program. Currently, some large districts continue to employ physicians, but many districts secure a physician only as a paid or
volunteer consultant to the health services program.

Interventions provided by this model include periodic screening for vision, hearing and scoliosis; sports physicals; emergency
care; direct services for special need students; individualized health
care plans; administration of medicine; monitoring of immunizations; and provision of health counseling and patient education.
Thirty-three states have legislated this type of school health services programming, but only twelve states have mandated specific
health facilities.

Expanded School Health Services

In a country where many U.S. children live in poverty, do not share equally in health and access to
health care, and are at risk for several adolescent

problems, health promotion has become the new
frontier in health care. (Giordano and Igoe, 1991)

Because of technological gains in medical care over the past
century, the focus of child health has shifted from medical care to
the promotion of health and prevention of disease. Many of the
problems facing today's youth—substance use, stress disorders,
suicide—can be ameliorated through health promotion interventions (Giordano and Igoe, 1991). The expanded health services
program builds upon the basic school health services foundation
and extends the range of services provided to students by the
health service staff and public health and community mental
health providers who are brought into the school on a part-time
basis (Schlitt, 1991).

One example of expanded services is the Student Assistance
Program. Because of the focus of the Department of Education on
substance abuse prevention, a number of schools have developed
student assistance programs for both elementary and secondary
students (Cohen, 1989). These programs, like their counterparts
in the adult workplace (Employee Assistance Programs), may be
administered by the school or by an outside mental health agency
contracted by the schools. If the school health services program is
not directly involved in the delivery of these services, it often
provides leadership in assisting teachers to recognize and refer
students with problems.

To implement a health promotion program, the American
School Health Association's School Nurse Study Committee suggests that an interdisciplinary school health service task force that
would include parents be formed in each school district. In addition to the customary health screening provided by school nurses,
the following additional assessments should be conducted: health
hazard appraisal, fitness screening, developmental evaluation and

nutritional history. From these screenings, school nurses could prepare annual individualized health plans that emphasize disease prevention measures. Special attention would be provided to students who have had no previous prevention health services and/or students who have special health problems or disabilities. Instructional programs in health and safety, along with environmental monitoring and use of the cafeteria as a nutritional learning laboratory, would complete the health promotion program (Igoe, 1990).

Comprehensive Primary Health Services

> Education requires undivided attention—possible only when children are free from discomforts caused by physical and emotional conditions that can be prevented, diagnosed, treated, or minimized through the provision of comprehensive primary health services. (Joint Statement of ANA, ASHA, NAPNAP, NASSNC, 1988)

The model which has generated the most interest recently is the comprehensive health service program in which primary health care is provided in school-based or school-linked clinics. The placing of clinics in schools has steadily increased since the first school-based clinic was established in 1970. By 1991, the Center for Population Options (CPO) had identified 306 school-based and 21 school-linked clinics operating in 33 states and Puerto Rico (Riessman, 1991). Typically, school-based clinics serve only one school while school-linked clinics serve students from more than one school as well as students from elementary through secondary schools and out-of-school youth. Of those school-based clinics identified by CPO in 1991, 51 percent operated in secondary schools, 13 percent in junior high or middle schools and

19 percent in elementary schools. Twelve percent served students from various levels (Riessman, 1991).

Within the past few years, comprehensive health care has expanded its focus from school-based clinics that provide only primary health care to full-service agencies that provide "one-stop shopping" for all health and social services including primary health care, mental health counseling, vocational services and social services. A movement to expand school-based health services to include primary health care has been advocated by leaders in education, business and government as well as health experts as a necessary strategy for improving students' academic performance. This interest has been stimulated by several factors: the increasingly complex array of unmet health care needs; the increase in premature sexual activity, substance use and violence among adolescents; lack of access to health care by uninsured families; increasing participation of mothers in the work force; and an increasing acknowledgment of the need to provide services to the children whose parents are addicted to alcohol and drugs (Fox, Wicks and Libson, 1992).

The medical services offered by school-based or school-linked clinics are quite similar. More than 90 percent of these clinics provide assessment and referrals to community health care providers or private practitioners, general primary care, acute and chronic illness management, routine and sports physicals, laboratory tests and mental health counseling. A number of clinics provide nonmedical services, including health education (96 percent), nutrition education (91 percent), mental health and psychosocial counseling (79 percent), drug and substance abuse programs (58 percent), family counseling (76 percent), sex education in a classroom setting (64 percent), as well as general health care, first aid and routine sports physicals. (See Figure 3.)

Administrative, medical and counseling personnel typically

Figure 3
Types of Medical and Counseling Services
Provided by SBCs and SLCs

Medical Services	SBC	SLC
General primary care	91%	87%
Routine or sports physicals	91	87
Diagnosis/treatment of minor injuries	92	93
Laboratory tests	87	93
Medications prescribed	83	87
Chronic illness management	78	60
Immunizations	71	86
Pregnancy tests	69	87
Medications dispensed	69	71
Diagnosis/treatment of STDs	57	87
EPSDT screening	41	67
Dental services	28	13
Pediatric care of infants of adolescents	19	33
Gynecological exams	56	80
Prenatal care on-site	24	33
HIV testing	14	33
Counseling Services		
Health education	96%	100%
Nutrition education	91	93
Mental health/psychosocial counseling	79	100
Job counseling	79	100
Sexuality counseling	76	100
Weight reduction	67	67
AIDS education in clinic	64	71
HIV counseling	61	67
Sex education in classroom	64	73
AIDS education in classroom	59	47
Support groups	58	53

Adapted with permission from Center for Population Options. C. Waszak and S. Neidell. 1991. *School-Based and School-Linked Clinics: Update 1991.* Washington, DC: Center for Population Options.

staff a school-based clinic (Waszak and Neidell, 1991). Approximately 80 percent of the clinics employed a physician, if only part-time; 50 percent of clinics employ nurse practitioners and social workers. The school nurse was present in approximately two-thirds of the school-based clinics and worked as part of the school-based clinic staff in one-third of the clinics. Figure 4 identifies the role of those school nurses who worked as part of the school-based or school-linked clinic staff.

Figure 4

Services Provided by School Nurses in SBCs and SLCs

Services	SBC	SLC
Performed screening	78%	75%
Provided follow-up services	73	75
Delivered direct services	68	38
Participated in staff meetings	60	50
Served on advisory boards	54	75
Supervised paraprofessional staff	30	13
Served as clinic manager/director	21	13

Adapted with permission from the Center for Population Options. C. Waszak and S. Neidell. 1991. *School-Based and School-Linked Clinics: Update 1991.* Washington, DC: Center for Population Options.

Fifteen states have recently enacted legislative or executive action that focuses on school-based clinics (Center for Population Options, 1989). Among the issues of concern at such clinics are consent, confidentiality and liability. While all clinics questioned by CPO required parental consent, this did not appear to be a problem in the delivery of care since only a very small percentage of parents withheld consent for services. Confidentiality laws vary considerably from state to state. School-based clinics can share information among clinics without a release but do not share information with other school personnel or community agency staff. Also, clinic records are not part of the "school health record." However, in some states, parents may have access to or authorize release of a minor patient's medical information. While there are a variety of reasons that a school-based clinic might face legal action, including failure to obtain consent, unauthorized disclosure of confidential information or failure to provide appropriate treatment, there has only been one lawsuit brought against a school-based clinic in the 18 years of their operation and that suit was dismissed as being without legal foundation (Center for Population Options, 1989).

Financing

The Council of Chief State School Officers made the following statement:

> At a time when many families across all income levels are experiencing greater stress and when child poverty is at record levels, the school cannot view itself as an isolated institution within the community, separate from family and community services. (Melaville and Blank, 1991)

The funding and sponsorship of school-based and school-linked clinics varies considerably. Three-fourths of school-based clinics are sponsored about equally by three types of agencies: community health clinics (28 percent), public health departments (26 percent) or hospital medical schools (24 percent); school-linked clinics are predominantly sponsored by public health departments (40 percent) (Waszak and Neidell, 1991).

Traditional school health services have been funded by three alternative models: (1) the provision of service by the public health department within the limitations of their operating budget; (2) the purchasing of services from the public health department by the school board; or (3) the direct employment of school health staff by the school board. In twenty states the school board has authority to hire health services personnel; in two states the public health department has authority to hire the health services personnel; 16 states allow both agencies to share hiring responsibilities and 12 states permit either agency to employ the health services staff (Lovato, Allensworth and Chan, 1989).

The Education and Health Services Consortium suggests that the key to large-scale delivery of comprehensive health services is interagency partnerships (Policy Studies Associates, 1992). Interagency partnerships offer the opportunity to (1) unite a broad spectrum of professional expertise and agency services on behalf of families and children; (2) secure funding from several institutional budgets; and (3) develop extramural funding requests for additional resources to create more effective prevention treatment and support services. Initiatives to expand interagency programming have occurred at both the service delivery level and at the system level. The names, purpose and contact person for selected examples of collaborative health services programming are provided in Figure 5.

Human Resources

The health services team, regardless of the delivery model used by the school system, may be comprised of a variety of specialists: physician, school nurse practitioner, school nurse, social worker, dentist, speech and hearing specialist, and health aide. At a minimum, health care experts suggest that a school nurse who works under the supervision of the public health director or a contrac-

Figure 5
Interagency Collaboration to Provide Health Services Programming—Selected Examples

Program	Purpose	Contact Person	Funding
Health Start, St. Paul	Combine adolescent medical health services and childcare	D. Zimmerman Director 640 Jackson St. St. Paul, MN 55105	Local budgets
Ensley H.S. Health Center	Provide primary health care and health education	D. Bailey, Director Department of Health 1400 6th Ave. S. Birmingham, AL 35202	Foundation grant
Communities in Schools	Provide health and social services at school site	D. Bine, Director Suite 150 4000 West Chase Blvd. Raleigh, NC 27607	Local budgets and private grant
School-Based Youth Services Program	Provide comprehensive preventive health and social services at school site	R. Knowlton, Director School-Based Youth Services Department of Human Services, CN 700 Trenton, NJ 08625	State funds and local funds
Joint Interagency Agreement	Mandated collaboration between state health and education agencies to provide health services	J. Battaglin, Coor. Comp. Health Services Department of Health and Rehab. Services 432 House Office Bldg. Tallahassee, FL 32399-2834	State funds

Reprinted with permission from the National Health/Education Consortium. Policy Studies Associates. 1992. *Creating Sound Minds and Bodies: Health and Education Working Together.* Washington, DC: National Health/Education Consortium, (202) 205-8364.

tual, part-time physician be employed (Hummel and Humes, 1984).

Physicians

Physicians serve in the school health services program in various ways, paid or volunteer, as full- or part-time staff to either the total program or to a specific element—for example, as the medical consultant for special education or an athletic team physician. Large metropolitan districts may employ more than one physician while smaller districts often contract for a physician consultant (American Academy of Pediatrics, 1987).

Responsibilities of the school physician include:

- examining students referred because of infectious disease, health problems detected through screening, or frequent absences
- conducting medical evaluations for special education placement
- conducting sports physicals
- contributing to the health education programs for students, school personnel and parents
- serving as a general consultant on health, environmental and safety concerns

Only three states provide opportunities for school physician certification. However, 17 states require school physicians to have either an MD or DO degree in order to practice as a school physician, and eight states require an MD degree (Lovato, Allensworth and Chan, 1989).

School Nurses

In most schools, the major provider of day-to-day health care is the school nurse (American Academy of Pediatrics, 1987.) Qualifications for school nursing vary; 32 states require a registered nurse's license while nine states allow licensed practical nurses to be employed. Eighteen states also require school nurse certification in order to practice (Lovato, Allensworth and Chan, 1989).

The five professional associations that promote school nursing have identified the following specific standards for the school nurse (Dleaf, Young and Hamilton, 1990):

- applying appropriate theory as the basis for decision making in nursing practice
- establishing and maintaining a comprehensive school health program
- developing individualized health plans
- collaborating with other professionals in assessing, planning, implementing and evaluating programs and other school health activities
- assisting students, families and groups to achieve optimal levels of wellness through health education
- participating in peer review and other means of evaluation to ensure quality of nursing care for students
- participating with other key members of the community responsible for assessing, planning, implementing and evaluating school health services and community services, including promotion of primary, secondary and tertiary prevention
- contributing to nursing and school health through innovations in theory and practice and participation in research

Each state defines the role and the responsibilities of the school nurse through legislative mandates, Department of Education guidelines, state board regulations and certification requirements. Figure 6 provides a listing of those responsibilities that the states mandate. The specific procedures mandated are discussed in the next section.

Figure 6
Responsibilities of the School Nurse

Level of Policy

Responsibilities	Mandatory Requirements N (%)	Recommended Requirements N (%)	No Policy N (%)
Help prevent/control disease	19 (37%)	26 (51%)	6 (12%)
Appraise health status of students	18 (35%)	26 (51%)	7 (14%)
Plan for students with special needs	16 (31%)	27 (53%)	7 (14%)
Provide emergency care	11 (22%)	31 (61%)	8 (16%)
Promote optimum sanitary conditions	11 (22%)	26 (51%)	14 (27%)
Counsel students/parents about health findings	8 (16%)	34 (67%)	8 (16%)
Coordinate student care with other agencies	6 (12%)	31 (61%)	14 (27%)
Provide health instruction	4 (8%)	30 (59%)	16 (31%)

Reprinted with permission from the American School Health Association. C. Y. Lovato, D. D. Allensworth and F. A. Chan. 1989. *School Health in America: An Assessment of State Policies to Protect and Improve the Health of Students.* 5th ed. Kent, OH: American School Health Association.

School Nurse Practitioners

The school nurse practitioner has completed an additional formal course in assessment, management of illness and injury, and health education in order to be prepared to assume the expanded role of providing primary care to students under the direction of a physician. Sixteen states have established school nurse practitioner certification (Lovato, Allensworth and Chan, 1989).

Health Aides

Because of the increased numbers of students with special health needs as well as decreased funding, which precludes employing additional nurses, health aides may be employed to assist the professional staff in delivering specific health services and/or recording health information (Snyder, 1991). Thirty-nine states employ health aides and nine states regulate the function of health aides (Lovato, Allensworth and Chan, 1989). In addition to paid health aides, some schools solicit the services of parent volunteer assistants and student volunteer assistants to aid in the delivery of designated aspects of the health services program (Snyder, 1991). Nonprofessional health personnel most often are supervised by a registered nurse.

Health Services Programming and Issues

The components of a comprehensive program include the assessment of student health status, prevention and control of communicable disease, care of the ill or injured, procedures for students with special health needs, screening programs, provision of a safe and healthful environment, health promotion, health counseling, maintenance and operation of the school health office, development of a school health advisory council, and program evaluation (Snyder, 1991).

For the health services program to function efficiently, the five professional organizations that promote school nursing suggest a nurse-to-student ratio for the general school population of one nurse for 750 students. For students with special needs who are mainstreamed within the general school populations, the ratio is 1 to 225. For severe and profoundly handicapped school populations, the suggested ratio is 1 to 125. Only six states have mandated a 1 to 750 nurse-to-student ratio (Lovato, Allensworth and Chan, 1989).

Continuing Education Needs

Physicians, school nurse practitioners and school nurses are being asked to provide more leadership in the promotion of health enhancing behaviors. One survey found that 73 percent of school nurses were asked to deliver instructional sessions within the classroom. While teachers judged the presentations as effective (3.62 on a five-point scale), the nurses perceived their presentations as less than adequate (2.76 on a five-point scale) (Dleaf, Young and Hamilton, 1990). A national survey of primary care physicians, nurses, psychologists and social workers found that 40 percent of these professionals believed that they were unprepared to treat adolescents who have alcohol or other drug use problems, who are depressed or who are at risk for suicide (Schwab, 1991). Both preservice and inservice programs could provide training to improve the instructional competence of the nurse (Dleaf, Young and Hamilton, 1990).

Screening Programs

An important aspect of managing school health services is screening for conditions that are amenable to treatment, identifying students with the problem, referring students for treatment, monitoring follow-up care, assisting students to adapt to the condition and consulting with school staff to ensure that educational accommodations have been met. The exact screening procedures conducted in any school are dependent upon state mandates, rate of incidence of the condition, staff resources, availability of time and facilities.

The *Implementation Guide for Standards of School Nursing Practice* identified a number of conditions that must be satisfied to ensure the screening program is valid (Snyder, 1991):

- Is the condition treatable?
- Will early treatment improve outcome?
- Is there sufficient time for screening?
- Is the condition relatively prevalent?
- Is the screening procedure simple and inexpensive?
- Is the procedure reliable, i.e., are there a minimum of false positives and false negatives?
- Can referrals to local community resources be handled in an efficient manner?
- Are financial resources available to assist needy families?

Two major problems that may affect learning—visual and hearing impairment—have been the mainstays of screening programs. Between 12 and 20 percent of all students suffer from a hearing loss. Approximately 15 of the children screened for vision will need corrective lenses for refractory errors, 5 percent for strabismus, and 2 to 3 percent for amblyopia (Lovato, Allensworth and Chan, 1989). Other conditions for which screening programs have been initiated include scoliosis, height/weight, physical exams, dental caries, speech impediments, TB tests and lead poisoning. The number of states that mandate or recommend these screening procedures is provided in Figure 7.

Liability
Until recently, risks of liability were not of great concern to school nurses, but legal actions against school nurses are increasing. Although the number of legal actions remains small to date, school nurses may be at particular risk because they are generally isolated from other health care providers, conflicts may occur between the policies of the board of education and professional standards of care for nursing, and conflicts exist between laws

Figure 7
States Mandating or Recommending Screening Procedures

Requirements	Recommended N (%)	Mandated N (%)
Hearing	14 (27%)	30 (59%)
Vision	15 (29%)	28 (55%)
Scoliosis	19 (37%)	20 (39%)
Height/Weight	19 (37%)	11 (22%)
Physical Examinations	15 (29%)	10 (20%)
Dental Examinations	21 (41%)	8 (16%)
Blood Pressure	15 (29%)	4 (08%)

Reprinted with permission from the American School Health Association. C. Y. Lovato, D. D. Allensworth and F. A. Chan. 1989. *School Health in America: An Assessment of State Policies to Protect and Improve the Health of Students.* 5th ed. Kent, OH: American School Health Association.

related to education and those related to health care. For example, parents are entitled to access to their children's educational records but some medical procedures protect minors' rights to confidentiality. To decrease liability, school health personnel must ensure that the policies and procedures of the school district reflect current standards of care (Schwab, 1991).

Students with Special Health Needs
Five to 20 percent of students have special needs, depending upon how disability is defined. The passage of PL 94-142 in 1975

ensured that all handicapped children would have access to free and appropriate public education. Students who have a chronic health condition or who are developmentally delayed require an assessment to determine the least restrictive educational environment. This information is conveyed to the school staff as the Individualized Educational Plan (IEP). The need for the participation of the school nurse in the development of the IEP was identified in PL 94-142. Seventeen states mandate that the school nurse be a part of the team that develops the IEP (Lovato, Allensworth and Chan, 1989).

In addition to the IEP, the Task Force on Standards of School Nursing Practice (1983) suggests that an Individualized Healthcare Plan (IHP) be developed to organize and document the delivery of services, procedures and technical assistance to students with health needs to promote their optimal well-being and functioning during the school day. The IHP documents the nursing process in the school setting. Included in the IHP are nursing assessments, nursing diagnoses, nursing interventions and outcomes (Hass, 1993).

Students who would benefit from an IHP include those with chronic and/or complex health problems and those with any special need that might impede learning. The objectives, performance standards and strategies for health and developmental screening are detailed in Figure 8.

Transitioning Students with Special Health Needs

As a part of the Individualized Educational Plan (IEP) developed for special education students, the Individualized Healthcare Plan (IHP) or Health Management Plan (HMP) documents the academic and physical program adaptations and health requirements needed for special education services. Essential to the IHP is a plan for transitioning youth as necessary. Examples of transitions common to many students with special health needs include

Figure 8
Goals and Objectives:
Health and Developmental Screening

Objective
- Assist in appropriate educational placement of children with special needs.
- Develop and implement individual Health Management Plan (HMP) to assist school personnel to consistently meet special care needs.

Performance Standard
- Comprehensive health and developmental history is on file.
- Current medical information is available regarding special needs.
- Parents involved in identification of needs and realistic intervention plans.
- Health professional available to monitor special care procedures.
- Interpret student's health data to staff and parents.
- Staff kept advised of changes in condition and of any need to change health plan.

Strategy
- Actively participate in staffing committee.
- Prepare summary of pertinent information from developmental history and medical records.
- Involve student and/or family in development of plan.
- Provide teacher/staff inservice regarding the student's health management plan.
- Assess home environment to determine students' usual coping behaviors.

Evaluation
- Children with health-related special needs are appropriately placed.
- Nursing care plan (IHP) or health component is on file and is reviewed at least annually.
- Teachers and staff demonstrate acceptance of health plan.

Reprinted with permission from the American School Health Association. A. A. Snyder, ed. 1991. *Implementation Guide for the Standards of School Nursing Practice*. Kent, OH: American School Health Association.

Figure 8 (continued)
Goals and Objectives:
Health and Developmental Screening

Objective
- Meet physical and psychological needs for students with handicaps to learning.

Performance Standard
- Policies covering medication and emergency needs are written and revised annually.
- Written emergency plans include details for handicapped students.
- Physical plant adapted for special needs.
- Student/nurse conferences are scheduled as needed.

Strategy
- Provide opportunities for students/families to share feelings regarding their handicapping conditions.
- Develop resources in health care community to help school meet special needs of students.
- Provide and/or supervise special health care procedures that will permit student to remain in the least restrictive environment.

Evaluation
- Students integrated into the least restrictive environment.
- Adaptations made to minimize effects of student's disability.

Objective
- Help student take the responsibility for managing his/her condition or providing self-care as soon as possible.

Performance Standard
- Written Health Management Plan exists for teaching self-care, which is revised as goals are met.

Strategy
- Provide opportunity for student to practice self-care under supervision.

Evaluation
- Student achievement of self-care practices that are attainable.

transition from hospital to school and school to hospital, from one school district to another, from elementary school to middle school to secondary school, and/or from high school to vocation or further schooling and adulthood (Hertel, 1991).

Knowledge of the disability and available community resources, as well as an understanding of the perceived needs of the student and his or her family, is essential to developing an effective program for transitioning youth with disabilities. Using a team approach to plan present and future care maximizes continuity of care, especially if the team consists of parental caregivers, health care providers, school administrator or designee, school nurses, other professional health care providers and the student, if appropriate (Hertel, 1991).

Parental Involvement

Ideally, school nursing has always viewed the family, not just the child, as the primary unit of care. The need for involving parents in the educational program of their children has been identified by a number of educational studies (Solomon, 1991; Perry, 1991; Werch et al., 1991; Perry and Crockett, 1987). The health services program also has recognized the need for renewed commitment to parental involvement (Rohrbaugh and Rohrbaugh, 1990).

Included within the definition of family are the child's caregivers as well as the "school family." Creating a bridge between these two families is essential when a health or behavior problem arises. This system's approach to school health assumes that a student's problem does not occur in isolation, but is embedded within the social environment. Rohrbaugh and Rohrbaugh (1990) provide the following guidelines to include families within the school health service program:

- Involve and empower parents as experts on their children.
- Emphasize parental competencies rather than deficits.

- When necessary, make home visits to involve disengaged or hard-to-contact parents.
- When parents are unavailable, look to extended family or neighbors as potential sources of support.
- Encourage teachers to deal with students and parents directly before turning a problem over to specialists such as the school psychologist, guidance counselor or outside therapists.
- Do not disqualify or contradict a parent or teacher in the presence of a child.
- Use a go-between role to defuse conflict and promote cooperation between parents, teachers and other helpers.
- With psychosocial issues, avoid challenging parents directly by pointing out dysfunctional family dynamics or defining your work as "counseling" or "therapy" (even when it is).

Medication

While drug use among children and youth has been the focus of many educational campaigns in the United States, the nation has overlooked another drug problem: improper use of legally prescribed, legally dispensed prescription medicines for school-age children. A 1989 report found that children of all ages take both a large volume and a wide variety of medicines. More than six million children have chronic diseases that require regular medicine. About 13 million children take prescription medicines in any given two-week period.

Unfortunately, up to half of the children who take medicines are not using them properly. In ten studies of children's medicine use, the average rate of adherence was only 54 percent, similar to that of the general population. The tendency not to follow treatment holds true even for chronic illness and life-threatening illnesses such as cancer and kidney transplants. Although medicine use problems exist among children of all ages, adolescents are more likely not to take medicines as prescribed (National Council on Patient Information and Education, 1989).

Four types of improper medicine use occur: (1) stopping a medicine too soon, (2) not taking enough of a medicine, (3) taking too much of a medicine, and (4) refusing to take a medicine. The consequences are serious and include dangerous health outcomes, inadvertent treatment errors, life-threatening adverse effects, unpleasant side-effects, unnecessary diagnostic and treatment costs, and great risk of accidental poisoning. Most medicine regimens necessitate taking medicine during the school day. As a result, school personnel face a number of important issues, including liability risks, designation of persons to administer medication, ability of school personnel to recognize medicine-related problems, and the role of staff in educating students in safe medicine use (National Council on Patient Information and Education, 1989).

A review of state mandates in school health revealed that no state mandates instruction in safe medicine use. Only 28 states had a policy that governed the administration of prescription medications, while 17 states had a policy that governed the administration of nonprescription medications (Lovato, Allensworth and Chan, 1989). Coherent policies that allow students to continue necessary medicine regimens, nurses and teachers who are competent to monitor medication use and recognize untoward effects, and instruction within the formal and informal curriculum on safe medication use are sorely needed.

Future Challenges and Opportunities

Oda (1991) describes school nursing as unique in that it occurs in an educational setting as opposed to a medical setting, treats a primarily well population, and may be provided with a professional staff of one nurse per building who may or may not work under the supervision of a physician. While many of these characteristics unique to school nursing may remain constant, Oda believes that school nursing practice in the future will be characterized by focus on prevention through collaboration, management skills, computer literacy, activism and research and that the services will be provided by a baccalaureate prepared nurse.

Collaboration between schools and local and state agencies, schools and parents is key to providing a single point of entry for essential services needed by students. Increased activism for the purpose of influencing health policy might be necessary if the school nurse is to serve as the children's health advocate and coordinate the needed services. Investigations documenting the effectiveness of school nursing interventions can provide the documentation needed to enable school nurses to become activists for child health locally.

The school health services component of the comprehensive school health program is evolving. There is interest shown by both health and education leaders in increasing the quantity and quality of health services provided to students. At one time, it was believed that locating a school-based clinic within the school would automatically solve some of the problems affecting children and youth—particularly those problems labeled as social morbidities.

There is no doubt that school-based and school-linked clinics can provide quality medical care to those students with no regular source of care (Donovan and Waszak, 1989). However, in reducing unintended adolescent pregnancy or substance use, multiple interventions by multiple disciplines within the school and community are more likely to be successful. The school-based or school-linked clinic is fundamental to programming, but it is only the first step. The clinic staff must join with students, parents and other professionals to develop proactive interventions based upon behavior change research (Allensworth, Symons and Olds, in press).

References

Allensworth, D. D., C. W. Symons and R. S. Olds. 1992. *Healthy students 2000: An agenda for continuous improvement in America's schools.* Kent, OH: American School Health Association.

American Academy of Pediatrics. 1987. *School health: A guide for the health professional.* Elk Grove, IL.

American Medical Association. 1992. *Guidelines for adolescent preventive services.* Chicago, IL.

American School Health Association, Association for the Advancement of Health Education and Society for Public Health Education. 1989. *National adolescent school health survey: A report on the health of America's youth.* Oakland, CA: Third Party Press.

Center for Population Options. 1989. *The facts: Legal issues and school-based clinics.* Washington, DC: Author.

Centers for Disease Control and Prevention. 1991a. Alcohol and other drug use among high school students—United States. *Mortality and Morbidity Weekly Report* 40 (45e): 776e-783.

Centers for Disease Control and Prevention. 1991b. Attempted suicide among high school students—United States 1990. *Mortality and Morbidity Weekly Report* 40 (37): 633-635.

Centers for Disease Control and Prevention. 1991c. Weapon carrying among high school students—United States 1990. *Mortality and Morbidity Weekly Report* 40 (40): 681-683.

Children's Defense Fund. 1990. *S.O.S. America! A children's defense budget.* Washington, DC.

Cohen, A. Y. 1989. *Hampton Intervention and Prevention Project (HIPP): An effective approach to school age substance abuse.* Hampton, VA: Alternatives, Inc.

Dleaf, D. V., A. S. Young and P. A. Hamilton. 1990. The educational role of the school nurse: Perceptions of school nurses and teachers. *School Nurse* 6 (4): 8-10.

Donovan, P., and C. S. Waszak. 1989. *School-based clinics enter the '90s: Update, evaluation and future challenges.* Washington, DC: Center for Population Options.

Fox, H. B., L. B. Wicks and D. J. Libson. 1992. *Improving access to comprehensive health care through school-based programs.* Washington, DC: Fox Health Policy Consultants.

Gans, J. E., and D. A. Blyth. 1990. *America's adolescents: How healthy are they?* Chicago: American Medical Association.

Giordano, B. P., and J. B. Igoe. 1991. Health promotion: The new frontier. *Pediatric Nursing* 17 (5): 490-492.

Hass, M. B. 1993. *The school nurse's source book of individualized healthcare plans.* North Branch, MN: Sunrise River Press.

Hertel, V. 1991. Transitioning students with special health needs. In *Implementation Guide for the Standards of School Nursing Practice,* ed. A. Snyder, 41-44. Kent, OH: American School Health Association.

Hummel, D. L., and C. W. Humes. 1984. *Pupil services: Development, coordination, administration.* New York: Macmillan.

Igoe, J. B. 1990. Beyond green beans and oat bran: A health agenda for the 1990s for school-age youth. *Pediatric Nursing* 16 (3): 289-292.

Inter-Agency Commission, WCEPA. 1990. *World Conference on Education for All: Meeting basic learning needs.* New York: UNICEF House.

Irwin, C. E., and S. G. Millstein. 1986. The health of America's youth: Current trends in health and utilization of health services. *Journal of Adolescent Health* 7 (65): 905.

Joint Statement of ANA, ASHA, NAPNAP and NASSNC. 1998. *Recommendations for delivery of comprehensive primary health care to children and youth in the school setting.* Kent, OH: American School Health Association.

Lavin, A. T., G. R. Shapiro, and K. S. Weill. 1992. *Creating an agenda for school-based health promotion: A review of selected reports.* Boston: Harvard School of Public Health.

Lovato, C. Y., D. D. Allensworth, and F. A. Chan. 1989. *School health in America.* Kent, OH: American School Health Association.

Melaville, A. I., and M. J. Blank. 1991. *What it takes: Structuring interagency partnerships to connect children and families with comprehensive services.* Washington, DC: Education and Human Services Consortium.

National Commission to Prevent Infant Mortality. 1992. *Troubling trends persist: Shortchanging America's next generation.* Washington, DC.

National Health/Education Consortium. 1990. *Crossing the boundaries between health and education.* Washington, DC: National Commission to Prevent Infant Mortality and the Institute for Educational Leadership.

Oda, D. S. 1991. The invisible nursing practice. *Nursing Outlook* 39 (1): 26-29.

Perry, C. 1991. Conceptualizing community-wide youth health promotion programs. In *Youth health promotion: From theory to practice in school and community,* ed. D. Nutbeam et al., 1-22. London: Forbes Publications.

Perry, C. L., and S. J. Crockett. 1987. Influencing parental health behavior: Implications of community assessments. *Health Education* 18:68-77.

Policy Studies Associates. 1992. *Creating sound minds and bodies: Health and education working together.* Washington, DC: National Health/Education Consortium.

Riessman, J. 1991. *The facts: School-based and school-linked clinics.* Washington, DC: Author.

Rohrbaugh, E. A., and M. Rohrbaugh. 1990. Kids, kin and context: Family nursing in an elementary school. *School Nurse* 6 (2): 18-22.

Ross, J., and G. Gilbert. 1985. Summary of findings: National children and youth fitness study. *Journal of Physical Education, Recreation and Dance* 1: 49-50.

Schlitt, J. J. 1991. *Bring health to school: Policy implications for southern states.* Washington, DC: Southern Center on Adolescent Pregnancy Prevention.

Schwab, N. 1991. Liability issues in school nursing. In *Implementation guide for the standards of school nursing practice,* ed. A. Snyder, 35-38. Kent, OH: American School Health Association.

Snyder, A., ed. 1991. *Implementation guide for the standards of school nursing practice.* Kent, OH: American School Health Association.

Solomon, L. P. 1991. California's policy on parent involvement: State leadership for local initiatives. *Phi Delta Kappan* 72 (5): 359-362.

Task Force on Standards of School Nursing Practice. 1983. *Standards of school nursing practice.* Kansas City, MO: American Nurses Association.

U.S. Department of Health and Human Services, Public Health Service. 1991a. *Child health USA '91.* DHHS Publication No. HRS-M-CH91-1. Washington, DC.

U.S. Department of Health and Human Services, Public Health Service. 1991b. *Healthy people 2000.* DHHS Publication No. (PHS) 91-50212. Washington, DC.

Waszak, C., and S. Neidell. 1991. *School-based and school-linked clinics: Update 1991.* Washington, DC: Center for Population Options.

Werch, C. E., et al. 1991. Effects of a take-home drug prevention program on drug-related communication and beliefs of parents and children. *Journal of School Health* 61 (8): 346-350.

Williams, B. C., and C. A. Miller. 1991. *Preventive health care for young children: Findings from a 10-country study and directions for United States policy.* Arlington, VA: National Center for Clinical Infant Programs.

Chapter 8

Integrating School Counseling and Health Education Programs

Nancy S. Perry, MSEd, NCC, NCSC

S chool counseling has changed dramatically in the last decade. The stereotypical high school guidance counselor, or dean of students, sitting in an office waiting for the next crisis, is slowly becoming a picture of the past. As our culture becomes character- ized by diverse and ever-changing values in the home, community and school, it is apparent that the societal structure of the past will not suffice to prepare students for their futures. This insufficiency is reflected in considerable increases in substance use, suicide, child abuse, teen pregnancy, truancy, school dropout and random acts of violence. For example (Children's Defense Fund, 1990):
- Every day, 100,000 children are homeless.
- Every school day, 135,000 students bring guns to school.
- Every day, six teenagers commit suicide.
- Every day, 2,989 American children experience divorce in their families.
- Every eight seconds of the school day, a child drops out.

- Every 47 seconds, a child is abused or neglected.
- Every 26 seconds, a child runs away from home.

Several years ago, school counselors, faced with the increasing multitude and severity of such problems, realized that the number of trained professionals available to help these children could never meet the demand. Therefore, a deliberate change took place that shifted the school counseling emphasis from treatment and remediation to prevention. The following parable illustrates the evolution of thinking that changed school counseling.

> A nationally recognized school of excellence was known for its many programs designed to save students. A wise man, hoping to learn from that success, decided to visit the school. As he approached, he saw that the school was by a river, and many children were being swept away by the strong currents. The principal was out by the river, pulling children out of the torrent, one at a time. The school counselor, the school nurse and the classroom teachers were also running out to help save the drowning children, one at a time. The wise man said, "Indeed, you do have many ways to save the children. But has anyone gone upriver to see who is throwing them in?"

"Going upriver" is prevention. School counselors realized that a systematic, planned program of prevention must be instituted in the schools, or increasing numbers of students would drown in the violent river of societal ills. They also realized that this program must be initiated at the child's earliest point of entry into the system. Thus was born the movement to place school counseling programs that emphasize prevention and early intervention into the elementary schools. This movement brought about the development of a comprehensive model of school counseling, based on developmental principles, that is slowly working its way through the intermediate level to the high school. This model will be described in detail later in this chapter.

Concurrently, health educators were feeling similar frustrations. Most formalized health education programs were placed at the high school level, usually in the form of a required, one-semester course. Health professionals knew that this was too little, too late.

A knee-jerk reaction to some of the biggest problems brought special programs into schools under categorical funding for drug and alcohol education, HIV/AIDS education, suicide prevention, teenage pregnancy prevention, dropout prevention, etc. Each program operated separately but used the same foundation—teaching the primary prevention skills of communication, decision making, responsibility, self-discipline and other facilitative skills that could help young people deal with everyday issues of life. Healthy self-esteem, built on a solid base of interpersonal skills, was seen as the foundation for success.

Health educators came to the same conclusion as school counselors. Prevention education, comprehensive in nature and encompassing the skills and information vital to wellness, is the only plausible strategy that holds any hope for the future. Health educators also realized that such a program must begin early and reach all students.

Opportunities for Cooperation

Two programs—counseling and health education—similar in nature and purpose, developed at approximately the same time. Integration of these two approaches avoids duplication of services and the risk of confusing the student. Cooperation and coordination between school counseling programs and health education programs will strengthen both approaches and benefit the student. Common areas of emphasis as well as support strategies can mutually enhance each program. For example, the topics listed in five comprehensive health education content areas have corresponding areas in comprehensive school counseling:

Foundations for Health. The topics of mental/emotional health, self-esteem, communication, relationships/friendships, responsibility, self-discipline, stress management, ethnic and cultural diversity and similarities, morals and values, refusal skills and decision making are all important topics for guidance curriculum.

Personal Health and Nutrition. Counselors stress the importance of body image as part of the total self-concept and encourage mental and physical fitness. They also refer students with eating disorders or other personal physical problems to agencies or private practitioners.

Substance Use and Abuse. This topic is one of the primary points of counselor intervention as well as education.

Family Life and Sexuality. School counselors are particularly sensitive to these issues as they help students relate their feelings to their choices.

Injury Prevention. Decision making is related to all kinds of self-destructive behavior. Suicide prevention is a major area of concern for school counselors when working with adolescents. Negotiation and mediation skills are often part of a curriculum to help students relate to the people and forces that put pressure on them instead of reacting in violent ways.

In other words, school counselors and health educators definitely agree on the areas of education necessary to help young people become healthy adults.

Because comprehensive health education programs and comprehensive school counseling programs share many goals, the two programs have many opportunities to reinforce and support each other. Comprehensive school health programs often emphasize the physical, mental and emotional factors affecting health. However, they cannot ignore the social context within which health decisions are made. Because school counseling programs approach student health from this social context viewpoint, they can offer valuable insight and support to school health programs.

For example: The family life and sexuality component of a comprehensive health education program would want to ensure that students have accurate information about reproductive health, pregnancy and birth. However, students must also understand the social consequences of teenage pregnancy and learn skills to resist peer pressure to become sexually active. This social context can be amplified by a comprehensive school counseling program. Both approaches are important to student understanding and provide a valuable opportunity for co-teaching.

The same type of cooperation could occur in the area of substance use prevention. A health education program might offer information on the effect of drugs on the body, but it would also need to help students understand why people take drugs and develop strategies to combat peer pressure around drug use. The school counseling program could augment and reinforce this understanding and skills learning.

A Developmental Comprehensive School Counseling Model

As school counseling and the new model of programming evolved, emphasis changed within the programs. The new assumption is that effective prevention requires that *all* students be reached, which cannot be done on an available service basis. The emphasis therefore changed from reactive to proactive. The counselor's responsibility now extends beyond "being there" for students with problems or special requests to establishing a comprehensive program to meet the needs of all students.

Even with excellent counselor/student ratios, seeing students individually is not always practical. The reality is that most counselors have ratios of 350 to 1 or more. Some elementary counselors have workload responsibilities of 1000 to 1 or more, usually in multiple schools. Therefore, for efficiency and effectiveness, counselors work more with groups, both classroom size and smaller, than with individuals.

Even in groups, it would be impossible to reach all students without additional help. School counseling programs therefore emphasize a team approach—a team that can include health educators, school social workers, school psychologists, school nurses, special education staff and classroom teachers. Using the "whole child" approach, school counseling programs endeavor to

---

Figure 1
Changes in Emphasis
Comprehensive Counseling Programming

Students with problems	⮕	*All* students
Services	⮕	Program
Reactive	⮕	Proactive
Sole provider	⮕	Coordinator/manager

The Comprehensive School Health Challenge

bring together all efforts to enhance the child's learning in an integrated, coordinated program. The school counselor, no longer able to be a sole provider, becomes a manager or coordinator of services.

A widely accepted model of the structure of the varied responsibilities of school counselors divides the program into three domains and four components (Gysbers and Henderson, 1988). School counselors work with the personal/social development domain, educational development domain and career development domain of all students. (See Figure 2.)

The personal/social domain, learning to live, is designed to help students become more aware of who they are and how they can effectively interact with others. The educational domain, learning to learn, involves efforts to help students become more aware of how to realize their achievement potential while in school. The third domain, career development or learning to work, helps the student become more aware of how to plan for life after school. These domains are interrelated and, being in an educational setting, are all aimed at the common goal of enhancing the learning of each student.

For example, educators know that a hungry child cannot concentrate on words in a book, or that a child under stress will not be receptive to learning that does not alleviate that stress. Therefore, personal/social issues are intricately entwined with educational issues. In the same sense, students need direction in their lives if school courses are to have any relevance to their futures. Career development, what they are going to do with their lives, is a motivator to learning. One model of implementation for school counseling programs is through the structure of the four components of guidance curriculum, individual advisement, responsive services and system support.

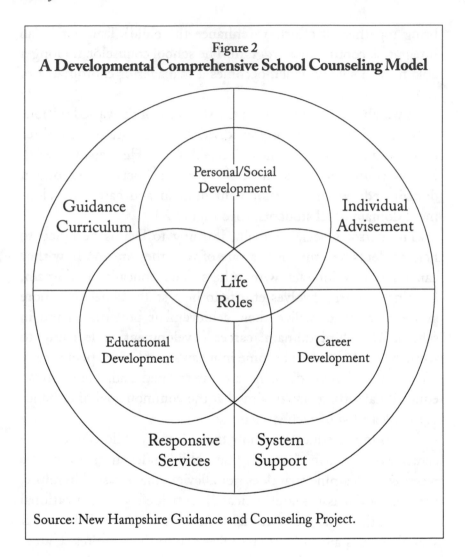

Figure 2
A Developmental Comprehensive School Counseling Model

Personal/Social
Development

Guidance
Curriculum

Individual
Advisement

Life
Roles

Educational
Development

Career
Development

Responsive
Services

System
Support

Source: New Hampshire Guidance and Counseling Project.

Curriculum

Curriculum refers to a planned program of teaching life skills, usually to classroom-sized groups. The purpose of the curriculum is to establish a continuum of skills and practices, based on developmental stages, that provides students with a sequential learning program of what are commonly known as the primary prevention life skills. These skills include self-esteem, communication, problem solving, critical thinking, dealing with peer pressure and relationships, stress management and decision making. For example, an elementary counselor might co-teach with a primary level classroom teacher, or perhaps the school nurse, a personal safety unit on "Good Touch, Bad Touch." At the intermediate level, that lesson would be centered more on appropriate touch, sexual abuse and ownership of one's body, while the high school student might be more involved with decision making regarding sexuality and relationships.

The developmental process goes from receiving information, to understanding, to application. The curriculum component of a school counseling program assumes that there is a planned, sequential delivery system to meet group objectives based on developmental stages. The methods used within the group may range from lecture to small group interactions and discussions. Although experiential learning is of great value with such topics, personal revelations are not encouraged because confidentiality cannot be ensured in a large group. However, classroom discussions can give students a common foundation for their own decision making.

Individual Advisement

The second component of a comprehensive school counseling program is individual advisement. Even though information can be given and processed in large groups, there comes a time when all of this information must be related to the individual. This function is most often related to choosing classes, career decision making, post-secondary education and/or training plans. The counselor works with students and/or their parents to interpret all of the information that is known about them to help them make informed educational or career decisions. This work often involves explaining forms of assessment as well as school records and self-reported information. Individual advisement, like curriculum, should be planned and purposeful. A schedule of individual appointments at critical points of a student's schooling should be a regular component of a student's educational experience.

Responsive Services

The area in which school counselors have traditionally been most active is that of responsive services. Responsive services are defined as those activities that are performed in response to a requested need. Strategies include individual and small group counseling, referral and consultation. This part of the comprehensive program cannot be planned because it is dependent on the needs expressed at any given time. For example, the death of a student might elicit a widespread need to help individual students handle their grief, to see students in small or large groups to process the event, to consult with teachers concerning class discussion of the death, to advise on appropriate memorials, or to relate the death to a learning experience. None of these activities could have been planned in advance, but they all take priority over any other activities.

Counselors often ask how they can be scheduled into classrooms for guidance curriculum when they must be available for such events. At this point, counselors must confirm their commitment to prevention strategies, because there will always be crises. With few exceptions, such as the one above, most "crises" can wait 45 minutes to be handled.

One junior high counselor has had to leave her classroom sessions fewer than a dozen times during ten years to respond to crises such as suicide attempts or threats, the death of a student or telling a student about the death of a family member, or a student's violent behavior. Nearly all other crises could be delayed by giving the student a quiet place in which to wait for the guidance class to end. If students were extremely upset, the secretary sat with them until the counselor could arrive. This waiting period often proved to be beneficial to students by giving them time to reflect upon the situation and perhaps resolve the problem themselves. The important issue for students is being assured that someone will respond to their needs.

System Support

System support involves those activities through which the school counseling program is managed and enriched and the total educational program—of which school counseling is an important part is supported. This support includes strategies related to planning, evaluation, professional development, public relations and committee functions.

Program Emphasis According to Educational Level

Although the goals and structure of a school counseling program may be similar at any level, the emphasis may change to meet the developmental needs of students. A truism of prevention is that the earlier a healthy behavior can be established, the better the chance of success in keeping it. The primary prevention skills must be taught to elementary school children.

Elementary Level

A majority of the elementary school counseling program is devoted to prevention through classroom guidance and early intervention in problems that may hinder learning. Very little individual advisement occurs at the elementary level.

The emphasis of system support is on the involvement of parents and classroom teachers in both the support and reinforcement of the teaching of primary prevention skills and attitudes and in attacking any problems that may be an obstacle to the child's learning. Parent education programs might be established to help parents help their children learn the lessons necessary to become responsible adults.

All efforts at the elementary level are focused on helping the child to develop healthy habits—physical, mental and emotional—through the supportive cooperation of the school and home. Elementary school counselors spend most of their time in cooperative teaching or consulting with teachers and parents.

Middle School Level

The early adolescent at the middle school level is beginning the journey from the dependence of childhood to the independence of adulthood. Relationships with parents, family, other adults and peers become the obsessive task of growing up. The push/pull of dependence and independence with the parents often causes tension in the home, as 12 and 13 year olds prefer to be thought of as orphans when hanging out with their peers.

James Garvin, a guru of middle-level education, described the process of adolescence as having one foot on the pier of family stability and the other in the boat of peer relationships. Much rocking and instability occurs before the adolescent is firmly in one place or the other. Therefore, the school counseling program at the middle level concentrates on helping young people understand what is happening to their feelings and their bodies and on building on the strong influence of the peer system.

Classroom guidance is usually less structured and small group interaction is the preferred method of delivering a message at this level. As students are trying to work out their new identities, they can try out different roles in the safe environment of a caring classroom. Earlier teachings can be reinforced at a deeper level of understanding.

Middle schools structured around teams provide ideal environments to involve the classroom teacher, counselor and students in meaningful discussions. Curriculum is still important, but the delivery may be through classroom teams, peer leaders or innovative forms of drama or music. For example, a group might write a rap to tell the story of how peers try to get a friend to smoke or drink and how the friend uses refusal skills, learned in the elementary grades, to assert his or her right to make decisions.

Individual advisement begins to take on more importance as the middle-level student considers both future academic and career choices. Self-analysis is an important part of the decision-making process as emerging adolescents begin to narrow the focus of their interests and recognize their talents. Information can be delivered in a large group, but students need to confer with a caring adult to relate the information relevant to their personal lives.

Responsive services also gain new importance as young people struggle to understand themselves in relation to the world. Lack of experience and fear of rejection magnify the smallest problem of the adolescent to gigantic proportions. The middle school counselor must be extremely patient and tolerant, remembering that the present issue is a very real problem to the student, even though it may seem trivial to an adult.

System support also takes on new meaning as young people communicate less with their parents. The school counselor can again offer parenting groups to offer understanding and support to parents of adolescents. Parents want to find out what is happening at school since their children may not be communicating with them. Continued parental involvement is important, although it may be done in less obvious ways. Parents and teachers also want to be assured that the time spent in life-skills learning and group work is valuable, so accountability and evaluation of the program become very important.

High School Level

The secondary school counseling program is the most familiar and the most tradition-bound of all levels. Classroom guidance is still an important part of the program, but it tends to center on application of previous learning to the real world of the student. For example, communication skills might be used to practice résumé writing or interviewing for jobs or college acceptance. Decision making is serious business as the young adult faces life decisions. Conflict resolution might mean the difference between a student living at home or running away. Students still need a forum in which to discuss their issues, but this is more often accomplished by the establishment of small groups of peers, led by a counselor and/or peer facilitator. Individual advisement becomes the primary emphasis of the school counseling program, as personal information and options are considered in assisting students to make informed decisions about their futures.

Responsive services take on more serious tones as one considers the statistics of adolescent suicide, violence, teenage pregnancy and school dropout. Individual or small-group counseling, combined with appropriate referrals, are common interventions. School counselors receive the same basic counseling preparation as mental health counselors in community agencies. However, because of time and/or priorities, school counselors are encouraged to refer students needing long-term counseling to private or agency counselors.

System support at the secondary level consists of planning, evaluating and promoting the programs that will benefit students most. Counselors can be effective advocates for students by using a systems approach to improving the overall learning environment in the school.

The functions most closely associated with the high school counselor have not yet been mentioned. Over the years, high school counselors have become schedulers and test administrators (administrative duties) and record keepers (clerical duties). School counselors should help students make decisions about their academic choices, but this task is different from the task of scheduling. School counselors are trained to interpret assessments and to assist students and their parents in using that information to make educational decisions, but test administration is a time-consuming, routine task. Records are important to the counselor in individual advisement, but keeping the records up to date does not require a master's degree in counseling.

One of the difficulties in changing secondary programs to direct greater effort toward prevention is the number of noncounseling duties that have often been assigned to the guidance department. As more and more counselors are trained in the comprehensive model, and as more and more administrators understand the depth of counselor training, high school programs will become more student-oriented and less administrative. Some state legislatures, impatient for change, have enacted laws requiring all school counselors to devote 75 percent or more of their time to direct services.

School counseling programs at all levels deal with the personal/social, educational and career development domains. All levels are structured to deliver comprehensive programs developmentally appropriate for all students. Most programs utilize the four components of guidance curriculum, individual advisement, responsive services and system support. The differences are in the degree of emphasis important at each level.

Guidance curriculum, teaching primary prevention skills and attitudes, is most important at the elementary level and decreases in time priority at the high school level. Conversely, individual advisement is negligible at the elementary level but is very important at the high school level. Responsive services differ in the severity of the issue and the primary recipient of the service—parent or student. System support remains important throughout all levels and may differ only in the degree to which each activity is practiced.

Working Together: Counseling and Health Education

There are basically three areas in which health educators and counselors can cooperate to develop a strong, integrated program to benefit each student. The main objective of any cooperative venture is to put together the most efficient and effective way of assisting young people to become healthy adults. Figure 3 illustrates three levels of integration between school counseling and health education programs.

Curriculum Delivery

One area is the delivery of curriculum. If the counselor and health educator co-teach a common curriculum, such as enhancing self-esteem through self-awareness, the unit could be jointly planned and the division of responsibility assigned. Both might be present for the session, with one person taking the responsibility of lead teacher, or they might decide to teach separately, but in a coordinated unit.

Another approach is to team teach a common curriculum by teaching together but from different perspectives. A prime opportunity to do this might be in the sexuality and family life unit. The health educator might teach about sexually transmitted disease—transmission, symptoms and steps for treatment. The school counselor could augment and reinforce the social context within the same unit. The counselor might work with the teachers to help

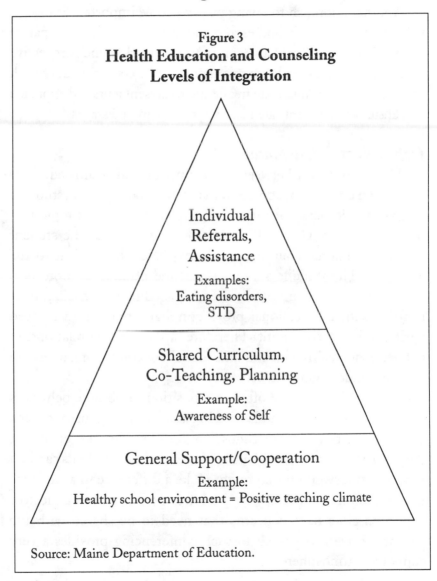

Figure 3
**Health Education and Counseling
Levels of Integration**

Individual
Referrals,
Assistance

Examples:
Eating disorders,
STD

Shared Curriculum,
Co-Teaching, Planning

Example:
Awareness of Self

General Support/Cooperation

Example:
Healthy school environment = Positive teaching climate

Source: Maine Department of Education.

students consider the types of decisions being made at each point in the process and how each decision could change the consequences, explaining the effect on the individual within the social context.

Another approach to giving young people important information concerning their bodies and themselves is to teach separate curricula but coordinate and communicate so that one perspective is reinforcing the other. With this approach, the counselor and health educator must communicate frequently to present a unified approach and ensure that students are receiving reinforcing messages.

Referrals and Assistance

The cooperation between the counselor and health educator can extend beyond collaboration in the classroom. Often, students might confide personal information related to a class topic to a health educator. The health educator may feel that the student needs professional counseling and may refer the student to the counselor. The student has the ethical and often legal protection of privileged communication when engaged in a counseling relationship with a professional, protection that cannot be guaranteed with another caring adult. Therefore, a cooperative relationship between the health educator and the school counselor can ensure that the student gets the necessary help.

Health educators are often in a position to observe behaviors when certain topics are addressed in class. They may suspect that a problem exists and may choose to consult with the counselor about their observations. Sharing concerns about students can be a powerful intervention that might make a difference in a student's life. Sometimes, especially in the lower grades, health educators and counselors have concerns that need to be shared with the parents. A team approach to such conferencing provides a very supportive atmosphere.

Occasionally, a health educator may introduce a topic in which a number of students show unusual interest. Because of curricular demands, the health educator may not be able to stick to that topic or may feel that continuation of the discussion may not be in the best interest of the entire class. The teacher may suggest to the counselor that this would be a good topic for small-group counseling.

Finally, if referral of a student to an outside agency is appropriate, the health educator and the counselor, working together, can coordinate with the agency so the student accesses necessary services with as little disruption to her or his educational program as possible. Since both positions may use outside agencies for education and referral, counselors and health educators can share information about services and staff that may be useful to the school.

Schoolwide System Support

System support is an area in which school counselors and health educators can be especially powerful working together. Schoolwide system support provides the broad base for cooperation, which can then extend to classroom curricula and referrals and assistance. Wellness in the workplace is an acknowledged benefit for employment, yet few schools make concerted efforts to establish such an environment for their staff. School counselors and health educators are logical staff to initiate healthy lifestyle activities such as before-school aerobics, nutritional lunches, lunchtime walks, meditation rooms, stress-reduction clinics and teacher support groups. Healthy employees have fewer absences and are more productive. School teachers, in particular, tend to work in isolation and need the encouragement and support of fellow workers. Wellness in the workplace for school staff is good business.

Of course, schools are supposed to be healthy places in which to learn. The creation of a healthy school climate should be the concern of all staff, but it is often overlooked in the hustle and bustle of everyday activities. School counselors and health educators are more often attuned to the big picture and can spot systemic problems that might be interfering with learning. For example, the strategy of assigning seats in the middle school cafeteria may be a good management decision, but it is depriving emerging adolescents of their great need to socialize with chosen friends at one of the few times when such behavior is acceptable in school. Helping administration and staff to understand the developmental needs of students is a step in creating a healthy learning environment.

Health educators and counselors can work together to provide inservice professional development for staff concerning topics such as adolescent sexuality or the effect on children of living in homes where substance abuse is prevalent. Those trained in such areas often lose sight of the fact that others may not be at their level of competency.

Since school counselors and health educators share so many common concerns and areas of instruction, they should also share support by serving on each other's advisory committees. A counselor on a health education advisory committee can be a supportive voice when sensitive issues arise. Parents and community members cannot be expected to understand all the subtleties and interrelatedness of health education topics. They may also not be aware of a need that exists within the student population. The health educator and school counselor can support each other in helping to educate noneducators.

This supportive relationship can reach beyond advisory committees. Every effort must be made to reach out to community members and help them understand the relationship of a healthy lifestyle to learning. Many parents feel that time taken for subjects such as health or guidance is of little value and would be better spent in math or science.

Without negating the importance of strong academics, it is important to demonstrate that increased time in a subject will not be productive if students feel that they cannot do the work or that they are stupid. Good math skills will not be of prime importance to a student who becomes HIV positive. The teenage mother who is facing overwhelming medical bills may not be able to concentrate on social studies. An angry adolescent, not knowing better ways to resolve problems, may become violent or self-destructive.

School counselors and health educators can be a powerful team in promoting the value of primary prevention to PTAs, Rotary Clubs and other community groups. In fact, the teaming of health educators and school counselors in collaborative and cooperative endeavors can create the synergy to help schools educate the whole child.

A Common Goal

School counselors and health educators share a common goal—assisting young people to develop the healthy lifestyles necessary to become productive adults. They share a concern for the "whole child" approach, realizing that all facets of a person must be developed in balance. Health educators and school counselors are well aware of the effect of personal issues on the academic performance of students. Therefore, they must team together to advocate for the nonacademic portion of the curriculum.

Although health educators and school counselors share many of the same areas of concern, they may approach the subject from different perspectives. If communication and cooperation are the basis for integration of the school counseling program and the health education program, the entire school will benefit. A wellness approach to both the work and learning environment will create a climate in which each person is free to reach his or her full potential. We have a serendipitous window of opportunity to combine two vital programs, health education and school counseling, into a powerful force to create a brighter future for our young people.

References

Children's Defense Fund. 1990. *Annual report*. Washington, DC.

Gysbers, N. C., and P. Henderson. 1988. *Developing and managing your school guidance program*. Alexandria, VA: American Association for Counseling and Development.

The New Hampshire Comprehensive Guidance and Counseling Project. 1991. *NHCG&CP Curriculum*. Hampton, NH.

Chapter 9

Health Promotion at the School Worksite

Judy C. Berryman, MA

W orksite wellness programming in schools can no longer be thought of as a luxury. With the alarming increase in health care costs in the United States, it is time to develop healthier lifestyles—lifestyles in which individuals assume a preventive stance and take more responsibility for their own health status. What better place to start this new thinking than in the schools?

If all the personnel employed by U.S. public schools were combined, this new "business" would be one of the largest corporations in the country. Improving the lifestyles and health habits of such a substantial portion of the work force can positively impact national health-care costs and stretch local taxpayer dollars. The faculty and staff of most school districts mirror the rest of the U.S. population, with similar health problems. Hypertension, obesity, cigarette smoking and sedentary living habits are common, and premature mortality, especially in men, is a major problem (Tager,

1985). Wellness programs that target these health areas can and will provide positive health benefits.

Since school districts usually provide medical care benefits, costs due to premature illness and death are borne by the districts. Coupled with the direct cost of health insurance are the indirect or hidden costs of absenteeism, disability, turnover, decreased productivity, and faculty and staff recruitment/replacement costs (Iverson and Kolbe, 1983).

Growing evidence now indicates that lifestyles associated with chronic disease in adulthood are the result of habits learned early in life. Programs designed to focus on changing these well-defined "bad habits" need increased attention if changes in the outcomes are desired.

School sites are ideal for the provision of health promotion and education for one simple reason: schools are where the children—the next generation—can be found. The many adult workers in the schools serve as role models for the children they teach, making schools ideal places for worksite health promotion. When these adults practice good health habits, they teach healthy living to their students.

Wellness programs in educational settings are on the increase in the United States largely because school personnel are voicing concerns about physical disability, burnout and perceived lack of emotional well-being. Wellness programs have been demonstrated to improve employee morale, reduce absenteeism, increase job satisfaction and generate greater productivity (Kaldy, 1985). School-based wellness programs can and do affect the bottom line by reducing health care costs and absenteeism while increasing productivity and school staff effectiveness. More important, these programs can improve the quality of life on and off the job (Blair, 1984).

The wellness concept assumes that we are born healthy and

usually stay that way unless we are unduly influenced by the home setting during infancy or by our own actions once we are old enough to be responsible for our behavior. Environmental factors and natural wear and tear of life also play a role, but often in the United States lifestyle has a significant impact on health. A 1980 W. K. Kellogg Foundation report discovered that 48 percent of U.S. mortality is due to unhealthy behavior or lifestyle, 16 percent to environmental hazards, 26 percent to human biological factors, including heredity, and 10 percent to inadequacy in the existing health care system (W. K. Kellogg Foundation, 1980).

Health promotion is defined as "any effort used to motivate, educate or provide resources that can improve individual and societal health by reducing health risk and increasing opportunities to satisfy personal, social and environmental needs" (Green and Krueter, 1991). The major areas of health promotion include wellness, risk reduction, self-care, self-help and fitness.

Health promotion and disease prevention may comprise the best opportunity to reduce the ever-increasing portion of resources spent to treat preventable illness and functional impairment. Smoking, for example, is the single most preventable cause of death and illness in the United States. Smoking-related illnesses cost our health-care system more than $65 billion annually (U.S. Department of Health and Human Services, 1991).

Today, most health promotion programs include physical fitness, but also address stress management, nutrition, smoking cessation, hypertension, control of alcohol and drug abuse, and safety. Some programs include professional development skills. Results of such programs in a Dallas independent school district demonstrated a 35 percent drop in absenteeism from 8.3 to 5.8 days (American Council of Life Insurance and Health Insurance Association of America, 1986). Other outcomes of school-based wellness programs include:

- reduced smoking
- decreased weight and body fat
- decreased systolic and diastolic blood pressure
- increased physical activity and exercise
- increased use of balanced diet principles
- decreased levels of anxiety and depression
- increased sense of personal well-being
- reduced health care claim costs
- improved morale
- increased productivity
- improved instructional quality and more time on task with students

The Healthy Lifestyles Program

In 1986, the Greater Battle Creek schools in Michigan (four public and four private) embarked on a project to improve the knowledge, attitudes and behaviors of 17,000 youth in kindergarten through twelfth grade in four target areas: substance use, fitness, nutrition and stress management. After months of research, the Healthy Lifestyles task force decided that in order to change the knowledge, attitudes and behaviors of youth, all school staff and parents needed to be included in the project. With that in mind, the staff and parents were targeted for wellness programs.

The task force offered worksite wellness programming to all school staff in the initial stages of project development. The basic message that launched the program was "Your students don't just listen to what you say—they watch what you do. Teachers' actions inside and outside the classroom teach hidden lessons to students—lessons about personal goals, values, habits and attitudes that influence them long after they leave the classroom. You teach what you are. If you model good health for your children, then you should *depict* good health" (American Council of Life Insurance and Health Insurance Association of America, 1986).

Healthy Lifestyles found that a base already in place in the schools was ready to be expanded. For example:

- Many public school personnel possess skills appropriate for participation in these programs because of their backgrounds in education.
- Public schools employ many qualified people, such as nurses, nutritionists, physical educators and counselors, who can serve as resource personnel.
- Most public schools have facilities—gyms, tracks, lunchrooms, classrooms and group meeting rooms—that are available to personnel.
- The public school can provide a more convenient and support-ive environment than other work settings that require busy professionals to travel across town to a fitness center.

The experiences of the Healthy Lifestyles Program demonstrate that certain steps help begin a school-based wellness program:

1. Introduce the concept to administration, board of education and union representatives.
2. Recruit and organize "wellness planning committees."
3. Research community health- and fitness-related agencies.
4. Announce the program to employees.
5. Conduct an employee interest survey.
6. Conduct committee review and select programs.
7. Develop a range of programs including evaluation and budget.
8. Review the program and establish means of financial support.
9. Announce schedule of programs.

10. Begin offering programs.
11. Evaluate the program.
12. Plan the maintenance of the program.

In the case of the Healthy Lifestyles Program, the board of education, superintendent and union representatives were convinced of the benefits of the program and supported those responsible for implementing it. Program staff held an orientation meeting with administration, board members and unions to demonstrate successful programs in other school districts. The worksite wellness program began with a letter of support from the board of education and administration to all employees.

The early involvement of represented employee groups was instrumental in the initial stages of development. The formal title for these groups eventually became "wellness committees." Membership included secretarial staff, maintenance staff, bus drivers, teachers, food service staff, administrators and board members. One individual assumed the role of program developer. Support or thanks for the efforts of the program developer came from the administration in the form of a one-year membership to a local fitness center. In one of the school districts, the administration allocated a faculty salary to support the efforts of the program developer. Committee members became the "cheerleaders" for the program. Committee tasks included program selection and planning, budget development, maintenance and evaluation.

Community Involvement
Involvement of community agencies is a significant plus in any wellness program. The use of community resources whenever possible ensures long-lasting ownership and development of personal and community pride in the wellness effort. Groups that can help include local hospitals, health departments, Y-centers,

American Red Cross, American Cancer Society, American Heart Association, local parks and recreation departments, and employee assistance groups.

In the Healthy Lifestyles Program, many organizations were anxious to offer programming for school staff, but did not have the means to reach this group through area schools. Organizations also discovered that additional programs for youth developed out of the initial efforts to create school staff programs.

The wellness committees' interaction with community resources created an advisory board that included members of the wellness committees, community health agencies, media, churches and local foundations. This board offered technical assistance, funding aid, support through the media, and coordination of services through community resources. The structure of this collaborative effort is illustrated in Figure 1.

Staff Participation

To assess their needs for wellness programming, school staff were surveyed. The assessment tool included questions related to staff's basic interest in participating in a wellness program, interest areas, ideal times to offer programming, and interest in participating in the development effort. These data were used to determine programs to be offered.

Motivating individuals to take part in health promotion programs may be the number one challenge for companies or schools. Often, the employees who are in the greatest need are the least interested in participating. The Healthy Lifestyles Program used several strategies to increase successful recruiting of not only those already interested in healthy behaviors, but also those who might be hesitant to initiate the health behavior change on their own.

First, the staff created a continual flow of information from administration to staff and back to administration. This top-down

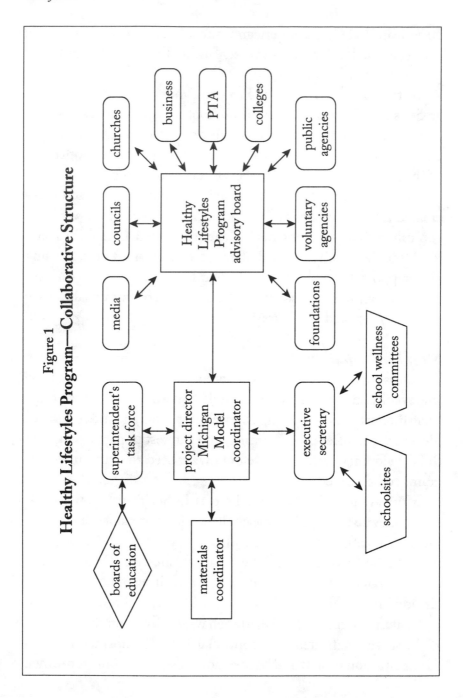

Figure 1
Healthy Lifestyles Program—Collaborative Structure

and bottom-up process of communication created an esprit de corps between administration and staff. Individuals from all levels in the schools found that they had a common interest—health. Other strategies included aggressive promotion and publicity, on-site activities, health screening for risk factors, peer-group support, and recruitment from one program to another.

The Healthy Lifestyles Program staff also published a monthly newsletter for all school staff. The newsletter included special topics in health, a profile of the "wellness person of the month" and a schedule of wellness events.

On-site activities included:
- fitness classes taught by staff personnel
- smoking cessation classes
- stress management sessions
- time management sessions
- "Over Forty and Fabulous" programs
- weight loss
- low cholesterol and fat-free cooking classes
- "Just for Secretaries"
- cross-country skiing

The project also sponsored a six-week competition called Staff Shape-Up. Staff in different buildings competed for total points. Staff accumulated points by practicing healthy behaviors, including:
- aerobic points according to level and length of the activity
- participation in wellness classes
- weight loss
- smoking cessation
- hugging a fellow employee
- having a healthy thought

Peer support encouraged many who would not otherwise have participated to join. Participants gained confidence in their ability to succeed in behavior change and were supported to sustain the changes. The winners received gift certificates to a local shopping mall.

Every School Can Afford a Wellness Program

Whenever a wellness program is presented, especially to school districts, the first question asked is Who pays for all this and what is it going to cost the schools? The answer is simple. Everyone can afford wellness programs. The programs implemented depend on the school district's ability to support programming. The Healthy Lifestyles Program used a pyramid approach to explain wellness program funding levels. (See Figure 2.)

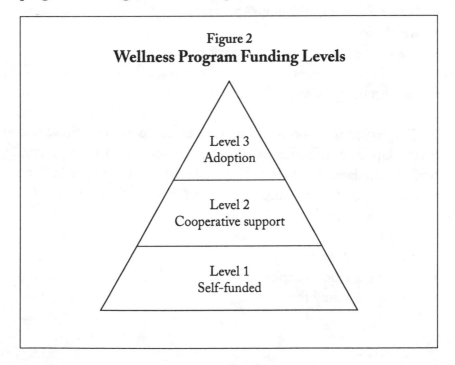

Figure 2
Wellness Program Funding Levels

Level 3
Adoption

Level 2
Cooperative support

Level 1
Self-funded

Level 1—Self-funded programming. At this level, all costs are paid for by the participant or an outside funding source. This type of programming can include discounts for fitness classes, employee-paid programming offered in school buildings, or free classes through area organizations. Program topics include fitness, nutrition, weight control, smoking cessation, relationships, time management, parenting, personal finance and life skills.

Often, a self-funded level may create what is called "the awareness phase." At this phase, individuals become aware of their health and may have an interest in further programs. If a program remains at this level without creating enthusiasm or offering additional programs, maintenance or continued participation may be threatened. Most of these programs have little follow-up. However, if awareness programs are used in conjunction with other programs or referrals—in other words, used to create an interest in continued programming—the results are beneficial. Eventually, schools should move into the next level of support to keep the participants interested and committed to health.

Level 2—Cooperative support. At this level, payment is shared by the employees, participants and/or outside funding sources. Programs may be offered on or off the school grounds, but fees are partially paid by the school district. Programs might include fitness assessments, lifestyle inventories, smoking cessation classes and others.

Level 3—Adoption. At this stage, financial support is provided entirely by the employer. Sometimes this level is called "institutionalization," because activities and beliefs become not only programs but policies. Employers recognize the benefits of wellness programs and are willing to develop policy to support them to create a healthy working environment. Financial support maintains ongoing programming.

Level 3 creates the supportive environment that brings about and sustains long-term change in the school culture. This level of funding contributes to the goal of creating a positive environment that encourages healthy lifestyles. Examples include but are not limited to the following:

- healthy foods in the cafeteria and vending machines
- no-smoking policies
- fitness facilities
- flexible benefits
- incentive systems
- employee assistance programs
- childcare

When considering a worksite health program, the school district should not assume that all financial support must come directly from the general fund. Contributions for funding can come from concessions, fundraising and grants. Eventually, long-term payment for such programs can be accrued from reduced health care costs and reduced absenteeism.

Once the means of financial support has been established, the planning committee can begin to set time lines for programming. It can also move to create an awareness of the worksite wellness activities as well as the importance of establishing a healthy lifestyle. Appropriate communication plays one of the most important parts in continuing high interest levels. Newsletters, mailings, memos, bulletin boards and paid inserts are just a few communication methods to use.

Evaluation

Worksite health promotion programs are implemented to attain specific goals. To assess the impact of health and fitness programs and the attainment of these goals, program process and results need to be evaluated.

During the process of program implementation, progress should be monitored through predetermined measurements, measuring success against previously established standards. Specific criteria (goals) should be selected and defined. Several types of program evaluation designs exist. The type used will be determined by time, staff and available funding. The most important objective is to determine the effectiveness of the program for the individuals involved.

According to Johnson (1981), the five major types of evaluation can be described as follows:

Nominal. This type of evaluation refers to the extent to which program activities were executed in accordance with the purpose of the program. The basic question answered is whether people did what they indicated they would do, and whether the health promotion program operated as planned. A nominal evaluation has the lowest level of sophistication and typically amounts to little more than contract compliance.

Effort. In an effort evaluation, the questions asked are How hard does this group work? and How many people do they reach? The prime issue is efficiency, i.e., reaching the maximum number of people with the least amount of program expenditure.

Process. Process evaluation is concerned with the effectiveness of administrative and operational procedures. The focus tends to be internal and descriptive. A process evaluation usually involves a logical examination of existing procedures, linkages and the flow of information and authority within an organization.

Cost-benefit. The cost-benefit approach to evaluation is an effort to compare various procedures and programs in terms of their rate of return, given an equal commitment of resources. Cost-benefit evaluations have inherent value because they pose the question of how much performance is received per dollar. Cost-benefit will always be an important piece of the program evaluation. It requires the accumulation of data related to absenteeism, health care costs, numbers of individuals who have stopped smoking, time on task, and support from the community (parents) for a worksite wellness program for staff.

Effectiveness. Effectiveness evaluation provides the necessary base for other evaluative efforts. This type of evaluation is concerned with the impact of the program on the population, both individually and collectively. Measurements would include biological data from fitness assessments or lifestyle inventories. Evaluation from screening programs involves testing of employees or identifying problems or conditions that may lead to health problems in the future. This evaluation usually is personalized and involves direct contact with employees.

Screening programs identify problems and refer the employee to other resources for treatment. Screening programs may examine hypertension, physical fitness, cardiovascular functioning and cholesterol levels. They may also include diet analysis and physical examinations. Screening programs should be voluntary and on-site. In one screening program, several volunteer substitute teachers relieve teachers so they can participate in on-site, all-day screening programs that include a comprehensive fitness exam and cholesterol testing.

In general, evaluation of programs and services provides information on whether a program is progressing as planned and what adjustments are needed to put the program on the correct course to meet the needs of the school staff.

The Ripple Effect

Because of the unique structure of a school and the growing evidence that lifestyles associated with chronic disease in adulthood are acquired early in life, the school site is ideal for health promotion and education of children. A worksite wellness program in local school districts could reach out to touch the lives of millions of American students and their families.

The Healthy Lifestyles Program found that when school staff actively worked on improving their own health, these efforts spilled over into the classroom. Teachers interested in walking began walking before class, and students started to follow them. The end result was walking maps inside and outside of all buildings. Walking groups also formed in cooperation with parents as after-school programs.

School staff interested in weight loss petitioned the administration to offer salad bars in the elementary schools. All area elementary school buildings added mini-salad bars, and the students loved them. In one school district, 10,000 more plates were served, with a gain of $50,000 to the local district.

Aerobic classes became an important component of high school physical education classes. The schools adopted a comprehensive health education curriculum for all elementary schools, kindergarten through grade six, and a pilot program for a preschool health curriculum was launched. This curriculum was added because the staff felt it was an important part of a child's education.

As a result of the intensive health education and promotion occurring in the classroom, parents became involved. As parents' awareness of the importance of health for their children grew, schools began to implement extensive sex education courses with little or no conflict from outside interest groups. The parents led the way to improve and support an increase of health initiatives in their schools.

Pitfalls

A pitfall in implementing any type of program, especially wellness in schools, is the expectation of "thermonuclear" change. Kaufman (1971), in describing the limits of organizational change, set forth two conditions: The environment changes slowly and organizations adapt, or the environment changes swiftly or unexpectedly and there is an anticipated slaughter of organization. He argued that numerous changes can result in "organizational death"—not necessarily the end of the organization, but changes so vast that "it makes no sense to consider the original system still in existence."

To avoid this pitfall of change, the values and expectations for such programs must be clearly communicated to all parents, school staff, administrators and board of education members. Public schools need to change slowly and not be overcome by unreasonable expectations associated with the announcement of unattainable goals.

Change is difficult; it should generally be slow. Change can destroy an organization if it comes too quickly or if it is forced. Program changes in the Healthy Lifestyles Program were elective; staff tried to sell health and healthy lifestyles, rather than dictating their adoption.

An Exciting Opportunity

Wellness programs are growing in popularity across the United States. Americans are beginning to understand that changes in our lifestyles over the past fifty years have been accompanied not only by more expansive waistlines but also by increased incidence of heart disease, hypertension, cancer and other stress-related illness. Schools across the United States can offer those working in their districts an exciting opportunity to break some bad habits.

The pay-off for adopting healthier lifestyles is a lifetime of health benefits. Not only will staff look and feel better, they will have taught children in their communities the most important lesson of all—that we are all responsible for our own health. Health promotion programming for school staff can be developed by using the strengths of existing personnel and existing community agencies.

Support of administration and the unions must be demonstrated throughout the programming. Time during the school day should be scheduled for orientation; buildings should be opened to accommodate programming; and program times need to be appropriate for all to attend. Policies must be developed to sustain the efforts over long periods of time. Volunteer or paid facilitators need to have leadership capabilities, schedule flexibility, and knowledge of the principles of adult wellness education in the areas of nutrition, fitness, stress and substance use.

Evaluation is essential to demonstrate the success of the wellness program. Evaluation will assist in gaining continuing support from administration and school boards. It will also help adjust programs to fit the needs of the staff. Schools play a special role in enhancing and maintaining the health of their communities. Allowing all those who are models for children to maximize their health through worksite health promotion and education is a valuable part of fulfilling this role.

References

American Council of Life Insurance and Health Insurance Association of America. 1986. Beyond an apple a day: Teachers and wellness. *Teaching Topics.* 33 (2).

Blair, S. N. 1984. *Health promotion for educators: Impact on absenteeism.* Dallas, TX: Institute for Aerobics.

Green, L. W., and M. W. Krueter. 1991. *Health promotional planning: An educational and environmental approach.* Mountain View, CA: Mayfield Publishing.

Iverson, D. C., and L. J. Kolbe. 1983. Evolution of the national disease prevention and health promotion strategy: Establishing a role for the schools. *Journal of School Health* 53 (5): 294-302.

Johnson, C. 1981. Audience assessment and effective evaluation. In *A technical manual on the planning, implementation and evaluation of utility communication programs,* ed. W. D. Crano, S. Ludwig, L. A. Messe and G. W. Selno, 9-41. Ann Arbor, MI: Michigan State University, Ann Arbor Press.

Kaldy, J. 1985. Schools shape up with employee wellness. *The School Administrator* (April): 12-18.

Kaufman, H. 1971. *The limits of organizational change.* Birmingham, AL: University of Alabama Press.

Tager, M. 1985. *Wellness at the school worksite: A manual.* Washington, DC: Health Insurance Association of America and American Council of Life Insurance.

U. S. Department of Health and Human Services, Public Health Service. 1991. *Healthy people 2000: National health promotion and disease prevention objectives.* DHHS Publication No. (PHS) 91-50212. Washington, DC.

W. K. Kellogg Foundation. 1980. *Viewpoint: Toward a healthier America.* Battle Creek, MI.

252   *The Comprehensive School Health Challenge*

Chapter 10

The Child Nutrition Program as a Partner in Comprehensive School Health

Priscilla Naworski, MS, CHES

The National School Lunch Program (NSLP) was first established in 1946 as an answer to an identified national defense problem—many of the draftees for World War II were poorly nourished. The government's response to this threat to national security was to fund a program that would provide free or low-cost vitamin-packed lunches to tens of millions of American school children.

The program also assisted the American farm industry, because it provided for the purchase and distribution of surplus farm products. Commodities such as wheat, rice, peanuts, butter and cheese were purchased from farmers who had over-production and were made available to schools for use in the preparation of the school lunch.

The program was successful in meeting both of its goals, and children were fed meals that were nutritionally balanced. Since its origin, many expansions, such as the School Breakfast Program, the Child Care Food Program and the Special Milk Program, have been added to the program, which is administered by the U. S. Department of Agriculture (USDA).

Today, with more single-parent households, more working mothers and more children living in poverty, school meal programs are more important than ever. Every school day, 24 million children sit down to food provided by their schools. For many children, this food has made the difference between going hungry and being satisfied, between being undernourished and being well fed, between academic failure and being ready to learn. For these reasons and many more, the school food service or child nutrition program is an essential, integral part of a school's comprehensive health program.

The Nutritional Content

USDA regulations establish a meal pattern that provides the student with a lunch containing one-third of the Recommended Dietary Allowances (RDA) for calories and essential nutrients for a 12 year old. The breakfast pattern provides approximately one-fourth of the daily RDA. These goals are achieved by a system that plans menus to contain prescribed numbers and serving sizes of different food groups.

The lunch pattern for a 12 year old dictates that the menu contain two ounces of protein, eight ounces of fluid milk (both whole milk and unflavored lowfat milk must be offered), a total of three-quarters cup of two or more fruits and vegetables, and eight servings of bread and bread alternative per week. (Refer to Figures 1 and 2 to find the recommended pattern for other age groups for lunch and breakfast.) The lunch pattern for the 12 year old is expected to contain approximately 550 to 600 kilocalories, with 21 to 24 grams of protein.

Figure 1
School Lunch Patterns for Various Age/Grade Groups

| | | Minimum Quantities | | | | Recommended Quantities |
| | Components | Preschool | | Grades K-3 | Grades 4-12 | Grades 7-12 |
Specific Requirements		ages 1-2 (Group I)	ages 3-4 (Group II)	ages 5-8 (Group III)	age 9 & over (Group IV)	age 12 & over (Group V)
• Must be served in the main dish or the main dish and only one other menu item.	**Meat or Meat Alternate** A serving of one of the following or a combination to give an equivalent quantity:					
• Vegetable protein products, cheese alternate products, and enriched macaroni with fortified protein may be used to meet part of the meat/meat alternate requirement. Fact sheets on each of these alternate foods give detailed instructions for use.	• lean meat, poultry or fish	1 oz	1-1/2 oz	1-1/2 oz	2 oz	3 oz
	• cheese	1 oz	1-1/2 oz	1-1/2 oz	2 oz	3 oz
	• large egg(s)	1/2	3/4	3/4	1	1-1/2
	• cooked dry beans or peas	1/4 cup	3/8 cup	3/8 cup	1/2 cup	3/4 cup
	• peanut butter or other nut or seed butters	2 Tbsp	3 Tbsp	3 Tbsp	4 Tbsp	6 Tbsp
	• peanuts, soy nuts, tree nuts or seeds	1/2 oz = 50%	3/4 oz = 50%	3/4 oz = 50%	1 oz = 50%	1-1/2 oz = 50%
• No more than one-half of the total requirement may be met with full-strength fruit or vegetable juice.	**Vegetables and/or Fruits** • two or more servings of vegetables or fruits or both to total	1/2 cup	1/2 cup	1/2 cup	3/4 cup	3/4 cup
• Cooked dry beans or peas may be used as a meat alternate or as a vegetable but not as both in the same meal.						

Figure 1 (continued)
School Lunch Patterns for Various Age/Grade Groups

Specific Requirements	Components	Minimum Quantities				Recommended Quantities
		Preschool		Grades K-3	Grades 4-12	Grades 7-12
		ages 1-2 (Group I)	ages 3-4 (Group II)	ages 5-8 (Group III)	age 9 & over (Group IV)	age 12 & over (Group V)
• At least 1/2 serving of bread or an equivalent quantity of bread alternate for Group I, and 1 serving for Groups II–V, must be served daily. • Enriched macaroni with fortified protein may be used as a meat alternate or as a bread alternate but not as both in the same meal.	**Servings of Bread or Bread Alternate** A serving is: • 1 slice of whole-grain or enriched bread • a whole-grain or enriched biscuit, roll, muffin, etc. • 1/2 cup of cooked whole-grain or enriched rice, macaroni, noodles, whole-grain or enriched pasta products, or other cereal grains such as bulgur or corn grits • a combination of any of the above	5 per week	8 per week	8 per week	8 per week	10 per week
The following forms of milk must be offered: • Whole milk • Unflavored lowfat milk *Note:* This requirement does not prohibit offering other milk, such as flavored milk or skim milk, along with the above.	**Milk** A serving of fluid milk	3/4 cup (6 fl oz)	3/4 cup (6 fl oz)	1/2 pint (8 fl oz)	1/2 pint (8 fl oz)	1/2 pint (8 fl oz)

Adapted from U.S. Department of Agriculture, National School Lunch Program.

Figure 2
School Breakfast Meal Pattern Requirements

Food Components/Items	Minimum Required Quantities		
	Ages 1-2	Ages 3, 4, 5	Age 6 & Up
Fluid Milk As a beverage, on cereal or both	1/2 cup	3/4 cup	1/2 pint
Fruit/Vegetable/Juice Fruit and/or vegetable or full-strength fruit juice or vegetable juice (A fruit, vegetable or juice that is a good source of vitamin C is recommended daily.)	1/4 cup	1/2 cup	1/2 cup

Select *one* serving from each of the following components or *two* servings from one component.

Bread/Bread Alternates One of the following or an equivalent combination:			
• whole-grain or enriched bread	1/2 slice	1/2 slice	1 slice
• whole-grain or enriched biscuit, roll, muffin, etc.	1/2 serving	1/2 serving	1 serving
• whole-grain, enriched or fortified cereal	1/4 cup or 1/3 ounce	1/3 cup or 1/2 ounce	3/4 cup or 1 ounce
Meat/Meat Alternates One of the following or an equivalent combination:			
• lean meat, poultry or fish	1/2 ounce	1/2 ounce	1 ounce
• cheese	1/2 ounce	1/2 ounce	1 ounce
• large egg	1/2	1/2	1/2
• peanut butter or other nut or seed butters	1 Tbsp	1 Tbsp	2 Tbsp
• cooked dry beans and peas	2 Tbsp	2 Tbsp	4 Tbsp
• nuts and/or seeds	1/2 ounce	1/2 ounce	1 ounce

Adapted from U.S. Department of Agriculture, School Breakfast Program.

Critics of this meal pattern say that it does not ensure nutritional quality in the meal. They suggest the meal should reflect the *Dietary Guidelines for Americans* (U.S. Department of Agriculture, 1990), which recommend that no more than 30 to 35 percent of the meal's kilocalories should come from fat and that no more than 10 percent of the total kilocalories should come from saturated fat.

Although there is no conclusive evidence that the health risks associated with eating too much fat originate in childhood, children do develop fatty streaks in their coronary arteries. Studies indicate that some of these fatty streaks are the precursors of atherosclerosis, one of the ten leading causes of death identified by the *Surgeon General's Report on Nutrition and Health* (U.S. Department of Health and Human Services, 1988).

Therefore, the call for menu planning based on the goal of lower total fat content is important to the future health status of children. A low-fat meal is also essential as a daily model of a healthful meal pattern. This lower-fat breakfast or lunch can be achieved by a conscientious effort to purchase foods and food ingredients that are low in fat and by using cooking techniques that will produce child-pleasing food items that have no added fat. For example, well-seasoned skinless chicken breasts can be offered instead of fried chicken; a baked potato rather than a high-fat hot dog can be topped with chili; and children will certainly eat oven-fried rather than deep-fat-fried potatoes.

The process for purchasing food needs to be structured around the nutrient content of the food. The food service director should require that the producer or vendor provide nutrient information about each processed food item. Progressive food service directors are now using computer nutrient database programs such as Food Processor II or Nutritionist 3 to analyze and plan their menus.

Many steps can be taken to modify cooking procedures to lower the total fat, sugar and salt content of foods. Kitchens everywhere are now modifying procedures by draining cooked meat before adding it to entrees such as chili or spaghetti, skimming fat from soups and stews, and preparing their own salad dressings, cutting down on the amount of oil and salt.

Other recommendations of the dietary guidelines can be implemented through meal planning, modified cooking techniques and thoughtful purchasing. The goal to provide more fiber in the meal is easily implemented. The menu can reflect an increase in fresh fruits and vegetables, using vegetables in main-course offerings and fruits as desserts. When a fresh fruit is used as a dessert, the amount of fiber in the meal goes up while the amount of simple sugars goes down. Pastas, desserts and breads should be made from fiber-rich whole grains. The kitchen baker can substitute whole-grain flour for half the amount of white flour in a quick bread recipe, and children will accept it. (See box.)

Healthy Menu Modifications

Plenty of Vegetables	Whole Grain Breads and Cereals
Low in Sodium (Salt)	Low-Fat Dairy Foods
Lean Meats or Legumes (Beans)	Low in Fats or Oils

The school menu has often been characterized as starchy, since it might feature a pasta dish, corn and bread on the same tray. This menu is in compliance with the meal pattern and the U.S. dietary guidelines, which suggest that daily intake should include much complex carbohydrates (starches) and few simple sugars. Education targeted to students, parents and staff can help them understand that this "starchy" menu is actually very healthy.

The USDA funds several training programs that help educate food service staff in better buying techniques and recipe modification methods. For example, the National Food Service Management Institute at the University of Mississippi currently provides both seminar and teleconference training. USDA also funds Nutrition Education and Training (NET) programs in each state. The state NET program is involved in both food service training and nutrition education curriculum and instruction. Many states have published excellent curriculum tools for both areas of responsibility.

Other Supportive Activities and Policies

Nutritional guidelines and menu modifications are one very important aspect of the effort to promote optimal nutrition and health for all children, but more needs to be done. Local school boards must write and adopt policies that support the concept of access to nutritious and appealing meals, served in pleasant surroundings and in an environment that fosters development of positive attitudes and social skills. These policies should ensure that the time set aside for students' meals is long enough to allow for a relaxed mealtime.

The lunch area needs adequate supervision so students will develop the habit of having lunch in an orderly, quiet manner. Some schools have implemented programs that use older students as lunch buddies who eat with younger students and model both positive attitudes toward lunch and social skills.

The nutritional policy for the school district should also contain guidelines for the sale of nonnutritious foods and the use of items donated by parents for classroom parties and schoolwide events. Such a policy is likely to be unpopular when first discussed, because often school programs such as athletics, student government and band make money by sponsoring candy and soda sales.

Congress allows schools to control the sale of foods of minimal nutritional value in the food service areas during meal periods.

The sale of competitive foods at other times and places is allowed only if the income is used by the school or by student organizations.

According to the USDA, "minimum nutritional value" means that a food provides less than 5 percent per serving of the U.S. RDA for each of eight specific nutrients. This definition bars the sale of soda pop, chewing gum and hard candy, but allows the sale of candy bars made with milk or nuts, and vitamin-fortified drinks, even though they have a high fat and sugar content. The sale of nonnutritious foods has been banned in Cincinnati, Ohio; Washington, D.C.; West Virginia; Louisiana; Arizona and Massachusetts.

Before a school board is ready to ban the sale of nonnutritious foods, it may need to address the financial problems that prompt school organizations to sell nonnutritious foods. Boards will also have a difficult time defining what such nonnutritious foods are if they are particularly interested in restrictions based on the fat, cholesterol and sodium content of the foods. The current USDA definition does not consider fat, sugar and fiber contents.

The school policy and program must make provisions for nutrition education as part of classroom instruction. This instruction should be based on a curriculum that has an appropriate scope and sequence and up-to-date instructional strategies. Inservice for the classroom teacher is essential to successful implementation of the program. A one-time inservice usually does not sustain the effort. Follow-up inservice and peer support teams help sustain a high level of quality and frequency of instruction.

The school child nutrition director can play a major role in assisting the school board to develop and implement policy. The director can also join forces with the district's curriculum staff to select and implement curriculum. The director will also be a valuable member of the inservice team. He or she will then be able to serve as an ongoing resource to classroom teachers for technical information and classroom support. Support may include allowing classes to use kitchen facilities or equipment for food preparation activities, opening the school kitchen facility for class field trips or visiting classes as a guest lecturer.

School policy should also call for ongoing professional development opportunities for both the child nutrition staff and the teaching staff. The ideal school is one in which the child nutrition staff has a career ladder and staff members receive promotions or pay increases based on the amount of continuing education that they receive. The American School Food Service Association conducts a certification program to promote continuing education for its members. The USDA strongly recommends that any school food service program involve an advisory committee comprised of students, parents, teachers and community representatives to advise them on nutrition issues, menu suggestions and program marketing.

Marketing

A school lunch program that serves well-planned, nutritious meals will not be considered successful until a large majority of the students eat the food. To achieve this goal, program managers must make conscious efforts to "sell" the program to students, parents, faculty and the community. This effort should not only market the availability of the program but also the nutritional quality of the food served.

Many families mistakenly feel that the school lunch program is too expensive. The typical price for an elementary school lunch is $1.50. A survey done in one California school district found that a typical lunch packed at home usually cost more than $2.20 and did not include all of the food categories that are part of the lunch pattern. The sack lunch is often an expensive, nutritionally unbalanced meal. Potato chips and soda are not a substitute for a baked potato and milk.

The school lunch program's information and sales campaign needs a multimedia approach to reach all of the essential populations. The child nutrition office can publish monthly menus with healthy menu modifications highlighted on the front and a fact sheet about nutrition on the back (see Figure 3). Many sources, such as the American School Food Service Association, the American Heart Association and the California Department of Education offer prepared fact sheets.

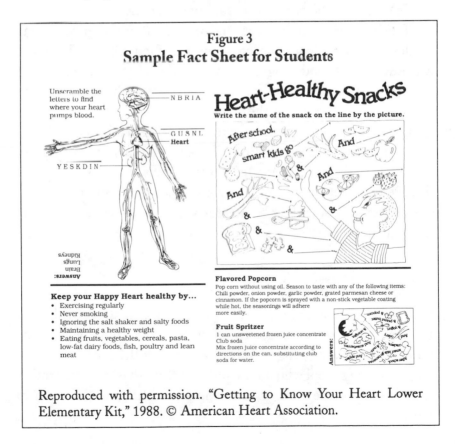

Figure 3
Sample Fact Sheet for Students

Reproduced with permission. "Getting to Know Your Heart Lower Elementary Kit," 1988. © American Heart Association.

If the school serves a multicultural population, the menu information should be provided in other languages. In many areas, local radio stations will broadcast weekly school lunch menus. Add notes to the menu to highlight the foods that are lower in fat or higher in fiber—take credit for the menu modifications that you have made.

Back-to-School Night or open house is a perfect time for the child nutrition program to market its activities to parents, with a display of school lunch trays and handouts about nutrition and the nutritional quality of the school lunch. When a lunch menu is analyzed by a computer nutrient analysis program, the resulting totals speak for the nutritional quality of the meal.

Teachers need to support the school program, encouraging students to participate and consume the food offered. Teachers' attitudes about food programs go a long way to encourage both participation and consumption. Supportive teachers can help to set norms for behavior in the cafeteria area, also.

Child nutrition programs across the country have used students as part of their marketing efforts by forming youth advisory councils. Such councils can help plan menus, serve as tasters for food items, plan and coordinate contests and events in the cafeteria and serve as sounding boards for students' concerns about the program.

The Feeding Relationship

From infancy, humans are conditioned to equate the providing of food as an act of caring for those who will receive the nourishment. This conditioning automatically places the team of professionals in the school who do the planning, purchasing, preparation and serving of the food on the school health team, the team of people who provide the instruction and support services designed to meet the physical and psychological health needs of the student.

The security of this relationship between the provider and the consumer can nourish both the hunger for food and the emotional need to be connected with people in caring relationships. Many adults still fondly remember the "food service lady" who smiled at them, called them by name and served them a lunch that was tasty and nourishing. It was a welcome interlude in the rigors of the school day.

In many schools, students are hired by the food service department to help in the serving line to speed up the lunch process. Student workers can derive a special sense of purpose from the work responsibility and a good feeling from the relationship with the adult staff. Many of these student workers are high-risk students who do not often receive social support and recognition for their contributions. For such students, the food service job can be a protective factor, helping them to build the self-esteem that can deter academic failure and poor health-related decisions.

The child nutrition program is an essential part of the school comprehensive health program. It gains its place on the school health team as a program that offers nourishment to students; nutrition education to students, parents, staff and community; and opportunities for students to practice what they've learned in health class as they make wise food choices.

References

American Cancer Society. 1990. *Changing the course: Manual for school foodservice providers*. Atlanta, GA.

American School Food Service Association. 1991. The healthy E.D.G.E. in schools: Eating, the dietary guidelines and education. *School Food Service Journal* supplement (March).

Citizens' Commission on School Nutrition. 1990. *White paper on school-lunch nutrition*. Washington, DC.

Collins, M. E. 1991. Promoting healthy body image through the comprehensive school health program. *Journal of Health Education* 22 (5): 297-302.

Farris, R. P., T. A. Nicklas, L. S. Webber and G. S. Berenson. 1992. Nutrient contribution of the school lunch program: Implications for healthy people 2000. *Journal of School Health* 62 (5): 180-184.

U.S. Department of Health and Human Services, Public Health Service. 1988. *The Surgeon General's report on nutrition and health*. DHHS Publication No. (PHS) 88-50210. Washington, DC.

U.S. Department of Agriculture and U.S. Department of Health and Human Services. 1990. *Nutrition and your health: Dietary guidelines for Americans*. 3d ed. Home and Garden Bulletin No. 232. Washington, DC.

Content Issues

Chapter 11

Personal and Social Skill Development Is Basic

Joyce V. Fetro, PhD, CHES

Risk taking is a part of normal psychological development. During their teen years, young people try a variety of "risky" behaviors with the expectation that they will not be permanently committed to or harmed by these behaviors. As they progress through this period of "storm and stress," adolescents typically acquire a variety of personal and social skills critical for dealing with a myriad of situations, problems and pressures. They make many choices, learn about appropriate and inappropriate risks and behaviors, and, ideally, emerge as functioning adults.

However, statistics related to adolescent health risk behaviors (using tobacco, alcohol and other substances, engaging in early and/or unprotected sexual intercourse, binging and purging to lose weight, drinking and driving, not using safety belts or safety helmets, carrying and using weapons, and committing suicide), are showing that typical adolescent experimentation is no longer harmless and may in fact have serious health consequences.

As a result, the Office of Disease Prevention and Health Promotion (1991) and the Centers for Disease Control and Prevention (1992) have targeted six priority areas for comprehensive school health education program focus:

- behaviors that result in unintentional and intentional injuries
- use of alcohol and other drugs
- tobacco use
- sexual behaviors that result in sexually transmitted disease, HIV infection and unintended pregnancy
- imprudent dietary patterns
- inadequate exercise

But how do we most effectively target these areas? Which program elements are necessary to effectively address these priority needs? And, once identified, how can these program elements be integrated within comprehensive school health education?

Over the past twenty years, a variety of prevention programs related to substance use and sexuality behaviors have been developed and evaluated. The most promising approaches are based on the results of these evaluation studies.

In the sixties, health education programs focused on the presentation of information about the physical and psychological effects of engaging in particular health-risk behaviors. In these programs, the underlying assumption was that if young people were aware of the short- and long-term consequences of using drugs, having sex and so on, they would choose not to engage in those behaviors. These programs typically used scare tactics to portray the negative personal, social and legal consequences of health-related decisions.

In the seventies, prevention programs incorporated more affective methods. They focused on eliminating interpersonal and intrapersonal factors that were thought to be associated with

particular behaviors. These programs included activities to enhance self-esteem, clarify values and strengthen decision-making
skills. Overall, information-based programs and affective education programs increased students' knowledge and attitudes, but
did not effectively delay onset or decrease incidence of health-
compromising behaviors.

Over the last decade, prevention programs have used a variety
of psychosocial approaches, including social learning theory, social
influences theory, social inoculation theory and cognitive behavioral theory, in hopes of decreasing adolescents' health risk behaviors. Such programs are based on the premise that young people
need a variety of generic skills that they can use in social situations
where they are confronted with making health-related decisions.

Evaluation of programs based on psychosocial theory have
identified several key elements necessary for program success.
First, accurate information is essential; effective programs examined short- and long-term physical, social, emotional and legal
consequences of health-related decisions and the internal and
external influences on personal health practices. Second, these
programs incorporated activities to increase self-awareness and
enhance self-esteem. Third, they used peer helpers in a variety of
roles and actively involved parents and other caregivers in the
program. Fourth, and most important, they included activities to
build personal and social skills. (For details about effectiveness of
specific prevention programs see: Alcohol, Drug Abuse and Mental Health Administration, 1990; Bell and Battjes, 1987; Botvin,
1987; Botvin and Wills, 1985; Eisen, Zellman and McAllister,
1990; Flay, 1985; Howard and McCabe, 1990; Glasgow and
McCaul, 1985; Kirby et al., 1991; Kumpfer, 1990; Lando, 1985;
Schaps et al., 1981; Schinke, Blythe and Gilchrist, 1981.)

Comprehensive health education is the most obvious forum for
targeting health issues and risk behaviors. However, to meet the

National Health Promotion and Disease Prevention Objectives, health education programs must be expanded to include personal and social skills that adolescents can use in making decisions about their health-related practices.

Four Generic Personal and Social Skills

Four generic skills have been identified as key to the development of personal and social competence: decision-making skills, communication skills, stress-management skills and goal-setting skills. The next section will provide an overview of each skill, including a discussion of essential information that should be presented in classroom discussions, as well as a list of subareas that should be addressed with classroom skill-building activities.

Making Informed Decisions
As young people pass through adolescence, they are confronted by a variety of personal, social, educational and career decisions they never had to make before. Some decisions are automatic and based on habit, such as deciding when to get up, what to wear, what to have for breakfast. Others are made on a hunch. Still others are made based on past experiences (i.e., "I did this before and it seemed to work") or by default (i.e., not deciding at all).

There are times, such as in an emergency, when there is not enough time to analyze the situation and examine the possible consequences of a decision. But in some cases, personal decisions are more important and must be given mindful consideration. If these situations and issues are not carefully thought through, their consequences could have far-reaching effects on a young person's health, future decisions and long-term goals.

Without strong decision-making skills to actively solve problems that may arise in personal and social situations, teens may feel unsure and overwhelmed. Understanding how decisions are made helps adolescents deal with difficult problems and makes these problems less overwhelming. Strong decision-making skills can increase adolescents' sense of control over their lives, thus enhancing their self-esteem and self-efficacy, and ultimately enabling them to take responsibility for their own decisions.

Class discussions about decision making should focus on internal and external influences on personal decisions. Young people often choose to use substances, have sex or engage in other health-compromising behaviors in an effort to feel important, be accepted, feel grown up, escape or take a risk. They make many choices in response to pressures from parents or other caregivers, teachers, significant adults and peers. In addition, teens can be strongly influenced by media, advertising, or behavioral norms that exist, or appear to exist, in the community.

A variety of other factors, including available information and resources, personal skills and experiences, personal values and beliefs, perception of risk, peer approval, availability and peer norm, may affect personal decisions. Students should examine these factors and influences as they relate to their own lives.

Finally, the steps to good decision making (define the problem; gather information; list possible solutions; list consequences of each solution; choose the best solution and try it out; evaluate the decision) should be discussed and applied to real-life situations.

Skill-building activities for making informed decisions should include:

- identifying decisions to be made or problems to be solved
- analyzing influences on personal decisions
- examining personal skills and capabilities as they relate to possible solutions
- distinguishing between things that can and cannot be changed

- identifying information sources and organizing available information
- personalizing risk of decisions to self and others
- correcting misperceptions of peer norms
- identifying positive and negative short- and long-term consequences of decisions
- identifying support systems
- analyzing real-life situations using the decision-making model
- understanding how one personal decision may affect subsequent decisions
- taking responsibility for personal decisions
- evaluating decisions and making necessary changes

Communicating Effectively

Every day, everywhere, we give and receive hundreds of messages. Think about a typical day. How many types of communication can you remember?—perhaps a baby's cry, laughter of young children playing during recess, a short note to an acquaintance, the wave of a hand, a pat on the back, signs, a frown on someone's brow, a lunchtime conversation with a good friend, an argument with your child or mother. The messages we give, how we give them (verbally or nonverbally), how well others understand what we meant and how well we understand what others mean directly affects the quality of our interpersonal relationships.

Communication—the ability to clearly express one's thoughts, feelings, beliefs, opinions, reactions, values, hopes and dreams—is a skill that must be learned. A young person's ability to communicate can have a direct effect on his or her level of self-esteem and the quality of his or her relationships with others. Poor communication can lead to misunderstandings and feelings of anger, mistrust and frustration with teachers, friends, family and others.

The ability to have successful interpersonal relationships

requires a broad range of communication skills, including the ability to initiate conversations, actively listen to others, express thoughts and feelings, agree or disagree with others' opinions, and give clear and consistent verbal and nonverbal messages. These skills are essential for self-efficacy—the ability to execute the behaviors necessary to produce a desired outcome (Bandura, 1977).

Young people must be taught how to send verbal and nonverbal messages that accurately describe who they are, what they think, how they feel and what they believe. Giving verbal and nonverbal messages that agree, as well as understanding the physical and emotional context of the message, are key to determining the overall meaning of communication.

Since people communicate on many different levels, class discussions should address how personal conversations can include cliches, information and facts, ideas and feelings, and finally, self-disclosure. Most often, levels of communication correspond to the level of intimacy in the relationship. The level of intimacy in a relationship, however, can change from day to day depending on the situation and the topic.

Understanding barriers and how to overcome them (e.g., the listener is not actively listening; the speaker and listener are "speaking" a different language; the listener's personal biases affect his or her response; the speaker makes assumptions about the listener) is critical to good communication. When a young person can recognize that a particular behavior is interfering with communication, he or she can take steps to replace old behaviors with new skills, resulting in more satisfying relationships.

Specific focus should be placed on assertiveness skills—helping students say what they think and stand up for what they believe and value, without hurting others or denying the rights of others. In learning the difference between passive, assertive and aggressive responses, students must understand the fine line between being assertive and being aggressive. In addition, they must be able to differentiate between situations where assertiveness may be helpful or harmful. Assertiveness skills learned in health education class help teens say no to friends, ask favors of others and express opinions when they differ from the rest of the group's. Strong assertiveness skills can increase the likelihood of getting what one wants, increase one's level of self-esteem, decrease frustration and stress, and decrease the likelihood of being taken advantage of by others.

Refusal skills, one type of assertiveness skill, help students clearly say no in a way that does not jeopardize peer and family relationships. Such skills can help young people avoid situations where they might be pressured or delay making a decision until they have had time to consider possible alternative actions. Refusal skills are based on the assumption that young people, if forewarned of internal and external pressures on health-related decisions, can develop and rehearse arguments in advance and successfully refuse to engage in health-compromising behaviors.

Skill-building activities for communicating effectively should include:
- initiating and maintaining conversations
- actively listening and responding to others
- following directions
- learning to communicate verbally and nonverbally
- identifying commonly used signs and body language that clarify or confuse a verbal message
- giving clear, consistent verbal and nonverbal messages
- identifying personal barriers to communication
- understanding how personal biases affect communication
- stating one's position whether it agrees or disagrees with that of others
- writing I-statements

- differentiating between passive, assertive and aggressive responses
- giving one-line refusals to peer pressure situations
- using scripted, half-scripted and nonscripted roleplays describing real-life scenarios to practice refusal skills
- resolving conflict in peer and family relationships

Managing Stress

Stress is a natural part of everyone's life. It can place people under pressure and make them feel uptight, or it can give them the drive and motivation to succeed. It can lead to conflict or can help solve conflict. It can make people tense and unhappy, or it can make their lives interesting and challenging. It can be helpful or harmful. Whether stress leads to growing or debilitating experiences is directly related to how well an individual deals with stressful situations.

Many students make unhealthy decisions because of stressful situations in school, at home and with peers. Young people need to know the difference between "good" and "bad" stress and how it can affect them physically, emotionally and socially. Class discussions should focus on identifying common stressors, the short- and long-term effects of stress and positive and negative ways of coping with stress (e.g., distraction, avoidance and escape).

Most important, students must learn effective ways of managing stress. Most people continue to use coping skills—short-term solutions—long after a stressful situation calls for more long-term strategies. For example, a young person may deal with a dysfunctional family situation by drinking or using other drugs rather than seeking help from friends, significant adults or professionals. A teen who feels unsuccessful at school may fake illness so that he or she does not continually face failure. Or a young woman, feeling unloved and unworthy, may choose to have unprotected sex and, ultimately, have a baby whom she can love and who will love her back.

Since stress is unavoidable, young people must learn to manage stressors and decrease the pressures they cause before the level of stress reaches a point where physical or emotional health is affected or before their way of coping becomes harmful (i.e., alcoholism or other drug addiction, withdrawal, suicide). Good stress-management skills, such as enhancing personal and emotional health, mental rehearsal skills, learning to relax and building a support network, can reduce overall feelings of stress or change a stressful situation into a healthy challenge.

Skill-building activities for managing stress should include:

* differentiating between "good" and "bad" stress
* identifying physical, emotional, social, family, school and environmental stressors
* monitoring stressful situations and ways of dealing with them
* examining physical and emotional reactions to stress
* clarifying expectations of self and others
* identifying ways to avoid stressful situations when feasible
* discussing personal strategies for coping with stress
* enhancing personal and emotional health
* learning relaxation techniques
* building and maintaining support systems at home, at school and in the community
* identifying sources of professional assistance

Setting Personal Goals

Some people set goals and accomplish them easily. Others talk about what they want and where they want to be but never really make anything happen. What makes these two types of individuals different?

People are not born with goal-setting skills. Nor do these skills magically appear as they grow older. In the process of growing up, teens attempt to move from dependence to independence, attempting to take responsibility for where they are going and who they will become. Many students, however, make choices based on their perceptions of the immediate rather than the long-term consequences of those decisions. In short, immediate gratification is the primary outcome of their decisions.

Short- and long-term goals can provide a framework for making personal decisions. They can be powerful motivators that help focus young people's energies so they can accomplish the things they set out to do. As young people develop—physically, mentally, emotionally, socially and spiritually they must first realize that they have the ability to influence who they are and what they can become. Subsequently, they can realize their full potential by taking charge, planning their futures, and taking small, yet important steps toward making their visions a reality.

Related to setting personal goals, class discussion should focus on the steps for achieving personal goals: examining "who you are" and "where you are," developing a vision, setting achievable goals, devising an action plan, establishing a support network and setting up a reward system. Personal awareness of strengths, capabilities, talents, skills and values will lead to the development of personal goals that are achievable. Short- and long-term goals evolve out of personal vision. If students compare who and where they are with who and where they want to be they can chart a course to get there.

Achieving personal goals is not as easy as it sounds. A number of factors may interfere. As they begin setting short-term goals, teens must become aware of numerous barriers, so they can overcome as many as possible and increase their probability of success. Finally, they must be able to predict the possible impact of health-related decisions on their short- and long-term goals.

Skill-building activities for setting personal goals should include:
- assessing personal strengths and weaknesses, capabilities and limitations, likes and dislikes
- clarifying personal values and beliefs
- identifying short- and long-term personal expectations
- predicting short- and long-term outcomes of personal behavior
- identifying support systems at school, at home and in the community
- identifying ways to reward personal achievements
- applying the steps for achieving personal goals
- identifying barriers to achieving personal goals
- analyzing the impact of personal decisions on future goals

Teaching Personal and Social Skills

Think back to any skill you have mastered (e.g., skiing, reading, swimming). What were some of the steps involved in learning that skill? First, someone may have told you how to do it. You might have read a book that described the skill step by step. At some point, another person may have demonstrated the skill to you. You practiced over and over and over again, until you got it. Finally, feedback from your friends, your family, and/or your teacher helped you perfect the skill.

Now, think about your own personal and social skill-building experiences. Were the steps to learning these skills the same? Learning how to make a decision, be assertive, set personal goals, and manage stress are actually very similar to learning how to swim, ski or read.

The previous section described the four generic personal and social skills. But simply presenting young people with information about personal and social skills is no guarantee that they will be able to make informed decisions, communicate effectively, manage stressful situations, or set and achieve personal goals, or that they will actually use the skills in their everyday relationships and situations.

No matter which personal and social skill students attempt to master, the likelihood that they will feel competent and will be able to use the skills once they leave the classroom involves five steps: introducing the skill, presenting the steps for developing the skill, modeling the skill, practicing and rehearsing the skill, and providing feedback and reinforcement.

Introducing the Skill

Discuss the importance of each new skill. Use simple, everyday examples to illustrate how the specific skill is used. For example, when introducing decision making, have students brainstorm a list of decisions they made before coming to school (e.g., deciding to get up, deciding not to eat breakfast, deciding what to wear). Or, after defining stress, have students identify things that are stressful to them in school, at home or with their peers and describe how they deal with these situations. These types of activities will help students realize that the skill is not new, that they in fact use the skill on a regular basis, often unconsciously.

Explain what makes each "generic" skill similar and/or different from the others. Identifying common elements among skills will serve as review and reinforcement of previously learned skills, ultimately increasing students' confidence in their ability to perform the new skill. For example, in the decision-making model, students are asked to identify consequences of possible solutions to a real-life situation. When setting personal goals, have students practice predicting short- and long-term effects of selected behaviors. Show your students how identifying consequences involves the same process as predicting short- and long-term effects.

Help students understand how the new skill builds on other skills. For instance, a young person may decide that he is not ready for sex (decision-making skills), so he must be able to say "no" to his partner (communication/refusal skills). Or another teen may decide not to take drugs (decision-making skills) because of her future plans to attend college and become a teacher (goal-setting skills). Linking one skill to another will increase students' understanding of how personal and social skills interrelate and cross over all aspects of their lives.

Finally, personalize information about the new skill. When you describe situations where the skill *is* or *can be* used, be sure to use examples that are real to your students. Encourage them to share their own experiences and think of situations in their lives where they could use the new skill.

Presenting the Steps for Developing the Skill

The first step in learning any new skill is knowing how to do it. Each generic skill has a series of specific steps necessary for successful performance. Present and discuss each step separately using a wide variety of activities.

For example, the steps for achieving personal goals include examining who you are and where you are, developing a vision, setting achievable goals, devising an action plan, establishing a support network and setting up a reward system. If, after introducing the skill and its importance, you proceeded to discuss these six steps concurrently, students would probably feel overwhelmed.

So, take it in small steps. Target one skill-building step at a time. That is, begin with activities that help students examine who they are—their strengths and weaknesses, capabilities and limitations, likes and dislikes, values and beliefs. Follow with activities that help students develop a vision—a picture of where they want to go and what they would like to be, and so on. Let the level of your students' responses be an indicator of whether or not they are ready to proceed to the next step.

Modeling the Skill

Modeling is critical to building personal and social skills. After students understand steps for building a specific skill, use one or more examples to model each step *and* the entire skill.

With cognitive skills such as decision making, present a simple but realistic problem and go through the process step by step: define the problem, gather information, identify possible solutions, list consequences of those solutions, make the decision and decide how to evaluate the success of the decision. Once students become familiar with the decision-making process, present a more complicated situation involving a variety of influences (e.g., a situation where peer influence is in direct conflict with parental or caregiver guidelines).

Similarly, with goal-setting, select a short-term goal that is realistic for your students and go through the steps, including listing the benefits of attaining the goal, identifying small steps toward reaching the goal, identifying obstacles that could prevent achievement of the goal and listing possible ways to overcome the identified obstacles.

With behavioral skills, such as assertiveness and refusal skills, present real-life situations using scripted, half-scripted and unscripted roleplays to demonstrate the skills in action. For stress-management skills, have students maintain a stress log, identifying daily stressors and the ways they deal with them. Using identified stressful situations, model alternative ways of coping with or managing the stressful situation with roleplays.

Personal and social skills should be modeled across all health content areas and all aspects of young people's lives. For example, refusal skills are most often associated with using substances and/

or having sex. These skills, however, are used in many everyday interactions with friends and family (e.g., refusing to help a friend cheat on a test, refusing to get in a car with someone who has been drinking, refusing to go to a movie that you really don't want to see).

Continue modeling different situations, alone or with students, until students' responses indicate that the majority of them understand. Whenever necessary, review the skill-building steps with realistic examples.

Practicing and Rehearsing the Skill

Related to academic, athletic, dramatic or musical ability, the phrase "practice makes perfect" is commonly used. The same phrase can be applied to personal and social skill building. Self-efficacy—young people's ability to actually execute a learned skill in their personal and social lives—depends upon the amount of practice and rehearsal they have had.

In almost all cases, however, the ability to perform a particular behavior (e.g., say no, be assertive, make an informed decision) is situation-specific. A young woman may be able to say no to smoking marijuana because she understands the personal risk, but she may not be able to say no to unprotected sex because she is afraid to talk about buying and using condoms. A young man may be able to express his feelings openly and honestly with his closest friends, but he may be unable to tell his parents he thinks the curfew they have set is unfair. A young couple may affirm their love for each other and plan their future together, but may be unable to talk about using protection to prevent disease and/or pregnancy.

Begin practice and rehearsal of new skills in small groups with nonthreatening situations. To ensure that all students participate, have them write their individual responses on worksheets. Shyer students can read their responses in small groups. When students feel comfortable and confident, use more complicated situations. Finally, practice in larger groups so that all students can interact and benefit from what was accomplished in small groups. Continued practice and rehearsal will empower students to think on their feet and respond to unanticipated issues and problems.

Providing Feedback and Reinforcement

Incorporate a process of feedback and reinforcement, beginning with skill modeling and continuing throughout the practice sessions. Encourage positive feedback by focusing on what has been done correctly and what could have been done differently, rather than what was done incorrectly.

Use observation worksheets to help students stay focused on specific skill-building steps during practice sessions. These worksheets will help students observe each other and give feedback about whether they have incorporated the key components of the specific skill.

In classroom discussion, elicit input from as many students as possible. Help students understand that they have different experiences and skills and that each situation can be handled in a variety of ways depending on the individual and the specific circumstances.

Promote the use of personal and social skills by asking students to share experiences where they used newly learned skills. This reinforcement will help young people personalize skill-building information. Daily logs, written assignments, small group interactions and large group discussions can be used to determine if students are actually using the skills and will help identify obstacles to using the skills on a regular basis. As a class, students can generate a list of ways to overcome common obstacles to using personal and social skills.

Empowering Students to Use Personal and Social Skills

In addition to understanding the skills themselves and the steps for developing them, several factors set the stage for whether students will actually practice and successfully use these personal and social skills: enhancing self-esteem, creating a supportive environment, putting yourself in your students' shoes, and involving students directly.

Enhancing Self-Esteem

Self-esteem is an evaluative term that reflects people's perceptions about their personal characteristics and abilities. In short, self-esteem refers to the way people think and feel about themselves. Levels of self-esteem change based on daily experiences and interpersonal relationships at home, at school, in peer groups and in the community.

Young people with high self-esteem are not only satisfied with themselves but are also able to take risks to try new things and develop new talents and abilities. They are not only satisfied with their existing relationships but are also able to meet new friends and develop more intimate relationships with old ones. They are not only confident of their ability to complete tasks successfully but are also able to accept additional challenges.

Most important, levels of self-esteem directly affect the ability to make informed decisions, communicate effectively, manage stressful situations and, ultimately, set and achieve personal goals. Thus, enhancing self-esteem is a critical first step toward empowering students to take charge of their lives and use personal and social skills.

According to Bean (1992), four conditions are essential to maintaining high levels of self-esteem: a sense of uniqueness, a sense of connectiveness, a sense of power and a sense of models.

Students with a strong *sense of uniqueness* have an accurate picture of themselves—what makes them special and what makes them similar to others. They recognize their capabilities and limitations, accepting the fact that they are not perfect. A sense of uniqueness can be developed through classroom and schoolwide experiences that help young people recognize and accept their unique attributes and qualities as well as those of others; express their ideas openly, without criticism and judgment; and be creative in a variety of ways.

Students with a strong *sense of connectiveness* identify with one or more groups of people, and, more important, are satisfied with their affiliations. They feel connected to their past and heritage and feel respected by others. A sense of connectiveness can be developed through classroom and schoolwide activities that provide students with opportunities to participate as functioning members of a group; share their ideas, interests and opinions with others; and gain personal recognition from peers, teachers and families.

Students with a strong *sense of power* believe they have the ability to affect what happens to them. They are able to take charge of things in their lives and make desired changes. They are able to distinguish between the things they can change and those they cannot. A sense of power can be developed through classroom and schoolwide activities that provide students opportunities to make choices that affect their personal and academic lives, take responsibility for those choices, demonstrate self-control and self-discipline, and acknowledge and increase their level of personal and social competence.

Students with a strong *sense of models* are confident in their ability to distinguish between right and wrong, are aware of the standards by which their actions will be evaluated, and, thus, are able to take responsibility for their actions. They are self-directed and motivated as they pursue personal goals. A sense of models can be developed through classroom and schoolwide activities that allow students to examine and express their personal, family, religious and cultural values and beliefs; identify future goals; and set and monitor achievable goals.

Wherever possible, to empower students to use the decision-making, communication, stress-management, and goal-setting skills they have learned, interweave activities to enhance self-esteem with skill-building activities. (For specific activities to increase a sense of uniqueness, connectiveness, power and models, see Fetro, 1992.)

Creating an Open, Supportive Environment

The classroom environment is critical to successful personal and social skill building. A forum that supports individual differences and enhances self-esteem will increase students' willingness to participate in discussions and share their thoughts, feelings, ideas and opinions with others. Students will be willing to take risks as they learn new skills and discuss sensitive health content areas. An open, supportive environment will give students a sense of security (I will not be harmed by trying this), a sense of belonging (We're in this together), a sense of respect (My opinion is just as valuable as anyone else's), and a sense of personal and social competence (I can do this!).

Young people are never quite sure how they are *supposed* to feel, what they are *supposed* to know, how they are *supposed* to react, and what they are *supposed* to believe. Setting and maintaining groundrules will allow students to share and explore personal and social skill building in an accepting environment. Typical groundrules include no put-downs; no question is silly or dumb; listen when others are speaking; everyone has the right to pass; all discussions are confidential. No matter which health content area is being discussed, student input is critical. With groundrules in place, students will have a clear idea of what is expected of them, their classmates and you.

Putting Yourself in Your Students' Shoes

Try to remember what it was like to be a teenager. Consider the choices you had to make; the pressures you had from your parents, teachers, and friends; and how you did or did not deal with them. Remember how difficult it was to say no to your friends because you wanted to be accepted, to be assertive with someone you really cared about for fear of losing them, or to tell your parents or caregivers that you didn't want to be what they wanted you to be.

Remember your internal confusion and insecurity as you made choices pitting your personal beliefs and values against your need for acceptance and love. Remember how totally overwhelmed you may have felt as you tried to meet the expectations of all those who were important to you. The more things change, the more they stay the same. Use your personal experiences to help tailor classroom activities and develop real-life scenarios and case studies that will be relevant to teens.

Involving Students Directly

Personal and social skill building cannot be successful without direct student involvement. As realistic as they may seem, the situations and examples you choose for classroom activities may need some fine-tuning from your own students. Challenge students to write their own roleplays, case studies and real-life scenarios. Then have them work together to act out their roleplays and make decisions for characters in their case studies.

Provide numerous opportunities for students to work together, formally or informally. Young people rely on each other for infor-

mation about health-related issues and concerns and discuss feelings openly and honestly with their peers (Cook, Sola and Pfeiffer,
1989). Use this built-in support system to enhance your skills-
based health education program. Have students present key information, facilitate small group work and model new skills. If
feasible, have your students make presentations to younger students, incorporating the skills they have learned and activities they
have developed.

Although it may require more organization and class time,
involving your students in the learning process will help them
personalize information and skills, leading to a higher probability
of success. They will begin to realize that the skills they have
learned can be used in any situation and that, with continued
practice, each of them can attain some level of personal and social
competence.

Training Health Educators to Teach Personal and Social Skills

Since personal and social skill building typically has not been
included in teacher preservice, inservice and professional preparation programs, training programs should be expanded to include
key information and skill-building activities related to decision
making, communication, stress management and goal setting. Just
as young people must learn the similarities and differences between the skills, understand the steps to skill development and
practice and rehearse each skill, so must the health educators who
will be teaching them.

Within the training, the sequence of activities necessary to
build each skill should be modeled and, subsequently, experienced
by health educators. In addition, follow-up discussions should
process each activity: What types of questions might students ask?

What situations might arise in the classroom to influence its success? What could be done to follow up or extend the activity? (For more information about preservice education, inservice training and professional preparation, see Chapters 27, 28 and 29.)

Integrating Skills Across All Health Content Areas
Health education has ten identified content areas: community health, consumer health, environmental health, family life, growth and development, nutritional health, personal health, prevention and control of disease and disorders, safety and accident prevention, and substance use and abuse (National Professional School Health Education Organizations, 1984). Think about how the four generic skills could be incorporated into all ten content areas.

Although decision making is often taught in relation to sexuality and substance use, young people make choices about the food they eat, the products they buy, the community resources they use and the safety precautions they take. Similarly, teens are taught to say no to substance use and sex, but they may find themselves saying no on a regular basis to a variety of other pressure situations (e.g., cheating, skipping school or fighting). Communication skills are not only important in maintaining interpersonal relationships with family members, friends and others, but are also essential to being a good health consumer.

Young people will not be able to transfer a skill they learned in one content area to another content area unless you show them that their newly-acquired skills are transferable.

Examining Your Existing Curricula
Most existing curricula incorporate some level of personal and social skill building. Use the information presented about each skill described earlier in this chapter to determine if key content areas and skill-building activities are included in existing curricula.

If more than one curriculum package is implemented (e.g., a published substance use prevention curriculum, a district-developed abstinence-based curriculum, and a community-based nutrition curriculum), examine each to determine gaps in key information and skill-building activities. Then select or develop new activities to fill the identified gaps.

Integrating Skills Across Health Content

Integrating generic personal and social skills across health content will accomplish two major goals. First, it will provide built-in practice, feedback and reinforcement sessions, regardless of which health education area is being discussed. And, second, it will save valuable curriculum time, since it will eliminate duplication and overlap that might occur from one curriculum to another.

Personal and social skills can be integrated one of three ways. In the first approach, rather than teaching a unit on substance use prevention, nutrition, family life or diseases and disorders, present each skill as a classroom unit. In other words, spend a designated number of days discussing decision making. Begin with the factors that influence personal decisions. Discuss how internal and external influences vary depending on the actual decision being made and how those influences may change as a person grows older. Identify sources of information. Incorporate activities examining perception of risk, correcting misperceptions of peer norms and predicting short- and long-term consequences of personal decisions. Finally, present the steps to making a good decision. Move from simple situations to more complex ones and continue practicing the specific skill until students become competent.

Throughout the decision-making unit, use examples and situations that relate to the six priority areas identified by the Centers for Disease Control and Prevention: (1) behaviors that result in unintentional and intentional injuries; (2) alcohol and other drug use; (3) tobacco use; (4) sexual behaviors that result in HIV infection, other sexually-transmitted disease and unintended pregnancy; (5) imprudent dietary patterns; and (6) inadequate physical activity. This approach may involve some curriculum reorganization, since the traditional ten content areas would be replaced by the six health-risk behavior areas.

The second approach involves integrating skill-building activities within existing content-specific curricula—that is, emphasize one or more skills within a specific content area to meet identified gaps and student needs. For example, decision making could be introduced and emphasized in a sexuality education lesson about why teens choose to have or not to have sex. The decision-making model could be presented in a lesson about whether to use protection to prevent STD, HIV and pregnancy. Communication skills could be introduced during a discussion about family roles, responsibilities and family conflict. And stress-management skills could be introduced during a mental health curriculum unit.

The most comprehensive approach involves incorporating all four generic skills in each health education content area. For example, if the first curriculum unit is substance use, introduce the decision-making model generically, but in class discussions and skill-building activities, use examples and situations specific to substance use. What are the internal and external influences on adolescents' use of substances? Where can students obtain accurate information about the physical and psychological effects of different substances? How harmful is tobacco, alcohol, marijuana, cocaine, etc.? What are the social norms related to substance use? What are the the short- and long-term consequences of substance use? Finally, apply the steps of the decision-making model, using real-life situations related to substance use.

If the second curriculum unit is sexuality education, review the generic skill-building model, but focus class discussions and skill-building activities on sexuality issues. Help students transfer what they learned in the substance use prevention unit by identifying similarities and differences. For example, are the influences on sexual behaviors similar to those of substance use behaviors? Discuss the physical and emotional effects of early sexual activity and the short- and long-term consequences of unprotected sexual intercourse. Similarly, in the nutrition unit, decision making will be reviewed with content-specific examples and situations.

Communication skills also can be presented generically and reinforced in each curriculum unit. But when practicing assertiveness and refusal skills, use content specific scenarios and case studies. Similarly, in a curriculum unit on family health, incorporate activities to strengthen listening and verbal or nonverbal communication skills and to identify communication barriers in the family. In sexuality education, develop roleplays in which young people negotiate the use of condoms for protection.

After presenting key information about goal setting, incorporate activities that predict immediate and long-range physical, emotional, social and legal consequences of substance use, unwanted pregnancy, HIV infection, crash dieting, or drinking and driving on an individual's health and future goals. Finally, related to stress management, describe the "fight or flight" response and follow with a discussion about healthy and unhealthy ways of dealing with stressful situations, such as drinking or using other drugs, overeating or committing suicide.

Whichever approach is used, integrating decision-making, communication, stress-management and goal-setting skills as often as possible will help young people realize that personal and social skills are not just something they learned in school, to be forgotten as soon as they walk out the door, but are an integral part of their lives.

Essential Skills

The development of personal and social skills—decision making, communication, goal setting and stress management—is an essential part of normal psychosocial development. Most often, teens learn these skills by observing and imitating adult role models who also provide opportunities for practice and feedback. For whatever reasons, young people are not mastering these skills before they are confronted with potentially health-compromising decisions. Inadequate skills affect adolescents' ability to have meaningful relationships, cope with daily stressors, make rational deci sions, maintain self-control, elicit social support, and, ultimately, succeed at school and achieve future goals.

To meet this need, comprehensive health education programs should be expanded to include personal and social skill-building approaches that have been effective in substance use and pregnancy prevention programs. Incorporating these skills across all content areas will create built-in practice and rehearsal sessions, enabling teens to use their newly developed competencies as they make choices about their personal lives.

References

Alcohol, Drug Abuse and Mental Health Administration, U.S. Public Health Service, Department of Health and Human Services. 1990. *Stopping alcohol and other drug use before it starts: The future of prevention.* Rockville, MD: Office for Substance Abuse Prevention.

Bandura, A. 1977. *Social learning theory.* Englewood Cliffs, NJ: Prentice-Hall.

Bean, R. 1992. *The four conditions of self-esteem: A new approach for elementary and middle schools.* Santa Cruz, CA: ETR Associates.

Bell, C. S., and R. J. Battjes, eds. 1987. *Prevention research: Deterring drug abuse among children and adolescents.* NIDA Research Monograph 63, DHHS Publication No. ADM87-1334. Rockville, MD: National Institute on Drug Abuse.

Botvin, G. J. 1987. Prevention research. In *Drug abuse and drug abuse research: The second triennial report to Congress from the Secretary, Department of Health and Human Services*. Rockville, MD: National Institute on Drug Abuse.

Botvin, G. J., and T. A. Wills. 1985. Personal and social skills training: Cognitive-behavioral approaches to substance use prevention. In *Prevention research: Deterring drug use among children and adolescents,* ed. C. Bell and R. Battjes, 8-49. Rockville, MD: National Institute on Drug Abuse.

Centers for Disease Control and Prevention. 1992. *Chronic disease and health promotion reprints from the MMWR: 1990 youth risk behavior surveillance system.* Atlanta, GA.

Cook, A. T., J. L. Sola and R. Pfeiffer. 1989. *Taking the lead with PACT: Peer education in sexuality and health.* New York: YWCA.

Eisen, M., G. L. Zellman and A. L. McAllister. 1990. Evaluating the impact of a theory-based sexuality and contraceptive education program. *Family Planning Perspectives* 22 (6): 261-271.

Fetro, J. V. 1992. *Personal and social skills: Understanding and integrating competencies across health content.* Santa Cruz, CA: ETR Associates.

Flay, B. R. 1985. What we know about the social influences to smoking prevention: Review and recommendations. In *Prevention research: Deterring drug use among children and adolescents,* ed. C. Bell and R. Battjes, 67-112. Rockville, MD: National Institute on Drug Abuse.

Glasgow, R. E., and K. D. McCaul. 1985. Social and personal skills training programs for smoking prevention: Critique and directions for future research. In *Prevention research: Deterring drug use among children and adolescents,* ed. C. Bell and R. Battjes, 50-66. Rockville, MD: National Institute on Drug Abuse.

Howard, M., and J. B. McCabe. 1990. Helping teenagers postpone sexual involvement. *Family Planning Perspectives* 22 (1): 21-26.

Kirby, D., R. P. Barth, N. Leland and J. V. Fetro. 1991. Reducing the risk: The impact of a new curriculum on sexual risk-taking. *Family Planning Perspectives* 23 (6): 253-263.

Kumpfer, K. L. 1990. Prevention of alcohol and drug abuse: A critical review of risk factors and prevention strategies. In *Prevention of mental disorders, alcohol, and other drug use in children and adolescents,* ed. D. Shaffer, I. Phillips and N. B. Enzer, 309-372. Rockville, MD: Office for Substance Abuse Prevention.

Lando, H. A. 1985. The social influences approach to smoking prevention and progress toward an integrated smoking elimination strategy. In *Prevention research: Deterring drug use among children and adolescents,* ed. C. Bell and R. Battjes, 113-129. Rockville, MD: National Institute on Drug Abuse.

National Professional School Health Education Organizations. 1984. Comprehensive school health education. *Journal of School Health* 54 (8): 312-315.

Schaps, E., R. DiBartolo, J. Moskowitz, C. Palley and S. Churgin. 1981. Primary prevention evaluation research: A review of 127 impact studies. *Journal of Drug Issues* 11:17-43.

Schinke, S. P., B. J. Blythe and L. D. Gilchrist. 1981. Cognitive-behavioral prevention of adolescent pregnancy. *Journal of Counseling Psychology* 28:451-454.

U.S. Department of Health and Human Services, Public Health Service. 1991. *Healthy people 2000: National health promotion and disease prevention objectives.* DHHS Publication No. (PHS)91-50212. Washington, DC.

Chapter 12

Preventing Teenage Pregnancy: The Necessity for School and Community Collaboration

Murray L. Vincent, EdD, CHES,
Brian F. Geiger, MS, and A. Sandra Willis, PhD

rank Furstenberg (1976) aptly describes the negative impact of early childbearing: "When parenthood occurs early in adolescence, it often creates a dilemma for the young mother and her child, threatening both their immediate and their long-range interests." The United States has approximately one million teen pregnancies annually, the highest rate of teen pregnancies of any developed nation (Jones et al., 1985; Brindis et al., 1991; Henshaw and Van Vort, 1989).

Sexuality Education: Purpose and Function

If parents and educators could identify the combination of sexual knowledge, attitudes and behaviors that precede first intercourse, it might be possible to interrupt the sequence to prevent unintended pregnancies. However, as Furstenberg notes, there is an "absence of normative boundaries for entering sexual relations."

Most professional educators believe that sexuality education seeks to do the following (Kirby et al., 1991):

- increase students' knowledge about human sexuality
- foster parent/child/teacher communication about sexuality
- encourage youth to abstain from coitus until adulthood
- improve reproductive health skills, including the correct use of contraceptives
- refer sexually active students to community health care and social service providers

Healthy People 2000 specified national sexual risk reduction objectives related to sexuality education, including:

> lowering the proportion of adolescents engaging in sexual intercourse, increasing the proportion of sexually experienced adolescents who have abstained from sexual activity for the previous three months, increasing use of contraception, especially combined methods, by sexually active people aged nineteen and younger, and increasing effectiveness of contraception as measured by decreases in the proportion of pregnancies that occur despite contraceptive use. (U.S. Public Health Service, 1992)

Availability of Sexuality Education

In the early 1980s, it was estimated that 80 percent of U.S. school districts in large urban areas offered separate sexuality education courses or included sex-related topics in other courses such as health and science classes. In 1987-88, an estimated fifty thousand secondary school teachers were providing sex education. Between 67 and 85 percent of U.S. teenagers received classroom sexuality education during the eighties; however, the components of instruction about human sexuality varied widely between schools and teachers (Marsiglio and Mott, 1986; Forrest and Silverman, 1989). Studies of school sexuality education have difficulty precisely assessing the quantity and quality of the instruction; thus, these estimations may be overstated.

Doug Kirby (1985) reviewed the health education research literature to determine the effects of sexuality education on sexual knowledge, attitudes and behaviors. Increased subject-specific knowledge gain was a common result of sexuality education; however, students' sexual attitudes did not significantly change with classroom-based instruction. Students' attitudes and comfort level concerning their personal sexual behaviors and their beliefs about premarital sex, contraceptive use and other sexuality issues are more resistant to change through health education instruction than is level of knowledge (Kirby et al., 1991).

A 1982 survey of 15- to 19-year-old females (Dawson, 1986) revealed that most (84 percent) discussed the menstrual cycle with their parents; 67 percent discussed the biology of reproduction and pregnancy with their parents; and 53 percent discussed contraception. Eighty-eight percent of the sample received formal instruction about the menstrual cycle in school.

Close to 70 percent of the 1,888 young women received classroom instruction on "how pregnancy occurs" and "methods of birth control." One-third of these young women said they knew the most likely time for conception during the menstrual cycle and knew how to use any of 14 methods of birth control. There was no statistically significant relationship between formal reproductive health education instruction and this knowledge.

Effects of Sexuality Education
According to National Survey of Family Growth (NSFG) data, sexuality education was positively related to adolescents' use of

contraceptives; however, the effect diminished with time. Of sexually active students who were educated about pregnancy and contraceptives, 62 percent reported current use of contraception, compared with 58 percent who did not receive sex education. Young women who were educated about contraceptive use were more likely to have used a contraceptive during sexual intercourse. Contraceptive education prior to first coitus was related to self-reported use of a contraceptive method during initial intercourse (Dawson, 1986). Length and quality of classroom instruction and student acceptance and comprehension were not available from these data.

During the eighties, classroom instruction in comprehensive health education in American public schools increased significantly (Metropolitan Life Foundation, 1988). Comprehensive health education should include instruction in the following sex-related topics:

• reproductive health education
• pregnancy prevention education
• prevention and control of sexually transmitted diseases
• family life education

Such instruction is not a matter of merely imparting subject-specific knowledge. School curricula for health should also include:

• communication and decision-making skills
• exercises for values identification
• strategies for decision making and problem solving
• education to enhance self-esteem and personal responsibility for health and behavior

The aim is to address both short- and long-term outcomes of health education; for example, increasing knowledge about alternatives to intercourse and reducing unintended pregnancy rates (Deputat and Pavlovich, 1988; Kirby et al., 1991; Saunders, 1991; South Carolina, 1988; Burleson, 1982).

Instructional programs actually have variable effects on students' values related to sexuality, incidence of sexual activity, self-reported use of contraceptives and pregnancy rates. One reason for a lack of correspondence between sexuality education and students' sexual activities is the timing of instruction. According to an editorial in *Family Planning Perspectives* (1986), one-half of adolescents who become sexually active do not receive school-based sexuality education until after first sexual intercourse.

Another determinant of the effect of sexuality education is the length and extent of classroom instruction. The national School Health Education Evaluation revealed that significant effects on students' program-specific knowledge were achieved after fifteen hours of classroom instruction; however, more than fifty hours of instruction were needed to demonstrate "large" effects on students' general health knowledge. Brief discussion of sex-related topics is insufficient to produce change in students' knowledge, attitudes and behaviors. To obtain "medium" changes in health-related practices and "small" changes in attitudes also required fifty or more classroom instruction hours (Connell, Turner and Mason, 1985).

Who's Teaching Sexuality Education?

A recent South Carolina survey queried 160 middle school teachers of health education in 34 urban and rural districts. It revealed that 83 percent of the teachers included instruction on reproduction, 74 percent on sexually transmitted disease, 73 percent on growth and development, 66 percent on pregnancy prevention and 37 percent on family life education. Most teachers (89 percent) used a curriculum guide for instruction on reproductive health. Three-fourths devoted 15 or fewer class periods to instruction on reproductive health during the 1990-91 school year; 8 percent devoted 26 or more classes to this topic. A minimum of 15 hours of reproductive health education, including pregnancy prevention, is mandated by state law for secondary school students at least once during the ninth to twelfth grades.

Less than 4 percent of these school health educators perceived opposition for reproductive health education from the community. School health educators reported greater levels of comfort than confidence in the following areas:
- teaching reproductive health information and skills
- answering students' questions
- using class participation activities
- identifying and using classroom resource materials
- interacting with parents and community agencies

In general, teachers felt less secure in their ability to identify and use community resources and interact with parents for reproductive health education than in tasks requiring internal contacts (inside the school), e.g., obtaining support and assistance from peer educators (Geiger and Saunders, 1992; South Carolina, 1988).

The results of a national survey of seventh- to twelfth-grade public school teachers were reported by Forrest and Silverman (1989). More than four thousand teachers from five areas—health education, physical education, home economics, biology and school nurses—answered questions about sexuality education, including content of actual instruction, topics they wanted to teach, and obstacles to sexuality education. Eighty-nine percent of these teachers had completed specific training for instruction in this content area. Almost all of the teachers surveyed (98 percent) stated that sexuality education is an appropriate area for student education.

More than three-fourths of these teachers reported current or previous experience as a school sexuality educator or had future plans to instruct students on this topic. Sixty percent devoted less than 10 percent of their instructional time to sexuality education. There were gaps between sexuality education content areas actually included in classes and areas teachers thought should be taught. The largest gaps were for sources of birth control, "safer sex" practices and homosexuality. Obstacles to sexuality education included:

- teachers' perceptions of parental pressure
- disinterested students
- lack of support from school administrators
- lack of curricular materials for the subject area

Sexuality Education and Comprehensive Health Education

Duration of instruction is not the only important variable related to health knowledge, attitudes and practices. Broad mandates for a minimum number of hours of public school sexuality education may fail to improve either the quality of health instruction or its effects on students' sexual knowledge and practices. Implementation of instruction on human sexuality requires a curriculum framework for comprehensive health education throughout the grades. Other necessary components include (Muraskin, 1986; Forrest and Silverman, 1989; Saunders and Geiger, 1991; Metropolitan Life Foundation, 1989):

- trained and enthusiastic teachers
- instructional guides for sexual and reproductive health topics
- age-appropriate learning materials
- support from parents, peers and administrators at the school and district levels
- procedures for evaluation and modification of instructional

programs based on progress made toward achieving clearly stated learning objectives

Sexuality education should not be presented in a piecemeal fashion, nor should sexuality textbooks or audiovisual materials be relied upon as substitutes for a comprehensive health education curriculum for the school district. Health education instruction must be sequenced from elementary to secondary grades (age-appropriate), interesting to the students, and integrated across the curriculum. Health education teachers must be trained to instruct students in health knowledge and practices, using standard curricula and instructional materials and creative learning exercises. To increase the effect of health education on students' health-related knowledge, attitudes and practices, instruction should not be limited to school settings. Adult and peer educators in different community settings (churches, youth clubs, recreational facilities, etc.) can teach about positive health behaviors, encourage practice of new health skills, and reinforce personal responsibility for health (Connell, Turner and Mason, 1985; Saunders, 1991; Muraskin, 1986).

School/Community Partnerships

Joy Dryfoos (1990a; 1990b) outlined characteristics of successful school and community partnerships to prevent high-risk behavior, including premarital intercourse and substance abuse among children and adolescents. "Innovative models that directly improved achievement levels included team teaching, cooperative learning, teacher and parent empowerment and school restructuring." When agencies and organizations that were external to schools became the catalyst for school change, both academic and social outcomes were improved. This does not imply that school personnel assumed a subordinate or passive role in the reform of educational efforts for youth; rather, agencies and schools formed a successful alliance or partnership for success (Dryfoos, 1990b).

Murray Vincent and colleagues reported the positive effects of a community-based health information and education intervention in a rural South Carolina county (Vincent, Clearie and Schluchter, 1987). The intervention was based on a collaboration between project researchers, school personnel and members of the community. Group and individual educational sessions focused on the following:

- communication and decision-making skills
- self-esteem
- family and community values
- knowledge of reproductive health, abstinence, pregnancy and contraception

These educational programs were offered to youth, parents, church members and community agency personnel; classroom teachers received sexuality education training. After two years of the program, estimated pregnancy rates (EPR) for 14- to 17-year-old females in the intervention area were significantly lower than for teens in the nonintervention portion of the county and for teens in nearby comparison counties. Adolescent EPRs in the comparison counties did not mirror the dramatic decline for EPRs in the intervention county.

The study was reported in the *Journal of the American Medical Association*. A comprehensive secondary evaluation of this project was completed by Research Triangle Institute (RTI) scientists (funded by the Centers for Disease Control and Prevention). The RTI report verified the accuracy of the original report in attributing the reduction in pregnancies to the combination of school/community programmatic interventions. However, the RTI report suggested that the journal article was lacking in not giving more weight to the impact of proactive school nursing services promoting access to contraceptives (Koo et al., 1992).

This community intervention model for teenage pregnancy prevention exemplifies the six components of successful prevention programs for high-risk youth identified by Dryfoos (1990b) in her review of the literature:

- individual attention
- early identification and intervention
- social skills training
- engagement of peers in interventions
- parental involvement
- link to the world of work

An intervention model based on community involvement and multiple interventions has more potential for success than isolated single interventions to alter the rates of health-compromising behaviors.

The Scope of the Problem

An estimated 10 percent of adolescent women between the ages of 15 and 19 become pregnant each year. Of these pregnancies, approximately 83 percent are unintentional. Seventy-five percent of unintended pregnancies occur due to nonuse or ineffective use of contraceptives (Trussell, 1988). Close to one-half of these pregnancies result in the birth of children, most of whom are raised by adolescent mothers. The remainder of the pregnancies end in miscarriage or abortion.

During the past decade, more unmarried American mothers ages 15 to 44 chose to raise their babies than place them for adoption (Bachrach, Stolley and London, 1992). Adolescent parenthood reduces optimal development of mothers and children by limiting opportunities for the mother's education and job training and by creating a less than optimal environment for the children (Hatcher et al., 1991; Mayer, 1982; Henshaw and Van Vort, 1989).

The U.S. Public Health Service's initiative *Healthy People 2000* specified objectives for sexual risk reduction, including decreased pregnancy rates among girls age 17 and younger, from 71.1 per 1,000 in 1985 to 50 per 1,000 by the year 2000. The estimated 1989 adolescent pregnancy rate was 72.4 per 1,000 (U.S. Public Health Service, 1992). The proportion of teenagers who are sexually active increases with age, with corresponding increases in adolescent pregnancies, abortions and births (Henshaw and Van Vort, 1989).

In 1981, 1.4 percent of 14-year-old girls became pregnant. The percentage of pregnant teenagers in America increased steadily to reach 15 percent of women at the age of 19. The percentage of live births to pregnant teens also increased with chronological age, from 39 percent for 14-year-old females to 60 percent at age 19. Birthrates for adolescent mothers fell to a record low in 1986 (National Center for Health Statistics, 1988). However, data from 1985 indicated higher birthrates for teens in southern states (e.g., Mississippi, Georgia and Louisiana) and the lowest birthrates for New England and Midwestern states (e.g., Connecticut, New Hampshire, Minnesota, and Iowa) (Henshaw and Van Vort, 1989).

Differences Between Racial Groups
Among young women ages 15 to 19, 1981 pregnancy rates for African-American adolescents (163 per 1,000) were nearly twice as high as those for White adolescents (83 per 1,000) in the United States. This trend continued in 1985. Differences in birth rates between racial groups are related to differences in adolescent pregnancy and abortion rates. For instance, in 1981, there were 97

births per 1,000 African-American adolescents versus 45 births per 1,000 White adolescents (Hatcher et al., 1991). In 1985, approximately 30 percent of total births to unmarried women younger than twenty were attributed to White adolescents, 26 percent to African-American adolescents and 7 percent to Hispanic adolescents (Children's Defense Fund, 1988).

The report on the fertility of American women (U.S. Bureau of the Census, 1991) shows 338,000 births to teen mothers during the year preceding June 1990. More than 200,000 of these births were to unmarried adolescent mothers; 40 out of every 1,000 adolescents ages 15 to 19 gave birth during that year. Substantial differences between racial groups for adolescent birth rates were evident: 33 per 1,000 for White females, 71 per 1,000 for African-American females, 50 per 1,000 for Hispanic females. In addition, there were significant racial differences in proportion of childbirths out of wedlock: 90 percent for African-American, 59 percent for White, and 65 percent for Hispanic females between the ages of 15 and 19.

There are also differences among racial groups in rates of adoption placements for women whose pregnancies were unplanned. Data from the 1982 and 1988 National Survey of Family Growth (NSFG) indicated that far fewer African-American or Hispanic mothers chose adoption following childbirth than did White mothers. Multiple factors relate to adoption decisions following unintended pregnancy among unmarried White, non-Hispanic women (Bachrach, Stolley and London, 1992). They include maternal age and level of education, school enrollment and academic performance at the time of conception, job experience and child's gender. Women whose "opportunity costs" of pregnancy and childbirth were greater—e.g., those who had not completed an educational program—were more likely to surrender their children for adoption. One determining factor for a pregnant adolescent's decision to surrender a child for adoption is a thoughtful phase of career exploration in which the teen has considered career options and the educational preparation necessary for those careers (Low, Moely and Willis, 1989).

Consequences of Teen Pregnancy

The consequences of teen pregnancy include multiple health, social and economic problems for the young mother, her infant and society in general. Individual differences in the mother's family background, race and economic status do affect childbirth outcomes; however, there are negative consequences for children and their teen mothers independent of these variables (Hayes, 1987). It is difficult to determine which adverse birth outcomes are due to young maternal age when many other variables are contributing factors. These variables include family income, access to health care and insurance, mother's education and work experience, and social support. Studies suggest that low-income women of any age lack access to adequate prenatal care and lack other resources necessary to the well-being of mother and child (e.g., limited residence and dietary choices) (Dryfoos, 1990a; Furstenberg, 1976).

The rates of perinatal and maternal morbidity and mortality are higher among teenage mothers, particularly for mothers younger than age 15. These outcomes include maternal anemia, hypertension and toxemia, shorter gestation period, miscarriage and stillbirth, prolonged labor, premature births and low birthweight.

Maternal age as a sole risk factor for negative birth outcomes may have been overstated in previous research studies. The effect of the mother's chronological age on birth outcomes is not independent of health and sociodemographic factors. Other significant determinants of poor maternal and child health include

(McAnarney, 1983; Makinson, 1985; Hayes, 1987; Ketterlinus, Henderson and Lamb, 1990):

- poverty
- level of education and vocational preparation
- inadequate prenatal and obstetrical care
- poor nutrition

According to Alexander and Cornely (1987), "prenatal care may serve a gate-keeper function, identifying and funneling expectant mothers to the appropriate level of medical care for delivery." Among adolescents who receive comprehensive prenatal care, health during pregnancy and birth outcomes typically do not differ from those of older women. Comprehensive prenatal care includes medical services, health education instruction and skills training, social support and nutrition assistance (Baldwin and Cain, 1980; Dollfus et al., 1990).

Cognitive Development of Children of Adolescent Mothers

Studies show a relationship between the age of the mother and the child's intellectual development. Children of younger mothers perform less well on standardized measures of intelligence and academic achievement and receive poorer performance evaluations from teachers. They are also more likely to be retained in grades and repeat an early childbearing pattern themselves.

However, the effect of maternal age on measures of academic aptitude is not significant. Poor educational achievement among children of adolescent mothers may result from parents' lack of social and financial resources, ability, willingness, and/or motivation to support and encourage their children's intellectual development (Baldwin and Cain, 1980; Card, 1981; Hayes, 1987; Mayer, 1982).

There is no reliable evidence showing a negative effect on social and emotional development based on the maternal age variable only. Economic factors are more influential. Adverse effects for children are more likely to occur when the adolescent mother raises her child without the aid and support of her parents or the child's father (Baldwin and Cain, 1980; Makinson, 1985).

Maternal Effects of Early Childbearing

Adolescent women who give birth at a young age are more likely to have multiple births and experience greater marital instability than those who postpone childbearing (Trussell and Menken, 1978; Mott, 1986). They tend to be more poorly educated and have lower incomes later in life (Hofferth and Moore, 1979; Marini, 1984; Mott and Marsiglio, 1985; Hayes, 1987).

Personal motivation, work skills and experience, and extent of career exploration also affect occupational success. Teen pregnancy and poor academic performance are not causally related in a simple way. The older the mother at first birth, the more education she is likely to complete. Also, "the more years of schooling a young woman has completed, the more likely she is to delay childbearing" (Hayes, 1987). It is difficult to assess directionality for the relationship between educational attainment and maternal age. A young woman who performs poorly in school may be more likely to drop out whether she is a parent or not. Certainly, parenthood does limit her ability to optimally benefit from educational experiences, and career motivational factors play substantial roles in determining long-term life success (Low, Moely and Willis, 1989).

Economic Outcomes of Adolescent Pregnancy

A longitudinal study conducted by Furstenberg, Brooks-Gunn and Morgan (1987) showed that during the five years after the birth of their first child, adolescent mothers performed more poorly in school than their nonparent peers. However, follow-up data collected seventeen years later revealed that a majority had received a high school diploma, found regular employment and did not have a lifelong dependence on welfare. Unfortunately, these women typically did not achieve the same educational and income levels as their peers who postponed parenthood until later ages. Women who performed well before their first childbirth, had high educational aspirations, and had economically secure and better educated parents were most likely to succeed. Approximately 25 percent of the original sample remained poor and welfare-dependent.

Approximately one-half of all adolescent mothers marry prior to their delivery date, although the percentage of teen mothers who choose not to marry has greatly increased during the past twenty years. Marital relationships between adolescent couples are frequently characterized by conflict, separation and divorce. Not surprisingly, family income is substantially lower among young divorced parents and never-married teen parents than among those with stable marriages (Hayes, 1987; Zelnik and Kantner, 1980; Furstenberg, 1976).

Adolescent mothers are more likely than older mothers to receive public assistance (Aid to Families with Dependent Children (AFDC), food stamps, Medicaid), due to lower educational achievement, less work experience and larger family size. It was estimated that one-half of the national AFDC budget in 1975 was allocated to families with mothers who delivered their first child as a teen. The financial allotments for young mothers are greater, due to a larger average family size (Block and Dubin, 1981; Hayes, 1987).

Historically, teenage childbearing is strongly related to higher completed fertility rates, repeated unintentional and nonmarital births, and closer spacing of births; however, these trends may be diminishing (Hayes, 1987). In 1985, $16.65 billion was spent on families in which children were born to parents in their adolescent years. Costs relevant to each teen birth register at approximately $18,000 (Vincent et al., 1988).

Factors Related to Adolescent Pregnancy

In 1986, it was estimated that 12 million out of 27 million American adolescents were sexually active (Johnson, 1986). In a survey of 36,000 Minnesota youth, 70 percent of the females reported having had sexual intercourse by age 18; most (75 percent) had done so three or fewer times (Blum, 1991). The national *Youth Risk Behavior Survey* (Centers for Disease Control and Prevention, 1992) revealed that 54.2 percent of all ninth-to-twelfth grade students reported having had sexual intercourse; 39.4 percent had sexual intercourse during the three months preceding the survey. African-American students (72 percent) were significantly more likely to have had sexual intercourse than White (52 percent) and Hispanic (53 percent) students.

Zelnik and Kantner (1980) compared the results of three national surveys of adolescents to determine changes in premarital sexual activity from 1971 to 1979. The proportion of 15- to 19-year-old metropolitan-area females who reported sexual intercourse before marriage rose from 30 percent in 1971 to 50 percent in 1979. The largest increase was among unmarried White females; however, African-American females were 40 percent more likely than Whites to be sexually active as teenagers. Among males ages 17 to 21, smaller differences in rates of premarital coitus were reported. Gender differences in proportions of teens who were sexually active were greater among Americans of European descent than among Americans of African descent.

Thompson's (1990) interviews of sexually active teenage girls suggest that a significant change has occurred in teenage romantic relationships. Petting, a practice commonly preceding intercourse as a part of foreplay, and the extent of some adolescents' shared sexual activity before the late 1960s, seems to have become less prevalent among teens since the late 1970s. Many teenagers who were interviewed thought that foreplay activities could be omitted in favor of sexual intercourse, which was perceived to be the mature, valuable part of sexual relations (Thompson, 1984; Haffner, 1988). This perception is unfortunate, since intercourse is the activity most likely to lead to pregnancy and infection with sexually transmitted disease.

Adolescents' Perceptions of Sexuality and Parenthood

Evidence indicates that most unmarried teens do not intend to become pregnant. National surveys of adolescents who became pregnant before marriage revealed a decrease in the proportion who intended to become pregnant from 1971 to 1979 and a corresponding increase in self-reported use of contraception to avoid pregnancy (Zelnik and Kantner, 1980). On the other hand, some adolescents perceive few or no benefits to postponing sexual intercourse and using contraception, particularly teens with limited life options and family role models of teen parenthood (Dryfoos, 1990).

Adolescent pregnancy and early childbirth have positive as well as negative outcomes. Dash (1989) described a decision-making process in which teen pregnancies are intentionally chosen because they represent a path to an alternative role status and environment. Pregnancy and parenthood may enhance a teen's sense of control over the environment and boost self-esteem. Approval by peers and parents for the pregnancy may diminish a teen mother's ability to accurately assess the potential educational, social and financial difficulties associated with delivery of her child (Furstenberg, 1976; Geiger and Morton, 1993).

Lack of Contraception

Adolescents with a strong need for privacy concerning their sexual behavior may find it difficult to communicate their feelings to peers and sexual partners, and particularly difficult to speak to parents and health professionals. One study (Zabin and Clark, 1983) reported an average of 11.5 months between adolescents' initiation of sexual activity and their seeking the services of a family planning clinic. Trussell (1988) reported that the majority of girls do not use reliable contraception for first intercourse and only one-third use contraception regularly. Others have reported that only one in two adolescent women used a contraceptive at first sexual intercourse (Pratt et al., 1984). Approximately one-third of adolescents do not report regular use of contraceptives: 27 percent of White teens, 35 percent of African-American teens, and 32 percent of Hispanic teens (Torres and Singh, 1986).

Why do so many sexually active adolescents not use contraceptives? Contraceptive use may be psychologically inaccessible for adolescents with romantic ideals. The advance planning necessary for effective contraception is inconsistent with the belief that sexual intercourse can only occur spontaneously with passion.

Another factor related to contraceptive use is knowledge about contraceptive methods and their effectiveness. Parents who discourage their adolescents from dating and all premarital sexual activity may also fail to discuss adult sexual relations and the need for contraception during intercourse. Parental values and norms regarding adolescent sexual activity influence teens' sexual behavior and contraceptive use. Opportunities to learn about their own children's sexual activities are lost when a family is silent on matters of sexuality (Hatcher et al., 1991; Baker, Thalberg and Morrison, 1988).

The retrospective 1982 NSFG results showed significant racial differences in adolescent contraceptive usage: 77 percent of Hispanics, 64 percent of African Americans and 45 percent of Whites did not use any protection the first time they had intercourse (Torres and Singh, 1986). National surveys of adolescent contraceptive use indicated that more sexually active White adolescents than African-American adolescents used contraceptives in 1976 and 1979 (Zelnik and Kantner, 1980).

These rates should not be misperceived to be the result of inherent racial differences. Other variables contribute to use of contraceptives among sexually active teens (Burke, 1987). They include:

- sexual knowledge
- access to contraceptives
- family income
- previous conception, educational and job experiences
- family history of premarital pregnancies
- degree of parental communication

Rivara, Sweeney and Henderson (1985) reported that a majority of poor African-American male adolescents they interviewed inaccurately assessed the risk of pregnancy during coitus. These males did not know the effectiveness of different methods of contraceptives. They frequently practiced unprotected intercourse and were unprepared for coitus. Teen fathers were more likely to have families that accepted teenage pregnancy than were nonfathers; premarital pregnancies were less common among mothers and siblings of the latter group.

The group of sexually active 14- to 19-year-old African-American males previously identified spoke of barriers to contraceptive use, including:

- belief that sex is less enjoyable with contraception
- negative responses from their female partners
- perceived health risks
- belief that they would be "hassled" at a health clinic
- previous negative experience obtaining contraceptives
- high cost

Perceived difficulties in obtaining and using contraceptives did not differ significantly between males who were fathers and those who were not.

Research conducted in other developed nations reveals reductions in teen pregnancy rates when contraceptive access is improved. In the United States, a vocal minority purports that adolescent sexual activity and pregnancies are legitimized by increasing teens' access to contraceptives and knowledge about human sexuality. Negative attitudes toward sexuality education and access to contraceptives for youth can be a significant obstacle for pregnancy prevention programs (Hatcher et al., 1991; Trussell, 1988).

Some adolescents are responsible contraceptive users. One study (Zelnik and Kantner, 1980) reported increased proportions of regular and occasional contraceptive use among metropolitan area adolescents from 1976 to 1979. Of the sexually active male and female youth surveyed by the Centers for Disease Control and Prevention (1992), close to 80 percent reported using contraception during their last sexual intercourse. Of sexually active adolescent females, 81 percent of Whites, 71 percent of African Americans, and 63 percent of Hispanics reported use of contraception. Condoms were chosen as a contraceptive by 40 percent of female and 49.4 percent of male sexually active ninth to twelfth grade students during their last sexual intercourse.

Community Opposition to Sexuality Education

Sexuality education is a controversial topic in many communities (Kirby et al., 1991). Some parents question sexuality education in the schools on legitimate dimensions: adequacy of training of sexuality teachers; opportunities for parental review of curricula, textbooks and instructional aids; and guidelines for selection and use of learning materials (Scales, 1982). A vocal minority of parent and community groups apply pressure to school systems to limit or eliminate student exposure to sex education on the basis that sex education undermines family values, promotes sexual promiscuity, or encourages toleration of "abnormal or deviant" sexual activities (Schlafly, 1981; McAuley, 1982). Is there evidence to show that education about human sexuality is linked to increased sexual activity, including coitus among youth?

Data analyzed in 1982 by NSFG showed that exposure to contraceptive education had no consistent effect on initiation of intercourse. A 1984 study, the National Longitudinal Survey of Work Experience of Youth, found that prior sexuality education had a weak effect on age of first sexual intercourse. The strength of the sexuality education effect on first coitus at ages 15 and 16 is weaker than effects exerted by other variables, e.g., church attendance, parental education and ethnicity. For example, youth whose church attendance was irregular, whose parents completed fewer than twelve years of school, and who were Americans of African descent were significantly more likely to have had first intercourse at age 15 (Marsiglio and Mott, 1986).

Other research findings negate the assumption that increased sexual knowledge results in increased sexual activity. Following student participation in an urban school-based program for pregnancy prevention, pregnancy rates were reduced, and students who were not sexually active at the start of the program postponed sexual activity (Zabin et al., 1986). The program combined sexuality education, counseling and contraceptive services.

A recent major study in California (Kirby et al., 1991) had similar results. An examination of the effects of *Reducing the Risk* (Barth, 1989), a curriculum based on social learning theory, social inoculation theory and cognitive-behavior theory, employed random assignment of classrooms to treatment and control groups in 13 California high schools. The use of the curriculum significantly increased participants' knowledge and parent/child communication about abstinence and contraception. Among students who were virgins at pretest, the educational intervention significantly reduced the likelihood that they would have had intercourse eighteen months later. Frequency of sexual intercourse or use of birth control among sexually experienced students, however, did not change during the program intervention. An assessment of six school-based clinics corroborates these findings (Kirby, Waszak and Ziegler, 1989) and provides evidence against the suggestion that sexuality education leads to sexual promiscuity.

Community surveys have indicated that a majority of parents support school sexuality education, particularly instruction related to abstinence from sexual intercourse and prevention of unintended pregnancy and sexually transmitted disease (Scales, 1982; Gordon, 1982; Forrest and Silverman, 1989). In one survey of rural southern parents in 105 households, 32 percent said sexuality education was "more important" and 53 percent indicated it was "about as important" as other academic subjects. More than one-third of these parents (37 percent) believed that sexuality education should begin by grade six or before. Seven out of eleven sexuality education content areas were acceptable to 90 percent or more of the householders (Vincent et al., 1985):

- pregnancy and childbirth
- birth control and family planning
- making sexual decisions

- physical and growth changes
- dating behavior
- venereal diseases
- marriage responsibilities
- rape and sexual assaults

Implications for the Future

This wealth of statistical evidence from reputable studies delivers a powerful message. American youth are sexually active at an early age, and there appears to be no evidence that this precocious behavior will change. These youth seldom use contraceptives at first sexual intercourse. They remain at high risk due to the absence of or episodic use of contraception in their continuing sexual encounters. Adolescents do not comprehend the realities of child-bearing and parenthood, and many of them become parents at a too-early age.

Confounding the situation is a parental and societal veil of silence and avoidance of these realities, which perpetuates ignorance and skills deficiencies among youth. Additionally, a vocal minority vigorously oppose efforts to educate youth to become problem solvers and critical thinkers. Resolving a major sociocultural problem such as teenage pregnancy will require an application of all the research findings addressed in this assessment of the pertinent issues.

Action Tasks for Communities

Communities must come to grips with the issues. Teen pregnancy is a problem of the entire community, and the community has a responsibility to resolve this dilemma through collaborative planning and delivery of educational programs and health services. Multiple interventions need to be directed to different targeted groups and organizations to provide a dosage level commensurate with the magnitude of the problem. "Magic bullets" do not exist, and isolated sporadic interventions will likely be doomed to fail.

The adults in a community influence youth. Aware and educated adults function as parents, teachers, religious advisors and medical providers. They need to set the following tasks for their communities:

- Involve representative organizations, agencies and community stakeholders in planning task forces and advisory groups.
- Hold public forums to develop community recognition and ownership of the problems of teen pregnancy.
- Foster the understanding that teen pregnancy is symptomatic of a community in need of education about the many dimensions of healthy human sexuality.
- Organize and assist religious organizations, agencies and others to provide sexuality-education-related programs for all adult citizens, including:
  — the elderly
  — midlife, empty-nest parents
  — parents of healthy and troubled adolescents
  — couples anticipating parenthood
  — persons anticipating marriage
- Cooperatively plan to provide medical and public health services that ensure confidential and easy access to contraceptive services, pregnancy testing, counseling and abortion services for all citizens, and especially for teens.
- Reaffirm the multiple contributors to teen pregnancy and provide for job-skills training, career planning, crisis intervention, well-baby care, prenatal care and other broad-based human services.

Action Tasks for Schools

Schools must be the lead organizations in community efforts. Children and adolescents from age four to eighteen attend school and are the recipients of the curricula provided. The curricula must be planned and sequenced so that graduates will be "sexually educated." Age-appropriate curricular content must be designed to develop the cognitive, attitudinal and behavioral skills necessary for wise decision making. "Too little, too late" curricula must be replaced by those that address the realities of the behavioral practices of youth. Abstinence and postponement of first sexual intercourse can be vigorously promoted; however, sexually active youth must also be educated to use contraceptives and available family planning services. The schools' tasks include the following:

- Assess the existing status and improve the K-12 sexuality education component of the school health education curriculum.
- Affirm that sexuality education is comprehensive and includes the biological, social, psychological, spiritual and family dimensions as focal points in the development of knowledge, attitudes and skills.
- Require all teachers, and especially those with specific responsibilities for sexuality education, to receive academic preparation to positively and correctly implement the chosen curricula.
- Solicit and involve outside agencies and organizations to enter the schools and provide sexuality education programs and services.
- Provide comprehensive school nursing services that include health status assessments, sexuality instruction and counseling, and pregnancy testing.
- Provide broad-based counseling and guidance services for healthy and troubled youth. Include life-options planning, social skills training and rehabilitative services.

- Establish linkages to medical and public health providers to allow easy access to services—especially those specific to reproductive health.

Prevention has never been more clearly needed. The potential talents lost among our teen parents, the personal suffering, and the cyclical debilitating effects on the innocent children born to children deserve our undivided attention and concentrated efforts. Community concern and commitment are essential. Yet success in reducing teen pregnancy is only likely to occur when financial resources are allocated to hire professionals with the ability to plan, manage and evaluate the collaborative interventions that a dedicated community can provide.

References

Alexander, G. R., and D. A. Cornely. 1987. Racial disparities in pregnancy outcomes: The role of prenatal care utilization and maternal risk status. *American Journal of Preventive Medicine* 3 (5): 254-261.

Bachrach, C. A., K. S. Stolley and K. A. London. 1992. Relinquishment of premarital births: Evidence from national survey data. *Family Planning Perspectives* 24 (1): 27-32.

Baker, S. A., S. P. Thalberg and D. M. Morrison. 1988. Parents' behavioral norms as predictors of adolescent sexual activity and contraceptive use. *Adolescence* 23 (90): 265-282.

Baldwin, W., and V. S. Cain. 1980. The children of teenaged parents. *Family Planning Perspectives* 12 (1): 34-43.

Barth, R. P. 1989. *Reducing the risk: building skills to prevent pregnancy.* Santa Cruz, CA: ETR Associates.

Block, A. H., and S. Dubin. 1981. *Research on the societal consequences of adolescent childbearing: Welfare costs at the local level.* Final report, No. 1-HD-92838. Bethesda, MD: Social and Behavioral Sciences Branch, Center for Population Research, National Institute of Child Health and Human Development.

Blum, R. W. 1991. Global trends in adolescent health. *Journal of the American Medical Association* 265 (20): 2711-2719.

Brindis, C. D., K. Pittman, P. Reyes and S. Adams-Taylor. 1991. *Adolescent pregnancy prevention: A guidebook for communities.* Palo Alto, CA: Stanford Center for Research in Disease Prevention.

Burke, P. J. 1987. Adolescents' motivation for sexual activity and pregnancy prevention. *Issues in Comprehensive Pediatric Nursing* 10:161-171.

Burleson, D. L. 1982. Integrating sex education into the K-12 curriculum. In *Discussing sex in the classroom: Readings for teachers*, ed. D. R. Stronck, 7-8. Washington, DC: National Science Teachers Association.

Card, J. J. 1981. Long term consequences for children of teenage parents. *Demography* 18 (2): 137-156.

Centers for Disease Control and Prevention. 1992. Sexual behavior among high school students—United States, 1990. *Morbidity and Mortality Weekly Report*, 40 (51 and 52): 885-888.

Children's Defense Fund. 1988. *Teenage pregnancy: An advocate's guide to the numbers.* Washington, DC: Adolescent Pregnancy Prevention Clearinghouse.

Connell, D. B., R. R. Turner and E. F. Mason. 1985. Summary of findings of the School Health Education Evaluation: Health promotion effectiveness, implementation, and costs. *Journal of School Health* 55 (8): 316-321.

Dash, L. 1989. *When children want children.* New York: William Morrow.

Dawson, D. 1986. The effects of sex education on adolescent behavior. *Family Planning Perspectives* 18 (4): 162-170.

Deputat, Z., and M. S. Pavlovich. 1988. School health programs: A comprehensive plan for implementation. *Health Education* October/November: 47-53.

Dollfus, C., M. Patetta, E. Siegel and A. W. Cross. 1990. Infant mortality: A practical approach to the analysis of the leading causes of death and risk factors. *Pediatrics* 86 (2): 176-183.

Dryfoos, J. G. 1990a. *Adolescents at risk: Pregnancy and prevention.* New York: Oxford University Press.

Dryfoos, J. G. 1990b. Community schools: New institutional arrangements for preventing high-risk behavior. *Family Life Educator* 8 (4): 4-9.

Family Planning Perspectives. 1986. Editorial. 18 (4): 150, 192.

Forrest, J. D., and J. Silverman. 1989. What public schools teachers teach about preventing pregnancy, AIDS and sexually transmitted diseases. *Family Planning Perspectives* 21 (2): 65-72.

Furstenberg, F. F. Jr., J. Brooks-Gunn and S. P. Morgan. 1987. Adolescent mothers and their children in later life. *Family Planning Perspectives* 19 (4): 142-151.

Furstenberg, F. F., Jr. 1976. *Unplanned parenthood: The social consequences of teenage childbearing.* New York: The Free Press.

Geiger, B. F., and K. Morton. 1993. Difference perceptions of pregnancy: Young pregnant women and health professionals in South Carolina. Paper presented at the Annual Conference of the South Carolina Association for Counseling and Development, Hilton Head Island, South Carolina.

Geiger, B. F., and R. P. Saunders. 1992. Reproductive health education in the middle grades: Implications of the 1991 survey of South Carolina health education teachers. Paper presented at the Annual Meeting of the South Carolina Public Health Association, Myrtle Beach, South Carolina.

Gordon, S. 1982. The case for a moral sex education in the schools. In *Discussing sex in the classroom: Readings for teachers*, ed. D. R. Stronck, 24-27. Washington, DC: National Science Teachers Association.

Haffner, D. W. 1988. Safe sex and teens. *SIECUS Report* 17:9.

Hatcher, R. A., F. Stewart, J. Tussell, D. Kowal, F. Guest, G. K. Stewart and W. Cates. 1990. Adolescent pregnancy. *Contraceptive Technology, 1990-1992.* 15th ed. New York: Irvington Publishers.

Hayes, C. D., ed. 1987. *Risking the future: Adolescent sexuality, pregnancy, and childbearing.* Vol. 1. Washington, DC: National Academy Press.

Henshaw, S., and J. Van Vort. 1989. Teenage abortion, birth and pregnancy statistics: An update. *Family Planning Perspectives* 21 (2): 85-88.

Hofferth, S., and K. Moore. 1979. Early childbearing and later economic well-being. *American Sociological Review* 44:784-815.

Johnson, K. 1986. *Building health programs for teenagers.* Washington, DC: Children's Defense Fund.

Jones, E. F., J. D. Forrest, N. Goldman, S. K. Henshaw, R. Lincoln, J. I. Rosoff, C. F. Westoff and D. Wulf. 1985. Teenage pregnancy in developed countries: Determinants and policy implications. *Family Planning Perspectives* 17 (2): 53-63.

Ketterlinus, R. D., S. H. Henderson and M. E. Lamb. 1990. Maternal age, sociodemographics, prenatal health and behavior: Influences on neonatal risk status. *Journal of Adolescent Health Care* 11:423-431.

Kirby, D. 1985. Sexuality education: A more realistic view of its effects. *Journal of School Health* 55 (10): 421-424.

Kirby, D., R. P. Barth, N. Leland and J. V. Fetro. 1991. Reducing the risk: Impact of a new curriculum on sexual risk-taking. *Family Planning Perspectives* 23 (6): 253-263.

Kirby, D., C. Waszak and J. Ziegler. 1989. An assessment of six school-based clinics: Services, impact and potential. Washington, DC: Center for Population Options.

Koo, H. P., G. H. Dunteman, C. George, Y. Green and M. Vincent. 1992. Reducing adolescent pregnancy through a school- and community-based intervention: Denmark, South Carolina, revisited. Manuscript.

Low, J. M., B. Moely and A. S. Willis. 1989. The effects of parental preferences and vocational goals on adoption decisions: Unmarried pregnant adolescents. *Youth and Society* 20 (3): 342-354.

Makinson, C. 1985. The health consequences of teenage fertility. *Family Planning Perspectives* 17 (3): 132-139.

Marini, M. 1984. Women's educational attainments and the timing of entry into parenthood. *American Sociological Review* 49:491-511.

Marsiglio, W., and F. L. Mott. 1986. The impact of sex education on sexual activity, contraceptive use and pregnancy among American teenagers. *Family Planning Perspectives* 18 (4): 151-162.

Mayer, W. V. 1982. Sexual ignorance is not bliss. In *Discussing sex in the classroom: Readings for teachers*, ed. D. R. Stronck, 4-5. Washington, DC: National Science Teachers Association.

McAnarney, E., and H. Thiede. 1983. Adolescent pregnancy and childbearing: What we learned during the 1970s and what remains to be learned. In *Premature adolescent pregnancy and parenthood*, ed. E. McAnarney, 375-395. New York: Grune and Stratton.

McAuley, J. A. 1982. Sex education in the curriculum: Opposed. In *Discussing sex in the classroom: Readings for teachers*, ed. D. R. Stronck, 5-6. Washington, DC: National Science Teachers Association.

Metropolitan Life Foundation. 1988. *"Health: You've got to be taught" survey.* New York: Metropolitan Life Insurance Company, Health and Safety Education Division.

Metropolitan Life Foundation. 1989. *"Healthy me" initiative to promote excellence in school health education: A compendium of award winning programs, 1985-1989.* New York: Metropolitan Life Insurance Company, Health and Safety Education Division.

Mott, F. L. 1986. The pace of repeated childbearing among young American mothers. *Family Planning Perspectives* 18 (1): 5-12.

Mott, F. L., and W. Marsiglio. 1985. Early childbearing and completion of high school. *Family Planning Perspectives* 17 (5): 234-237.

Muraskin, L. D. 1986. Sex education mandates: Are they the answer? *Family Planning Perspectives.* 18 (4): 171-174.

National Center for Health Statistics. 1988. Advance report of final natality statistics, 1986. *Monthly Vital Statistics Report* 37: 16-33.

Pratt, W., W. Mosher, C. Bachrach and M. Horn. 1984. Understanding U.S. fertility: Findings from the National Survey of Family Growth, Cycle III. *Population Bulletin* 39 (5): 1-42.

Rivara, F. P., P. J. Sweeney and B. F. Henderson. 1985. A study of low socioeconomic status, black teenage fathers and their nonfather peers. *Pediatrics* 75 (4): 648-656.

Saunders, R. P. 1991. *South Carolina School Health Leadership Conference Report.* Columbia, SC: School of Public Health.

Saunders, R. P., and B. F. Geiger. 1991. Integrating the Comprehensive Health Education Act: A survey of CHE coordinators. *Palmetto Administrator* 6 (1): 14-17.

Scales, P. 1982. The new opposition to sex education: A powerful threat to a democratic society. In *Discussing sex in the classroom: Readings for teachers*, ed. D. R. Stronck, 19-22. Washington, DC: National Science Teachers Association.

Schlafly, P. 1981. What's wrong with sex education? *The Phyllis Schlafly Report* 14 (7): 1-2.

South Carolina. State Senate and House of Representatives. 1988. *Comprehensive Health Education Act.* Amendment to Title 59 of 1976 Code of Laws of South Carolina by adding Chapter 32. Columbia, S.C.

Thompson, S. 1984. Search for tomorrow: On feminism and the reconstruction of teen romance. In *Pleasure and danger: Exploring female sexuality*, ed. C. S. Vance, 350-384. Boston, MA: Routledge and Kagan Paul.

Thompson, S. 1990. Putting a big thing into a little hole: Teenage girls' accounts of sexual initiation. *The Journal of Sex Research* 27:341-361.

Torres, A., and S. Singh. 1986. Contraceptive practice among Hispanic adolescents. *Family Planning Perspectives* 18 (4): 193-194.

Trussell, J. 1988. Teenage pregnancy in the United States. *Family Planning Perspectives* 20 (6): 262-272.

Trussell, J., and J. Menken. 1978. Early childbearing and subsequent fertility. *Family Planning Perspectives* 10 (4): 209-218.

U.S. Bureau of the Census. 1991. *Fertility of American women: June 1990.* Current Population Reports, Series P-20, No. 454. Washington, DC.

U.S. Public Health Service. 1992. *A Public Health Service progress report on Healthy people 2000: Family planning.* Washington, DC.

Vincent, M. L., A. F. Clearie, C. G. Johnson and P. A. Sharpe. 1988. *Reducing unintended adolescent pregnancy through school/community educational interventions: A South Carolina case study.* Atlanta, GA: U.S. Department of Health and Human Services, Public Health Service, and Centers for Disease Control and Prevention.

Vincent, M. L., A. F. Clearie, N. Obanor and J. B. Dannelly. 1985. Old wine in new bottles: Parent receptivity to school-based sex education. *South Carolina Journal of Health, Physical Education, Recreation and Dance* 17:14-16.

Vincent, M. L., A. F. Clearie and M. D. Schluchter. 1987. Reducing adolescent pregnancy through school and community-based education. *Journal of the American Medical Association* 257 (24): 3382-3386.

Zabin, L. S., and S. Clark. 1983. Institutional factors affecting teenagers' choice and reasons for delay in attending a family planning clinic. *Family Planning Perspectives* 15 (1): 25-29.

Zabin, L. S., M. B. Hirsch, E. A. Smith, R. Street and J. B. Hardy. 1986. Evaluation of a pregnancy prevention program for urban teenagers. *Family Planning Perspectives* 18 (3): 119-126.

Zelnik, M., and J. Kantner. 1980. Sexual activity, contraceptive use and pregnancy among metropolitan-area teenagers: 1971-1979. *Family Planning Perspectives* 12 (5): 230-237.

Chapter 13

Tobacco Use Prevention

Nathan Matza, MA, CHES,
with Ric Loya, MS, CHES

I n 1964, the first Surgeon General's Report on Smoking and Health suggested that smoking was related to lung cancer and other diseases. This report led to the warning label that began to appear on cigarette packages in 1966. The label read: "Cigarette smoking may be hazardous to your health."

More recent statements from the Surgeon General's office are very specific. C. Everett Koop, Surgeon General of the United States from 1981 to 1989, has written many times about the health hazards of tobacco use. One of his summaries includes the following statement: "Cigarette smoking is associated with more deaths and illness than drugs, alcohol, accidents and AIDS combined" (Koop, 1991). By the early nineties, deaths due to cigarettes were estimated at more than 434,000 each year. That works out to about 1,200 deaths each day, fifty each hour.

Nicotine, the drug in tobacco, is a powerful, addictive drug, as addictive as heroin and crack cocaine. Many experts believe that cigarettes serve as a gateway drug to allow children and teenagers to experiment with other illegal drugs such as marijuana, cocaine and heroin. It is much easier for a youngster to smoke marijuana or crack after having smoked cigarettes (Jacobs, 1990).

The High Costs of Tobacco Use

Ample research supports the conclusion that tobacco can kill. Tobacco use causes cancer of the mouth, tongue, face, lips, larynx, esophagus, stomach, pancreas, bladder and kidneys. Tobacco use is also responsible for chronic bronchitis, emphysema, chronic obstructive pulmonary disease, heart disease, strokes and wrinkles.

Other studies have linked tobacco to a variety of other health problems, including back pain (due to decrease of oxygen levels to lumbar disks), cervical cancer, diabetes (due to poor absorption of insulin), drug interactions, ear infections, gastrointestinal cancer, infertility, low birth rate, leukemia (carcinogens, such as benzopyrene, are found in tobacco), occupational lung cancer, osteoporosis, premature aging, slow recovery from surgery, poor nutrition, tooth loss and fires (*Bottom Line*, 1992).

Tobacco takes an economic toll as well. In California alone, smoking costs more than $7.6 billion a year in health care expenditures and lost productivity due to disease and early death (Rice and Max, 1992). Nationwide, Action for Smoking and Health estimates that smoking costs the American economy more than $100 billion a year (Banzhaf, 1993).

Secondhand Smoke

Environmental tobacco smoke (ETS), also called secondhand smoke, is also a health concern. Thousands of deaths annually can be attributed to environmental exposure to tobacco smoke (Glantz and Parmley, 1991). A person in a smoke-filled room for eight hours a day will smoke the equivalent of one cigarette each hour just by being in the room, according to recent research. Unborn fetuses take in the smoke their mothers consume. Children whose parents smoke have more respiratory infections, colds and general childhood illness as a result of their parents' smoking habits (Glantz, 1992; Koop, 1989; U.S. Department of Health and Human Services, 1986).

The World Health Organization (1991) has issued a summary of the proven health effects of exposure to ETS. These effects include respiratory problems; irritation of eyes, nose and throat; and lung cancer. Children also suffer the effects of ETS. Children whose parents smoke have up to 300,000 lower-respiratory infections such as pneumonia and bronchitis each year, up to one million asthma attacks, and up to 15,000 hospitalizations. They also suffer increased middle ear effusion and reduced levels of lung function (U.S. EPA, 1992).

Glantz and Parmley (1991) estimate that ETS is associated with 53,000 deaths each year in the United States. Of these deaths, 37,000 are related to heart and blood vessel disease, 4,000 to lung cancer and 12,000 to other cancers.

More than two million California nonsmokers were exposed to secondhand smoke in the workplace in 1990. As part of the 1990 California Tobacco Survey, Ron Borland reported on 7,162 adult nonsmoking, indoor workers (California Department of Health Services, 1990). The rate of ETS exposure decreased with increasing education. Workers with less than a high school education reported an exposure rate of 43.1 percent, while only 18.6 percent of those with at least a college education reported ETS exposure. The survey concluded, "For industries and other institutions in which the employees are likely to be in these [high risk] demographic groups, high priority should be given to establishing ordinances mandating smokefree worksites."

The report also states, "Our data indicate that the only way to protect nonsmokers' health is with a smokefree worksite. The available evidence indicates that bans are accepted by smokers once the bans are implemented. Although these facts alone will motivate many employers to take further action, we also must work toward establishing local smoking ordinances that require smokefree work sites to protect the health of nonsmoking workers" (California Department of Health Services, 1990).

Children's Risk Factors

Today, most of the American population acknowledges the health hazards of cigarettes and tobacco products, but few see the implications of tobacco's pervasiveness in our society for children, school settings, businesses, cities and states throughout the United States. Nicotine is an *addictive drug*. Cigarette smokers are drug addicts. As with any drug, children are at risk if they have a high number of the risk factors for drug use (Hawkins, Lishner and Catalano, 1985). These factors include:
* economic and social deprivation
* low neighborhood attachment and high disorganization
* community norms and laws favorable to the use of tobacco, alcohol and other drugs
* availability of tobacco, alcohol and other drugs
* family management problems, including lack of clear expectations for children's behavior, lack of monitoring, inconsistent or excessively severe discipline, lack of caring
* use of tobacco, alcohol or other drugs by parents
* parents' low expectations for children's success
* family history of alcoholism
* lack of a clear school policy regarding tobacco use

- availability of tobacco, alcohol or drugs on campus
- changing schools often
- academic failure
- lack of involvement in school activities
- little commitment to school
- alienation and rebelliousness
- antisocial behavior in early childhood and early adolescence
- favorable attitudes toward drug use
- early first use of tobacco products
- greater influence by and reliance on peers than parents
- friends who use tobacco, alcohol and other drugs or sanction their use.

Children from Asian, Hispanic, Middle Eastern and other backgrounds may be at high risk for tobacco use because smoking is not only accepted, but promoted in their cultures. For example, Southeast Asian families often use cigarettes as party favors at weddings. Many new immigrants have been influenced by Western tobacco companies' advertising in their countries to believe that smoking is a valued aspect of American society. In addition, they may not be aware of the health hazards of tobacco use.

The American Cancer Society is now providing health education materials in many languages to help recent arrivals to the United States learn more about smoking and health risks. Classroom teachers may easily convince preteen and high school immigrant students of the health risks, but their parents are not as easily won over. However, students may serve as health educators for their parents while they become acculturated to the United States.

Business and Politics

Tobacco companies are businesses. As in any business, the ultimate goal is to turn a profit and stay in business. Tobacco companies spend in excess of $7 million every day on advertising and promotion. That means they spend more than $3 billion per year, or about $100 every second. For every dollar spent opposing tobacco use, the tobacco industry spends $4,000 to refute the warnings.

Most tobacco companies are huge international corporations. These companies have recently sought to obtain political and economic influence by acquiring subsidiaries of non-tobacco-growing companies. While diversification of any business makes good sense, the political impact of tobacco companies' diversification can wield a powerful influence on other businesses as well as governmental agencies. For example, if a publisher who is sensitive to tobacco-related health problems refuses to carry tobacco advertising in a magazine, the tobacco company can cancel advertising for its other products, such as food products, in that publication.

During the 1989/1990 election cycle, tobacco and alcohol lobbies were big spenders. Eighty percent (420 out of 525) of the members of the Congress received money from the tobacco industry, either in campaign contributions or "honoraria." Although honoraria may no longer be used in this way, the tobacco lobby has had a strong influence in Washington. One result has been that the United States ranks last among industrialized countries in the amount of tax collected on tobacco products.

The Los Angeles Daily News reported in 1991 that tobacco lobbyists were among the biggest spenders in Sacramento, California's state capital. "They buy dinners, concert tickets, limousine service, trips to New York and a grab-bag of other gifts for legislators and their staff members, and at the California State Capitol, the tobacco industry seldom loses" (U.C. San Diego, 1992). Diane Kaiser, a lobbyist for the American Heart Association, described the situation: "All the tobacco lobbyists have to do is walk into a committee room and the message is clear to legislators: Don't vote against them."

The California Experience

In January 1989, California implemented a voter initiative (Proposition 99) that added a tax of 25 cents per package on cigarettes sold in California. By the end of the first year, more than one billion dollars had been raised by the new tax, despite a $21 million counterattack by the tobacco industry. Funds collected under the new law go toward health education, hospital services, physician services, research and public resources. Research indicates that action resulting from the passage of Proposition 99 reduced tobacco consumption in the state by 17 percent in the first three years (Burns and Pierce, 1992).

Raising cigarette taxes appears to be an effective public health intervention, as demonstrated not only in California but also in Canada. Canadians pay more for cigarettes—in excess of $3.00 a pack—and the tobacco sales decline in Canada is faster than that in the United States (Peterson et al., 1992; Kaiserman and Rogers, 1991).

Most California cities, government offices and even private businesses either restrict or completely ban smoking indoors. Many universities do not allow any smoking indoors, and even some outdoor sports stadiums have banned smoking or confined it to a special section. Many county detention facilities have also banned smoking.

Many California communities have passed laws that ban smoking even in restaurants. Despite restaurant owners' concern about loss of business due to the smoking ban, data indicates no such loss (Smith and Glantz, 1992). Studies have shown that no-smoking ordinances actually benefit restaurants by increasing slightly the fraction of total retail sales that go to restaurants. The research counters the tobacco industry claim that no-smoking ordinances cause a 30 percent reduction in business.

"The overall conclusion is that 100 percent smokefree restaurant ordinances do not adversely affect restaurant sales within a community or lead to a shift in patronage to restaurants in communities with no such ordinances," says Stanton A. Glantz, professor of medicine at the University of California, San Francisco, and investigator at the Institute for Health Policy and Cardiovascular Research. In four cities with 100 percent smokefree restaurants, the fraction of total retail sales that went to restaurants in those communities *increased* from an average of 12.7 percent to 13.9 percent after the laws were in force (Smith and Glantz, 1992).

The Youth Market

Tobacco companies insist that their advertisements are merely designed to encourage adults to switch brands and flatly deny any targeted efforts toward youth. Doctors Ought to Care (DOC), an antismoking activist organization of doctors, has been countering this message around the United States and the world.

A well-publicized edition of the *Journal of the American Medical Association* (December 11, 1991) was able to explain that not only have tobacco companies been targeting youth, but some kids were able to recognize the Camel cigarette "Old Joe" character more readily than Disney's Mickey Mouse (Fischer and Schwartz, 1991).

When children played a game in which they were asked to place 22 product logos—including products for adults and children—on a game board featuring twelve products—including Mickey Mouse, pizza, hamburgers and automobiles—30 percent of the three year olds were able to match the Old Joe cartoon with Camel cigarettes.

In 1984, the Tobacco Institute produced a booklet called "Helping Youth Decide." The purported intent was to help children look at adult smoking behaviors. However, the booklet was attacked by the American Lung Association and others for lack of information on the health hazards of smoking. The document was being promoted through the National Association of School Boards. In response to public pressure, the school board group broke their affiliation with the Tobacco Institute.

In 1992, the Tobacco Institute produced a booklet called *Helping Youth Say No*. The authors claim that students need to recognize that only adults should decide about smoking. While this may *seem* to be a positive step in antitobacco education, the guide may actually encourage youth to look up to and emulate adult behaviors—i.e., smoking. The booklet also avoids any mention of cancer, lung disease, heart disease, emphysema or death; it focuses only on the misleading message that smoking is an adult decision. As educators are well aware, most teenagers want nothing more than to be adults, making adult decisions.

Ironically, this booklet can serve as an excellent teaching tool. Teachers can have their students carefully read the booklet to locate any messages related to the health problems of smoking and determine the real message of the Tobacco Institute. With careful discussion and analysis, educators can use this booklet to illustrate to students the institute's false and misleading message.

RJR Nabisco has also disseminated a program called *Right Decisions, Right Now*. In San Diego, California, the San Diego

City Unified School District rejected this program, stating, "We consider it a conflict of interest and of our philosophy to have your name associated with any comprehensive health education and tobacco use prevention program" (Tobacco Education Oversight Committee, 1993).

In recent years, DOC has focused attention on the pervasiveness of tobacco advertising at televised sporting events. In 1971, television advertising for tobacco products was banned. However, tobacco companies continue to sponsor televised events such as the Virginia Slims tennis tournaments and the Winston Cup racing circuit. Tobacco advertisements and sponsorships in sports stadiums are also widely televised.

Dr. Eric Solberg, writing in *DOC News and Views*, called for efforts "to get the U.S. Justice Department to act on these televised tobacco promotions masquerading as sports events." "If the Attorney General of the United States were to enforce the Public Health Cigarette Smoking Act of 1969," Solberg wrote, "complete with a $10,000 fine for each violation of the law, televised sports sponsored by cigarette and other tobacco product manufacturers would become extinct in the United States" (Solberg, 1992).

Educating Our Youth

In 1989, 2.6 million children between age 12 and 17 smoked cigarettes, and 1.5 million (57.5 percent) bought their own cigarettes; 85 percent of the purchases were from small stores. Tobacco-related diseases occur at higher rates for persons who start smoking at younger ages. As Altman et al. (1991) state, "Access to tobacco is conducive to developing and maintaining a tobacco addiction. In field trials around the country, minors' attempts to purchase tobacco from stores and vending machines have been successful more than 50 percent of the time." Despite laws in 44 states and the District of Columbia that prohibit the sale of tobacco products to minors, underaged youth usually have been successful in their attempts to purchase tobacco. In fact, their success rate in purchasing from vending machines is almost 100 percent (STAT, 1991).

As laws prohibiting sales of tobacco products to minors are passed and enforced, children who cannot purchase cigarettes will be at much less at risk for health problems. Educational interventions directed at vendors to decrease or eliminate tobacco sales at the retail level have resulted in some temporary reduction of sales to minors, but the greatest decrease of sales to underage buyers has been documented in communities that have active supervision or surveillance of retail stores accompanied with substantial penalties for noncompliance (Feighery and Altman, 1991). Law enforcement officers need to be as vigilant with tobacco sales and use by minors as they are with alcohol.

From November 1990 until June 1991, the American Lung Association worked with the Latino Tobacco Free Coalition in the Los Angeles area to implement a student "sting" operation (with parental consent and approval) that was able to dramatically lower sales of tobacco to minors. The operation began by posting California Penal Code 308 at locations where cigarettes were sold. The penal code section states: "Unlawful to sell to persons under 18 years of age tobacco, cigarette or cigarette papers, or any preparation of tobacco, or any other instrument or paraphernalia that is designed for the smoking or ingestion of tobacco, products prepared from tobacco, or any controlled substance." Minors were then videotaped purchasing cigarettes. Later, vendors who had sold cigarettes to minors were visited by police officers and tactfully reminded about the law.

The program produced a significant decrease in purchases of cigarettes by minors. A follow-up study of 1,400 vendors found that while 70 percent were selling to minors before the sting, only 30 percent sold to minors after the sting. This represents a 57 percent reduction in the number of vendors selling tobacco products to minors. At the end of one year, the ratio was about 50 percent of vendors selling and 50 percent not selling to minors (Loya, 1993). A teacher's guidebook based on the program, "Kicking Butt," has been produced for teachers to use (Loya and Vidstrand, 1990).

Despite the continued efforts of health educators to help young people understand the dangers of tobacco use, many children and youth are not concerned with statistics about chronic problems such as cancer, emphysema and heart disease. Information about other drawbacks of tobacco addiction, such as yellow and brown stains on teeth, bad breath, smelly hair, stinky clothes, wrinkles and a smelly house, may be more relevant, particularly if it's suggested that such effects are a turn-off for most potential dating partners. The use of humor and music may also help students be more receptive to the message.

Statistical data about deaths from tobacco use are often hard to visualize. A simple way to dramatize the hundreds of thousands of deaths a year in the United States due to tobacco use is to ask a typical, large middle or high school class of 38 students to gaze at the seats they vacate at the end of a one-hour session. Statistically speaking, everyone in that class will die as the bell rings. At least this many deaths occur twenty-four hours a day, seven days a week, in the United States alone.

Students can be empowered to become activists in the crusade against tobacco use. In the summer of 1990, during a year-round school session at a predominantly Hispanic Los Angeles middle school, the makers of Skoal chewing tobacco were advertising their deadly chew to sixth graders. A large sign, written in Spanish, was in direct view across the street from the school. The sign's ethnically related focus suggested that chewing tobacco gave men a macho image.

Classroom teachers, along with the American Lung Association, American Cancer Society, California Association of School Health Educators and other antismoking groups, called a press conference, attended by students, at the school. The resulting media coverage lead to the sign being removed within five days. Students watched the sign removal, cheering and waving at the camera crews. Students also make very effective speakers at public hearings on tobacco use prevention.

Recommendations for Action

The health risks of tobacco use are very clear today. The tobacco industry, with its well-organized and heavily funded marketing staff, both in the United States and overseas, presents a major health challenge to Americans today. The passing of laws to increase taxes on cigarettes does result in the decline of cigarette sales. Combined with efforts aimed at the prohibition of sales to minors, such taxes could serve to dramatically reduce smoking in America and help citizens to reach the public health objectives for the year 2000 set by *Healthy People 2000* (U.S. Department of Health and Human Services, 1991). Objectives 3.1, 3.2 and 3.3 relate to tobacco use and the reduction of deaths due to coronary heart disease, lung cancer and chronic obstructive pulmonary disease.

The following recommendations for interventions at all levels, from early childhood education to community action, including state and national political action, could help eliminate the problems of tobacco addiction.

Education

- Provide comprehensive health education for kindergarten through grade six in all U.S. schools. Include a full year of comprehensive health education in middle school and high school. Classes should be taught by certified health educators. Even preschool children benefit from comprehensive health education and antismoking campaigns.

  Comprehensive health education addresses all health-compromising behaviors, including tobacco use. It helps foster healthy attitudes and behaviors about substance use, including tobacco, and promotes healthy lifestyles. In addition to offering information about the effects of tobacco and other substance use, a comprehensive health program helps students develop skills to avoid risky behaviors (Fetro, 1991).

- State-of-the-art classroom methods, such as computer-assisted interactive instruction and videodisc interactive teaching based on cooperative learning techniques, may have an additional impact on students. Intensive prevention programs using roleplaying and refusal-skill techniques should start at grade four, if not sooner, and continue through grade twelve.

- Train students as health education peer counselors to help classmates overcome smoking addiction. Offer smoking cessation programs for adults and students, funded by tobacco education taxes, at both business and school sites.

- Develop special classes in health education to promote health advocacy. Students could present data at city council meetings and school board meetings and advocate to eliminate smoking in the school setting.

- Community antismoking coalitions can involve high school students, civic leaders and community health agencies. Students could earn community service credits toward graduation. These groups could work with law enforcement to develop sting operations to eliminate tobacco sales to minors.

- Promote a smokefree environment in all schools, not only for students but for visitors, faculty and other staff. Use outreach programs to teach parents and other family members the importance of being role models for their children, especially in relation to tobacco use. Train students from families with limited English skills to act as health educators for their parents and family members to teach them the health risks of smoking and tobacco products.

Legislation

- The Secretary of Health and Human Services has made the following recommendations (U.S. Department of Health and Human Services, 1990):
  - Institute 19 years as the minimum age for legal tobacco sales.
  - Create a tobacco sales licensing system similar to that for alcoholic beverages.
  - Establish a graduated schedule of penalties for illegal sales, with separate penalties for failure to post a sign regarding legal age of purchase.
  - Place primary responsibility for enforcement with a designated state agency, with participation and input from local law enforcement and public health officials.
  - Use civil penalties and local courts to assess fines.
  - Ban cigarette vending machines.

- In addition to banning the sale and distribution of tobacco products through vending machines, outlaw the sale of single cigarettes from any location.
- Pass and enforce laws that prohibit the purchase, distribution and use of tobacco by minors. Support laws such as those in

California that discourage the use of tobacco products through taxation. Following the Canadian model, taxes could be raised to as much as 75 percent of the retail sales price of cigarettes.

- Eliminate tobacco subsidies while providing incentives for tobacco farmers to produce other edible crops. Ban the exportation of tobacco products to other countries.
- Ban smoking in all indoor public places such as restaurants, bars, shopping malls and sports arenas. Prohibit smoking on all public transit, including but not limited to taxis and buses and the ticket, boarding and waiting areas of public transit depots.
- Prohibit tobacco advertising and promotion in any facility owned by a city or any agency of a city, county or state government that hosts athletic events, as well as other government-owned premises, including facilities and parks. Prohibit tobacco advertising and promotion within a two-mile radius of schools, community centers and churches.
- Develop company or governmental policies to hire only non-smokers, especially as police officers and firefighters, and offer nonsmoking employees lower rates on health insurance and life insurance. Products such as "Smoke Check," an ETS monitoring badge, can be worn by individuals to measure daily exposure to environmental smoke products.

Looking Forward

"I do not believe the United States will ever again be a growing market for tobacco products," Dr. Koop has stated. "The curve is going down at an accelerated pace. But the tobacco companies have not given up" (Koop, 1991). Koop believes there are three major battles to be fought:
- cigarette vending machines
- cigarette advertising
- the international power of the tobacco companies

As the United States approaches the year 2000, we look forward to a time when the national health objectives on tobacco use are met or exceeded. Children, teenagers and young adults will no longer accept cigarette and tobacco products as normal, sensible behavior.

Tobacco companies will eliminate the glitzy advertising and promotion of tobacco products and concentrate on other products for which death is not the end result of product usage. Government will recognize and reinforce the scientific data related to complete freedom from tobacco use. Families will develop positive models for their children to emulate while living in a healthy environment. American homes, cars and hotel rooms will no longer be permeated with the smell of tobacco smoke. Americans will live longer, healthier lives—tobacco free.

References

Action on Smoking and Health. n.d. Involuntary smoking: The factual basis for action. *ASH Smoking and Health Review,* Special Report.

Alcohol and tobacco lobbies are big spenders. 1992. *Prevention File: Alcohol, Tobacco and Other Drugs.* Vol. 7, No. 2. University of California, San Diego.

Altman, D. G., L. Rasenick-Douss, V. Foster and J. B. Tye. 1991. Sustained effects on an educational program to reduce sales of cigarettes to minors. *American Journal of Public Health* 81:891-893.

American Heart Association. 1991. News Release, November.

Banzhaf, J. F. III. 1993. Personal communicatio, 17 June.

Bottom Line/Personal. 15 August 1992.

Burns, D., and J. P. Pierce. 1992. *Tobacco use in California 1990-1991.* Sacramento, CA: California State Department of Health Services.

Escobedo, L. G., and P. L. Remington. 1989. Birth cohort analysis of prevalence of cigarette smoking among Hispanics in the U.S. *Journal of the American Medical Association* 261:66-69.

Feighery, E., and D. G. Altman. 1991. The effects of combining education and enforcement to reduce tobacco sales to minors. *Journal of the American Medical Association* 266:3159-3161.

Fetro, J. V. 1991. *Step by step to substance use prevention: The planning guide for school-based programs.* Santa Cruz, CA: ETR Associates.

Flewelling, R. L. 1992. First-year impact of the 1989 California cigarette tax increase on cigarette consumption. *American Journal of Public Health* 82:867-869.

Fiore, M. L., and T. E. Novotny. 1989. Trends in cigarette smoking in the U.S.: The changing influence of gender and race. *Journal of the American Medical Association* 261:49-55.

Fischer, P. M., and M. P. Schwartz. 1991. Brand logo recognition by children aged 3 to 6 years. *Journal of the American Medical Association* 266:3145-3148.

Glantz, S. 1992. *Tobacco, biology and politics.* Waco, TX: Health EDCO.

Glantz, S., and W. Parmley. 1991. Passive smoking and heart disease: Epidemiology, physiology and biochemistry. *Circulation* 83 (1): 1-12.

Hawkins, J. D., D. M. Lishner and R. F. Catalano. 1985. Childhood predictors of adolescent substance abuse. In *Etiology of Drug Abuse: Implications for Prevention,* ed. C. L. Jones and R. J. Battjes. Washington, DC: U.S. Department of Health and Human Services.

Jacobs, E. 1990. Marijuana and tobacco update. Paper presented at the Annual Conference of California Association of School Health Educators, Pacific Palisades, California, 18 November.

Kaiserman, M. J., and B. R. Rogers. 1991. Tobacco consumption declining faster in Canada than in the U.S. *American Journal of Public Health* 81:902-904.

Koop, C. E. 1989. Smoking: Everything you and your family need to know. Home Box Office Productions. Video broadcast, July 1989.

Koop C. E. 1991. *Koop: Memoirs of America's family doctor.* New York: Random House.

Loya, R. 1993. Personal communication with author, 14 February.

Loya, R., and E. Vidstrand. 1990. "Kicking Butt Curriculum Guide." American Lung Association. (Available from American Lung Association of Los Angeles County, 5858 Wilshire Blvd., Suite 300, Los Angeles, CA 90036.)

Peterson, D. L., S. L. Zeger, P. L. Remington and H. A. Anderson. 1992. The effect of state cigarette tax increases on cigarette sales, 1955-1988. *American Journal of Public Health* 82:94-96.

Rice, D. P., and W. Max. 1992. *The cost of smoking in California, 1989.* Sacramento, CA: California State Department of Health Services.

Smith, L., and S. Glantz. 1992. Smoke free restaurants ordinances don't reduce business. *Prevention File: Alcohol, Tobacco and Other Drugs.* Vol. 7, No. 2. University of California, San Diego.

Solberg, E. 1992. *DOC News and Views: The Journal of Medical Activism* 7:2-6.

STAT. 1991. Questions and answers about the Tobacco Institute's program for preventing youth smoking. Springfield, MA.

Tobacco Education Oversight Committee. 1993. *Toward a tobacco-free California: Exploring a new frontier 1993-1995.* Sacramento, CA.

U.S. Department of Health and Human Services. 1986. The health consequences of involuntary smoking: A report of the Surgeon General. DHHS Publication No. (CDC) 87-8398. Washington, DC.

U.S. Department of Health and Human Services, Public Health Service. 1990. *Model sale of tobacco products to minors act.* Washington, DC.

U.S. Department of Health and Human Services, Public Health Service. 1991. *Healthy people 2000: National health promotion and disease prevention objectives.* DHHS Publication No. 91-50212. Washington, DC.

U.S. Environmental Protection Agency. 1992. *Respiratory health effects of passive smoking: Lung cancer and other disorders.* EPA/600/6-90/006F. Washington, DC.

World Health Organization. 1991. World No Tobacco Day. Geneva.

Chapter 14

Alcohol and Other Drug Use Prevention Education

B. E. "Buzz" Pruitt, EdD, CHES

The quality of life of today's adolescents is not what it should be. Drug use by children and adolescents inhibits, perhaps even blocks, their potential to grow to healthy adulthood, to meet life's challenges and to be satisfied human beings. Drug use by a small but significant percentage of the student-age population robs this country of productive, contributing citizens. It delays emotional maturity, social development, and in some cases, even physical growth of young people. It robs a crucial segment of our population of a secure, carefree and enjoyable youth. Drug use often robs young people of life itself.

The Congress of the United States acknowledged these effects in its *Adolescent Health* report, compiled by the Office of Technology Assessment (1991). The report presented an appropriate vision of adolescence as "the beginning of the productive phase of life where young people are contributing members of society, meet commitments to families and friends, and accept the responsibilities of citizenship."

The literature of both education and health in general recognizes the threat of drug use among school-age populations. During the last two decades, thousands of papers have been written about drug use prevention. Entire journals have been devoted to the subject; successful businesses have been built around the need for drug education curriculum materials; and extensive research has been conducted, much of it accurately documenting trends in use patterns.

The National Education Goals for the year 2000 include the following:

> Every school in America (by the year 2000) will be free of drugs and violence and will offer a safe, disciplined environment conducive to learning. (National Education Goals Panel, 1991)

The governors who authored this goal acknowledge the significant problems our country faces related to drug use among youth. *Healthy People 2000* (U.S. Department of Health and Human Services, 1991) presents more than two hundred objectives addressing health threats ranging from communicable disease to violent acts. Several of the objectives directly relate to drug use by student-age populations, for example:

> Increase the proportion of high school seniors who associate risk of physical or psychological harm with the heavy use of alcohol, regular use of marijuana, and experimentation with cocaine. (Objective 4.10)

These goals are direct challenges to professional educators, educational administrators, and public and school health professionals. Those who work with youth have an obligation to give every student an opportunity to learn. They are also obligated to work toward solutions to the drug-use problems children face. No one can stand by and assume that someone else will do it; all must get involved. Several challenges face public school and public health personnel as they confront the problems stemming from drug use among the nation's youth. There is much to consider concerning educational intervention in one of the greatest challenges facing the United States—drug use by its young people.

The Scope of the Problem

Much information about drug use among school-age populations is available. The National Adolescent Student Health Survey (ASHA, AAHE and SOPHE, 1989) indicated that students of this age group do use drugs. According to the National Commission on Drug-Free Schools (1990), when alcohol is included in the definition of illegal drugs, more than 90 percent of high school graduates have used illegal drugs.

Alcohol is, in fact, illegal for school-age populations. It is also the drug of choice among students, with more than 90 percent of high school seniors reporting consumption of alcohol. Students as young as grade three have used alcohol and tobacco, and many even younger children have been exposed to illicit drugs through peers, older siblings and parents (National Commission on Drug-Free Schools, 1990).

Student attitudes concerning the use of drugs, including alcohol and tobacco, have changed. The perception among students that all drugs are harmful was at its highest point in over a decade in 1990 (National Commission on Drug-Free Schools, 1990). With the exception of alcohol, the rate of most illicit drug use is falling. Illegal drug use by high school seniors decreased from a high of 66 percent in 1981 to 51 percent in 1989 (Johnston, O'Malley and Bachman, 1989).

However, increased use of all drugs is seen among disadvantaged youth (Newcomb and Bentler, 1989). Heavier use is also found in disturbed families in which there are drug-use role models (Hawkins et al., 1986). Programs to address the family factors have become more prolific and claim more success. Yet in some homes, drug use, particularly the use of alcohol and tobacco, remains common.

Younger students look to the home and to family members as sources of values and information related to drug use (Hawkins et al., 1986). Upon entering adolescence, these same students turn to peers for information and for positive reinforcement of their behavior (Pruitt et al., 1991). This change underscores the Carnegie Commission's characterization of the middle school years as a "turning point" in a child's life—a point at which decisions about the present dramatically affect the future (Carnegie Council on Adolescent Development, 1989).

Institutional responses to drug-use problems have been significant. Health educators and administrators in schools now, even more than in the past, recognize that drug use is a problem. They are developing programs to help students understand and resist pressure to use drugs. Professionals in public health fields are doing the same.

Federal funding for drug education and prevention efforts increased substantially in the 1980s, to a great extent due to laws such as the Drug-Free Schools and Communities Act of 1986 and the Anti-Drug Abuse Act of 1988. The National Commission on Drug-Free Schools found that the majority of schools in the United States had some type of drug education and prevention programs by 1990.

In many communities, even without local or federal financial support, parents have taken the lead in fighting drugs by forming community action committees, pressuring public officials and lobbying for local action to combat drug use. In many other communities, however, school policies have limited the role of volunteers and parents in fundraising and similar tasks related to drug-use prevention. Overall, participation in parental groups is increasing, and tolerance of the problems associated with drug use, crime and violent behavior is decreasing.

Although tremendous energy and resources have been focused on addressing the drug-use problem, much remains to be learned. Bonnie Benard states, "It's fair to say that educators have had more experience than success with substance abuse prevention programs" (Benard and Perrone, 1987). Not enough is known about why school-age populations use tobacco, alcohol and other drugs.

Students remain, for the most part, cynical about school drug education programs (National Commission on Drug-Free Schools, 1990). Educators don't yet know how to effect changes in areas such as parental standards and advertising policies, factors that relate to the use of tobacco, alcohol and other drugs. Too little is known about the students who drop out of school and, thus, comprise a cohort that is not included in most surveys of drug use among older students.

More attention needs to be paid to program effectiveness. Most schools now conduct some form of prevention program, but there is a need to invest more time and effort in determining what works and what does not. Such efforts would help identify how best to spend the considerable resources now directed toward the problem of drug use. Efforts should be made to understand where students get their information about drugs and how their attitudes are influenced. This information can help identify the type of school policies needed to combat drug use by school-age populations.

Much remains to be learned about these complex issues. However, ignorance is not an excuse for inaction. To the credit of educators and health professionals, many well-intentioned attempts to address drug-use problems have been made over the years.

Prevention Efforts

School-based drug-use prevention dates back to the 1800s when the Women's Christian Temperance Union successfully lobbied every state of the United States to implement educational programs on the dangers of alcohol. Since that time, numerous efforts have been made to persuade children to stay away from drugs, to scare them about drugs, and even to give them simplistic answers to the problems associated with drugs.

In the 1990s, a variety of drug-use prevention programs exist. Some have a national focus, while others have a highly localized focus; some focus on a single drug, others on all drug-use behavior; some are very personal in approach, while others are totally focused on social interaction. The specific objectives of drug-use prevention programs vary as widely as the program designs. However, several basic objectives are found in most drug-use prevention educational programs. These basic objectives serve to categorize drug education efforts to date.

Knowledge-Based Programs
Most programmatical efforts to prevent drug use have set a goal of increasing students' knowledge about drugs. Generally, this means increasing knowledge of the dangers of drug use, the effects of specific drugs on the body, drug laws and the consequences of getting caught using drugs. Some programs include some historical background on drugs and drug culture.

This "knowledge" goal is an appropriate role for schools because transfer of information is their primary business. But research on the effectiveness of programs that focus on knowledge transfer is disturbing and compelling (Tobler, 1986; Bangert-Drowns, 1988). Knowledge increase alone does not positively correlate with a reduction in drug-use behavior.

This finding is not recent. In the early 1970s, warnings were issued about programs that focus only on knowledge transfer. These warnings suggest that such programs might actually increase curiosity about and experimentation with drugs, thus prompting results opposite to those intended (National Commission on Marijuana and Drug Abuse, 1973).

Attitude-Based Programs

Some programs are considered more "affective" than knowledge-based programs. These programs focus on attitude change as a primary goal. They accomplish change through activities designed to build self-esteem, clarify personal values, encourage responsible decision making and warn of the dangers of drugs. Programs using scare tactics are an extreme example of this type of program, some of which are notable in the history of drug education. What health educator has not seen clips from the film *Reefer Madness,* in which the effects of drugs were exaggerated? The connection between attitudinal change and drug-use behavior, however, remains unclear (Tobler, 1986; Bangert-Drowns, 1988). And, in light of fervent political opposition to many aspects of this type of approach (such as values clarification), such programs have a tenuous status among accepted drug education efforts.

Skill-Based Programs

Another goal often found in drug prevention programs is enhancement of personal and interpersonal skills, particularly skills used in interaction with peers. These peer resistance skills have become the central theme of many programs, including some of the most widely used drug-use prevention programs of the nineties. Such skills help students avoid all kinds of negative situations that can lead to problems, while at the same time allowing them to maintain their self-respect and their friends. Skill-based programs are especially appropriate for adolescent students, for whom interaction with peers is crucial and often awkward.

Not surprisingly, the timing of skill-based education is critical. The middle school years appear to be the best time to provide peer-resistance training. During these years, success in resisting pressure to use drugs holds the greatest promise for life-long impact.

Alternatives-Based Programs

A final category of drug abuse prevention program aims to increase an individual's participation in positive alternatives to drug use. These programs advocate becoming involved in activities that are fun, emotionally stimulating, and involve experimentation and risk taking in a safe or controlled environment. Alternative programs stress participatory activities such as art, special health courses and outdoor education courses. Outside the formal school setting, Boys and Girls Clubs or Scouting are examples of this type of program.

Measuring Success

The continued levels of problems associated with drug use among school-age populations seem to indicate that efforts to alleviate the problems have not yet been very successful. An objective review of drug education efforts to date indicates only limited, qualified success. Lack of success may suggest that the right programs have not yet been developed. Or it may indicate that existing programs have not been rigorously evaluated. Perhaps no one has asked the questions, Which programs work? and, Why?

Almost every drug use prevention program includes an evaluation component of some sort. The purpose of the evaluation varies from program to program. Some are designed to determine if the program had an effect on the drug-use behavior of the target population; others are designed to justify the continuation of the program in an environment of competing financial interests. Attempts to compare program evaluations are fraught with problems, primarily because of design differences.

One research method, however, that does address the overall effectiveness of program types is meta-analysis research. In this method, a researcher accumulates as many studies as possible, then combines or integrates the results of those studies. The most extensive analysis of school-based drug-use prevention programs was completed in 1986 by Nancy Tobler, who studied 143 drug-use prevention programs. Her research was followed two years later by Robert Bangert-Drowns. These analyses of drug-use prevention efforts revealed a great deal about the effectiveness of drug education prevention programs. They also provided some encouraging findings concerning the types of efforts currently underway.

According to Tobler, programs that focus only on knowledge change demonstrate little effectiveness in drug-use behavior change. Likewise, programs that focus only on attitude change demonstrate little effectiveness when actual drug-use behavior is evaluated. Even in the case of programs that combined both knowledge and attitudes objectives, effectiveness was minimal.

The programs that demonstrated the most success with low-risk populations, the "average teenager," and other students who were not considered likely to experience drug problems were peer resistance programs. Labeled as refusal skills, peer resistance skills or peer pressure resistance, these programs have documented success in preventing or delaying drug experimentation.

Newcomb and Bentler (1989), however, point out that it is misleading "to bask in the success of some peer programs that have reduced the number of youngsters who experiment with drugs and ignore the tougher problems of those youngsters who are at high risk for drug abuse as well as other serious difficulties." Tobler's research indicates that alternatives programs demonstrate reason for optimism in dealing with high-risk youth, who are the ones most prone to drug-use problems.

Programs providing drug-free activities have demonstrated success in reducing drug use on the part of these populations. A logical explanation for this success is that high-risk youth rarely have opportunities to be involved in drug-free experiences. Thus, when opportunities are provided, success is easily achieved.

Taken as a whole, the findings of these two meta-analyses should not be surprising. The studies show that high-risk youth who are not being raised in a drug-free environment benefit greatly from activities that remove them from their normal environment and place them in a positive, drug-free environment. Findings also indicate that students from drug-free environments who hear, sometimes every day, about the dangers of drug use respond favorably to peer pressure training related to drug use refusal. What is more difficult to accept, though it is repeated often in the literature, is the lack of demonstrated effectiveness of knowledge-based and attitude-based programs.

What Does Work?

Some success in drug-use prevention education has been documented. Many other efforts remain unproven. Many challenges remain.

Challenge: Change the Focus of Drug Use Prevention from Drugs to Children

Students do not have drug problems; they have problems, and they use drugs. This significant distinction points to the complexity of the issue of drug-use prevention. Over the years, many have paid lip service to this challenge, but to date most programs fail to take into consideration the complexity of the drug-related problems that students face.

This failure is evidenced by the success of peer programs and alternatives programs, and the lack of success of more traditional drug education efforts. Though it may be easy to say and difficult to do, the question of focus begins with the planning stage of drug-use prevention efforts.

Planning involves all constituents of a community in the policy and practice of the school. Good planning mandates the informed involvement of teachers, parents, community representatives and students. It involves writing philosophical statements that keep students in the forefront, setting goals about student needs and behaviors rather than about drugs, and measuring the accomplishments of students, not those of teachers, administrators or law enforcement officers. Most important, planning involves the development of a unified vision of a drug-free educational institution devoted to students.

Dwight D. Eisenhower once said, "The plan is nothing, planning is everything." This wisdom is basic to shifting concerns away from drugs and toward children. The final published plan is not as important as is the strength gained from the involvement, goodwill, and program ownership felt by a local community, a professional team and the students themselves. By focusing the planning efforts of drug-use prevention on children—their special needs, their special problems and their special circumstances—school administrators, teachers and public health officials can change the entire nature of drug-use prevention efforts.

Challenge: Ensure a Drug-Free School Environment

Perhaps the most difficult challenge facing school and administrative personnel is to provide a drug-free environment that reinforces the value of drug avoidance through positive role models and consistent organizational decision making. While the need for this environment may seem obvious, not all schools have policies and practices that ensure a drug-free learning environment.

In many schools, tobacco is freely used by teachers, administrators and the adult public. However, enough is known about the dangers of tobacco smoke, both to the smoker and to those who inhale secondhand smoke, to suggest the restriction of the use of tobacco products on all school property and at all school functions. Such a restriction can also be justified on the basis that tobacco is considered a "gateway" drug. Schools that provide drug-use space (smoking lounges) and drug paraphernalia (ashtrays) paid for with tax dollars might be considered to promote the use of this drug.

In addition, when the National Commission on Drug-Free Schools submitted its final report, one of its major findings was that students in every school the commission visited confirmed what many had feared—that all drugs, from alcohol to crack cocaine, are readily available to anyone who wants them. Actual sales may take place off school grounds, but the campus provides an avenue of marketing, communication and access to the drug market.

Providing a drug-free environment means more than lining the halls with police to deter the illicit drug trade. It means instituting policies and practices that acknowledge the negative impact of all drugs, including tobacco and alcohol, on the learning environment. The most appropriate drug policy for schools is quite simple: a total ban on the use of tobacco, alcohol and other drugs on school property.

School policy can firmly restrict any drug trade on campus. And it can enforce these restrictions by cooperating with law enforcement agencies to prosecute offenders fully. Weak school policies, or policies that remain unenforced, enable young people to begin and continue down the path of drug use.

An example of a firm discipline management plan designed to address drug offenders on campus was developed by a regional educational service center in a mostly rural area of Texas. (See Figure 1.) The plan is firm but compassionate. It emphasizes

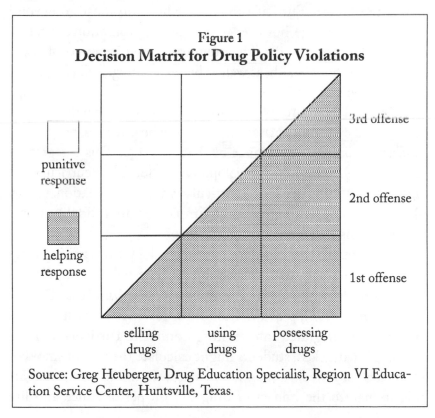

Figure 1
Decision Matrix for Drug Policy Violations

Source: Greg Heuberger, Drug Education Specialist, Region VI Education Service Center, Huntsville, Texas.

helping and punitive responses to violations. By simplifying policy, the students, parents, administrators and teachers all are well aware of the results of drug possession, use or trade on campus.

Challenge: Provide Both Categorical and Integrated Drug Education as a Part of Comprehensive School Health Programs

Even though effectiveness data on programs that focus on knowledge about drugs and the dangers of drug use are discouraging, it essentially remains the role of the school to provide information that students can use as the basis for quality decision making. Deliberate education about drugs through health education remains important. Curricula for drug education must go beyond knowledge exchange, however, to include the promotion of healthy attitudes and social skills. The program should be a part of comprehensive school health, as well as being an integrated element of other subjects.

Repeated exposure to the "no-use" message in English, social studies and even math classes, as well as in health class, only serves to underscore the importance of that message. This integration may mean the continued development of localized curricula designed to meet the needs of a particular student population. It may also mean using, with attention to implementation fidelity, existing programs that have proven effective.

The state of Texas has developed a model for integrating drug education messages with other subjects. The publication, *Education for Self-Responsibility II: Prevention of Drug Use* (Texas Education Agency 1992), provides lessons for teachers of most subjects that can be integrated into existing nonhealth curricula. For example, in math class, students might calculate the cost of smoking cigarettes for a week, a month and a year. In music class, students might analyze the impact of drug use on performance and life expectancy. In vocational education, students might identify the skills needed in the workplace and speculate on the impact alcohol would have on those skills. The Texas model has now been adopted by the state of Oregon, is supported by the U.S. Department of Education, and has been extremely well received by the teachers of Texas.

Even programs using scare tactics may have a place in drug prevention education efforts. Experts in health communication are reevaluating such programs and are finding that scare tactics actually do have an effect on behavior if, and only if, they are accompanied by efficacious means of addressing the threat.

In other words, if a child is given frightening information on the deadly effects of alcohol along with skills on how to avoid an alcohol overdose, the scare may be effective in reducing alcohol consumption. On the other hand, if a child is given frightening information about alcohol without information on avoiding the dangers, the child may deal with the fear by denying its existence.

This denial may be an underlying reason for many adolescents' false belief that "it could never happen to me." These findings present a challenge to health educators who have for years rejected any form of scare tactics when dealing with drug use. Perhaps the time has come to reconsider the value of such tactics (Witte, 1992).

Challenge: Target the Middle School Years

Educators have just begun to understand how important the middle school years are in determining the quality of life of young people. The Carnegie Foundation's 1989 publication *Turning Points* prompted considerable excitement on the part of educators nationwide. That excitement arose from a growing confidence that an informed leadership in education and health could not continue to ignore the special needs of middle school youth.

The document was named *Turning Points* because many educators believe the middle school years represent a "turning point" toward either a diminished future or a productive life. Studies on the initiation of drug use bear out this thesis; many students begin using drugs during this period. (See Figure 2.)

Turning Points concluded, among other things, that "a volatile mismatch exists between the organization and curriculum of middle-grade schools and the intellectual, emotional, and interpersonal needs of young adolescents." As might be expected, this

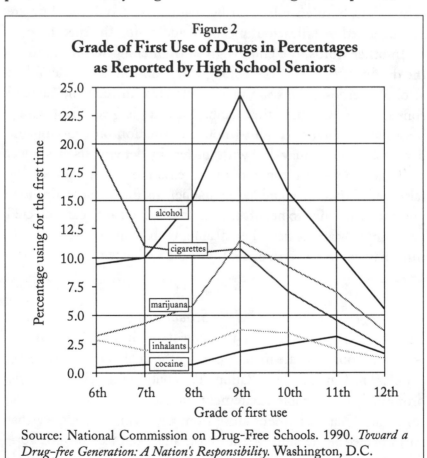

Figure 2
Grade of First Use of Drugs in Percentages as Reported by High School Seniors

Source: National Commission on Drug-Free Schools. 1990. *Toward a Drug-free Generation: A Nation's Responsibility.* Washington, D.C.

publication and several companion publications gave particular emphasis to the need for drug-use prevention efforts targeted at this age group.

Several other reports and publications from highly respected professional and governmental organizations also call for change in our response to the health needs of middle school youth. *Code Blue* (National Commission on the Role of the School and the Community in Improving Adolescent Health, 1990), *The Health/ Education Connection* (American Association of Colleges for Teacher Education et al., 1991), and *Healthy People 2000: National Health Promotion and Disease Prevention Objectives* (U.S. Department of Health and Human Services, 1991) represent collaborative efforts by health and education professionals to study and recommend future directions for serving the needs of our youth.

In sum, these publications detail a crisis situation for today's middle school child and suggest that we have little choice but to reform education. The momentum for middle school educational reform is great. The challenge is to keep the health of the child, and particularly drug-use prevention goals, in the forefront as these reforms come about.

Challenge: Provide Alternatives to Drug Abuse

A challenge to communities as a whole is to provide drug-free alternatives to youth who are most at risk for drug abuse. As school budgets shrink and as teachers and administrators come under increasing pressure to improve student scores on standardized examinations, it may be easy to cut programs that are considered extracurricular or are specially designed to target high-risk students.

But research suggests that instead of cutting extra programs, the number and type of drug-free extracurricular activities available to young people should be increased. Some of the greatest

Pruitt

documented successes in drug prevention education have provided opportunities for academic achievement and extracurricular involvement as alternatives to drug abuse. This challenge presents an opportunity to involve community organizations, local health departments, churches, civic groups, and ad hoc organizations in the effort to prevent drug use.

Challenge: Honestly Examine Effectiveness

One of the most interesting findings of the Bangert-Drowns (1988) meta-analysis was not what was included in the study, but what was missing. In an analysis of drug prevention programs that spanned more than fifteen years, Bangert-Drowns found that fewer than twenty programs qualified for inclusion, because so few programs had collected precise effectiveness data. During that period, hundreds, perhaps thousands, of programs were in use, many sponsored with tax dollars, but very few apparently stopped to consider whether they were accomplishing anything.

Health education researchers must ask, Do these programs work? Current findings raise more questions concerning the effectiveness of drug-use prevention efforts. Some of these efforts are known to be basically ineffective in changing drug-use behavior, but they continue to be promoted because they are appropriate school activities or because they are endorsed by a strong political faction within a community. Some are thought to be effective if presented appropriately, but upon close examination are often found to have been presented inappropriately. Some are known to be effective with low-risk students, yet are used extensively with high-risk populations. Some are known to be effective with high-risk youth, but are not available due to high program cost.

Some drug-use prevention efforts tend to reinforce the protective factors that are already in place; those based on the simplistic concept "just say no" may reinforce what many children are hear-

368

The Comprehensive School Health Challenge

ing at home. For high-risk children, however, who are hearing and seeing just the opposite at home, such programs may be laughable. Obviously, the evaluation of drug-use prevention programs is complex. It does not lend itself to simple methods, any more than the problems related to drug use lend themselves to simple answers.

An examination of program effectiveness is of no use unless sustained efforts are evaluated. Long-term vision is needed to address the drug-related problems of the nation's schools. The patchwork, emergency-like programming that has characterized drug education and prevention over the years is not enough.

There is a need to collect data, implement programs and collect more data over a period of years. Then programs can be revised to make them more effective, instead of relying on the "purchase and discard" approach that currently typifies drug education.

Nothing can be gained by ignoring research on program effectiveness. Likewise, nothing can be gained by saying drug education simply cannot be evaluated. Assessing the effectiveness of drug education programs will not be easy, but it is a challenge that health education must face. Educators must accept the challenge and work to find new ideas and new programs along the way.

Challenge: Have Realistic Expectations

Everyone has an opinion about drug education, and quite often that opinion includes the idea that schools should do more to prevent children from using drugs. But is it realistic to place the burden of drug-use prevention entirely on schools? All too often, public opinion, the opinion of program planners, public health officials, and even drug educators reflects unrealistic expectations of drug education.

School-based substance-use prevention programs, including drug education curricula, should be examined in a societal context. Drug problems are not unique to the young. Adults, including parents, are clearly a part of the environment that supports drug use. Schools cannot control the behavior of parents.

Consequently, both educators and the public need to recognize that drug prevention programs in the schools are not a panacea for society's drug problems. While we can aspire to "drug-free" schools, we cannot continue to expect that school-based drug-use prevention programs will change society as a whole.

Looking Forward

Educators are beginning to understand both how drug-use prevention efforts have failed and how they have succeeded. It would be wrong to abandon programs simply because ill-conceived evaluation strategies suggest their ineffectiveness. Likewise, it would be wrong to deter creative energies directed only toward demonstrated success.

Successes in this area have not been so great that anyone can claim to have found the answer. However, the failures have not been so dramatic as to suggest giving up on traditional drug prevention programs. The challenge remaining for health and education professionals is immense. As we continue our endeavors in this relatively uncharted field of drug-use prevention education, perhaps our best strategy is a simple one: Keep going.

References

American Association of Colleges for Teacher Education, American Academy of Pediatrics, and the Maternal and Child Health Bureau, U.S. Department of Health and Human Services. 1990. *The health/education connection: Initiating dialogue on integrated services to children at risk and their families.* Alexandria, VA.

American School Health Association, Association for the Advancement of Health Education and Society for Public Health Education. 1989. *National adolescent student health survey: A report on the health of America's youth.* Oakland, CA: Third Party Press.

Bangert-Drowns, R. L. 1988. The effects of school-based substance abuse education: A meta-analysis. *Journal of Drug Education* 18:243-264.

Benard, B. F., and J. Perone. 1987. Knowing what to do—and not to do— reinvigorates drug education. *ASCD Curriculum Update.* Alexandria, VA: Association for Supervision and Curriculum Development.

Carnegie Council on Adolescent Development. 1989. *Turning points: Preparing American youth for the 21st century.* Washington, DC.

Carnegie Council on Adolescent Development. 1990. *At the threshold: The developing adolescent.* Washington, DC.

Carnegie Council on Adolescent Development. 1992. *Fateful choices: Healthy youth for the 21st century.* Washington, DC.

Hawkins, J. D., D. M. Lishner, R. F. Catalano and M. O. Howard. 1986. *Childhood predictors of adolescent substance abuse: Toward an empirically grounded theory.* New York: Haworth Press.

Johnston, L. D., P. M. O'Malley and J. G. Bachman. 1989. *Drug use, drinking, and smoking: National survey from high school, college, and young adults populations 1975-1988.* Rockville, MD: National Institute on Drug Abuse.

National Commission on Drug-Free Schools. 1990. *Toward a drug-free generation: A nation's responsibility.* Washington, DC.

National Commission on Marijuana and Drug Abuse. 1973. *Drug use in America: Problem in perspective.* Washington, DC.

National Commission on the Role of the School and Community in Improving Adolescent Health. 1990. *Code blue: Uniting for healthier youth.* Alexandria, VA.

National Education Goals Panel. 1991. *The national education goals report: Building a nation of learners.* Washington, DC.

Newcomb, M. D., and P. M. Bentler. 1989. Substance use and abuse among children and teenagers. *American Psychologist* 44:242-248.

Office of Technology Assessment, Congress of the United States. 1991. *Adolescent health: Summary and policy options.* Washington, DC.

Pruitt, B. E., P. M. Kingery, E. Mirzaee, G. Heuberger and R. S. Hurley. 1991. Peer influence and drug use among adolescents in rural areas. *Journal of Drug Education* 21:1-11.

Texas Education Agency. 1992. *Education for self-responsibility II: Prevention of drug use.* Austin, TX.

Tobler, N. S. 1986. Meta-analysis of 143 adolescent drug prevention programs: Quantitative outcome results of program participants compared to a control or comparison group. *Journal of Drug Issues* 16:537-564.

U.S. Department of Health and Human Services, Public Health Service. 1991. *Healthy people 2000: National health promotion and disease prevention objectives.* DHHS Publication No. (PHS) 91-50212. Washington, DC.

Witte, K. 1992. Putting the fear back into fear appeals: The extended parallel process model. *Communication Monographs* 59:329-349.

Chapter 15

Nutrition Issues

Gail C. Frank, DrPH, RD, CHES

An overriding issue in child nutrition is the lack of acceptance of two concepts—first, that eating behavior influences health, and, second, that eating behavior in childhood initiates adolescent and adult eating patterns. Many parents and other adults are responsible for food services to children. They must understand and acknowledge the benefits of good nutrition, which include prevention of cancer, heart disease, obesity and osteoporosis, for the long-term health of a child. Adults must integrate facts and recommendations about nutrition into their meal planning and nutrition education programs.

The major child nutrition responsibility of schools is two-fold: first, to protect the health and well-being of students with whole-some foods, and, second, to provide an enjoyable environment that makes healthful foods accessible to all children. Coordinating classroom learning with cafeteria decision making and supporting inservice training for child nutrition employees and teachers are of paramount importance.

The following groups are key national players in child nutrition at schools:
- the U.S. Department of Agriculture (USDA) and its Nutrition Education and Training Program (NETP), National School Lunch Program (NSLP), School Breakfast Program (SBP) and commodity programs
- the American School Food Service Association (ASFSA)
- the School Nutrition Services Dietetic Practice Group of the American Dietetic Association (ADA)
- state child nutrition directors
- food manufacturers

These groups are responsible for informing legislators of the needs and priorities for effective and efficient child nutrition programs across the United States. As child nutrition is integrated into comprehensive school health, the Centers for Disease Control and Prevention and other national survey and professional organizations become more and more important.

The complications and real challenges for child nutrition programs include:
- integrating national nutrition directives into programs
- developing and structuring programs for success
- targeting modifiable variables

Direct services must be incorporated for children at high nutritional risk, from the hungry to the obese. These services must address the needs of children in all ethnic groups and in all age groups from lower elementary through high school. Evaluations must be planned into all programs and reported in a timely fashion.

Key Terms and Acronyms

ADA — American Dietetic Association
ASFSA — American School Food Service Association
NETP — Nutrition Education and Training Program
NSLP — National School Lunch Program
SBP — School Breakfast Program
USDA — U.S. Department of Agriculture
RDAs — Recommended Dietary Allowances
cancer
cholesterol
iron deficiency anemia
obesity
primary prevention
the Food Guide Pyramid
reimbursable meal pattern

Schools' Responsibility for Sound Nutrition

In 1946, Public Law 79-396 created the National School Lunch Act for the purpose of protecting the health and well-being of the nation's children. The act directs local school districts to serve lunches without cost or at a reduced cost to any child who is unable to pay the full cost. Schools use surplus commodities when possible in meal planning and do not discriminate against any child who is unable to pay a full price.

The Child Nutrition Act of 1966 (Public Law 89-642) authorized the School Breakfast Program as a pilot program. The program was extended to all schools using grants-in-aid in 1975. During the 1970s, legislation improved the quality of meals, emphasized nutrition education and enlarged coverage of programming. The Omnibus Budget Reconciliation Act of 1981 (Public Law 97-35) targeted benefits based on need and improved program management and accountability at the local schoolsite level.

The Food and Nutrition Service (FNS) of the USDA implements programs legislated by Congress. It establishes regulations, policies and guidelines about school foods and monitors program performance. In addition, the service provides program and administrative funds to states via seven regional offices. States generally assign the responsibility for program administration to the state educational agency, e.g., the state department of education, which assists local school districts by establishing fiscal recordkeeping systems and monitoring performance. The individual school is responsible for the actual preparation of nutritious meals and serving those meals to children.

The Reimbursable Meal Pattern

The National School Lunch Program has nutritional requirements for lunches served to children. Generally, lunches provide one-third of a child's age-specific RDAs. RDAs are set for energy, protein, ten vitamins and seven minerals. Minimum requirements are set for sodium, chloride and potassium. RDAs are the quantitative standards for planning nutritionally adequate breakfast and lunch menus, but other government directives, such as the *Surgeon General's Report on Nutrition and Health* (U.S. Department of Health and Human Services, 1988) and *Nutrition and Your Health: Dietary Guidelines for Americans* (U.S. Department of Agriculture and U.S. Department of Health and Human Services, 1988), provide the qualitative canvas for planning meals for children.

Recent federal directives identify the *Dietary Guidelines for Americans* as the basis for all child nutrition program menu-planning activities. The *Menu Planning Guide for School Food Service* and the new publication *Nutrition Guidance for the Child Nutrition Programs* identify the guidelines as the basis for the *quality* of the menu and recommend, "Keep fat, sugar, and salt in school lunches and breakfasts at a moderate level."

USDA program guidelines define a four-component meal pattern that must be offered to children in the minimum amounts for their age. The components are meat or meat alternate, vegetables and fruits, whole-grain or enriched bread or bread alternate, and fluid milk. This regulation must be met at all meals, and is the basis of partial reimbursement to the school.

Schools can add foods to the required servings at their own discretion. An "offer vs. serve" parameter is now extended to all elementary, junior and senior high students (Public Law 97-35). Under this parameter, schools must offer five items but students can select three. New FNS regulations allow students to request smaller portions of food items than the amount defined in the five-item pattern. Previously, this request was not allowed.

The School Breakfast Program (SBP) regulations do not define specific nutrient goals, but planning is guided by the RDAs. The accepted nutrient content for breakfast is one-fifth to one-fourth of the student's RDAs. Menu planners choose portions of the meal components—meat or meat alternate, fruit, whole-grain or enriched bread or bread alternate, and fluid milk—to meet nutrient requirements.

Nutrition education has been a mission of school food service since the 1940s, when a total school program was defined as one in which students learned the relationship between food, nutrition and health. Public Law 91-248, enacted in 1970, was the first federal legislation to specify nutrition education provisions that authorized training school food service workers in nutrition. Public Law 95-166 established the Nutrition Education and Training Program (NETP) in 1977. This program gave new impetus not only to teaching children the value of a nutritionally balanced diet through positive daily lunchroom experience and classroom reinforcement, but also to training teachers and school food service personnel to implement programs. The NETP funding is decentralized; state departments of education direct the awarding and evaluation of programs. (See Chapter 10 for more discussion of school food services.)

The School Eating Environment

Students may have 12 to 25 minutes for lunch. In this time, they must obtain their meal, find a place to sit, eat, socialize and discard waste. This rushed environment decreases chances for optimal food intake.

Meal monitors are employed in some schools as "traffic" and "time keepers." If their efforts are positive and not demeaning for students, a receptive environment occurs. Some schools even present lunch as a pleasant social time with music and citizenship awards for clean-up and manners.

Student meal acceptance has usually been based on plate waste. To lower plate waste, menu planners have developed potato, salad and sandwich bars as enticements to participate. Youth advisory groups have been devised by the ASFSA to bring students into the planning, tasting and decision-making process (American School Food Service Association, 1990).

The multicultural environments of many schools today require school foods that are diverse in taste and enhance the cultural pride of the students. To increase acceptability, cultural foods should be incorporated into school menus. However, with Westernization, many of the benefits of nutritious foods from different cultures have been lost. For example, tofu may be deleted from Asian dishes, and high fiber ingredients may be left out of salads and vegetables of the Middle East. Individual student tastes and cultural practices have been shaped by societal norms and food preparation practices.

Children are receptive to change. To see the association between children's reported acceptance of foods and the frequency
with which they ate them, a study identified the top five school
lunch entrees for fifth and sixth grade students in the ABC
Unified School District in Los Angeles County (Hong et al.,
1992). The 172 students were 30 percent Hispanic, 30 percent
Asian, 30 percent White and 10 percent Portuguese, East Indian
and other. A significant Pearson correlation coefficient was noted
between both the acceptance and the frequency of eating certain
routine entrees and a new recipe for a lowfat Chinese meat bun
that substituted tofu for beef. As the data in Figure 1 indicate, the
new recipe was as acceptable as the routine entrees. When given
culturally diverse foods, culturally diverse children select and eat
them, as noted by the high "r" values, or correlations, and the high
"p" values.

Several education/demonstration studies have successfully reduced the fat and saturated fat content of school recipes. The "Go
for Health" program focused on influencing the student environment by enhancing physical activity classes and by lowering the fat
and sodium content of school lunches. In select schools, total fat
was lowered by 16 percent, saturated fat by 32 percent and sodium

---

Figure 1
Association Between Acceptance and Frequency of Eating
Pearson Correlation Coefficient

Entree	r Value
nacho beef and cheese	0.739
pepperoni pizza	0.753
spaghetti	0.739
chicken chunks	0.717
diced turkey	0.786
Chinese meat bun	0.850
(All p < 0.001)	

by 54 percent. Dietary recalls óf students indicated that they consumed fewer calories, total fat and sodium than students not offered the modified menus (Simons-Morton, 1991).

The "Heart Smart" program developed a complementary approach for cardiovascular health promotion. The school cafeteria and classroom were effective vehicles to translate reduced fat, sodium and sugar content of menus into acceptable foods (Frank et al., 1989a).

Food Service and Classroom Education

In a survey of 407 fourth- to eighth-grade students, 94 percent thought that the food they eat can affect their future health. Ninety-nine percent understood the importance of exercise for good health, 80 percent could identify three of the four food groups then being taught, and 98 percent recognized the importance of eating plenty of fruits, vegetables and high-fiber foods (National Center for Nutrition and Dietetics and International Food Information Counicl, 1991c).

Simply knowing about fruits, vegetables and fiber isn't enough to make individuals eat more of these foods, however. Since students report that their primary sources of nutrition information are schools (95 percent), parents (86 percent) and health professions (73 percent), schools need to be actively involved in nutrition education (National Center for Nutrition and Dietetics and International Food Information Counicl, 1991d). Surveys support nutrition education as an acceptable method for reducing population risk factors for chronic disease. Such education provides a less expensive approach to improving nutrition than medical and clinical strategies (Levy, Iverson and Walberg, 1980). In a 1989 survey, 76 percent of the grocery shoppers surveyed stated that nutrition is a very important factor when they choose food. Fat, salt and cholesterol content were their major concerns (Food Marketing Institute, 1989). High interest in nutrition emphasizes the relevance of nutrition education for children about healthy food selections.

The "Food for Thought, All About Nutrition and You!" program in a Palm Beach school district revealed that 10 percent of children were either underweight or overweight. Age-appropriate nutrition education activities were placed in the curriculum, and students prepared healthy snacks in the classroom. An increased acceptance of vegetables, skim milk and other foods that had been used during class were noted by the child nutrition employees in the cafeteria. The majority of teachers, principals and students wanted to continue the program the following year, and test packets were distributed to other district schools (Dubinsky and Bodner, 1991).

The earlier we integrate nutrition education into the classroom, the more likely students will practice healthy eating behaviors. The "FUN KIT" developed in the Portland Public Schools packages nutrition education for preschoolers with puppets, music cassettes and stickers. The aim of the FUN KIT is to coordinate classroom nutrition education, healthful school meals and family participation (Portland Public Schools, 1989).

Training Food Service Personnel and Classroom Teachers
The ability of school cafeterias to link with classroom education is often determined by the skill of the child nutrition employees and the food service delivery system. A centralized service provides preparation of all food in a central kitchen, often using a "cook-chill" process. Food is transported daily to specific school sites, where it is refrigerated and then heated prior to serving. This system provides a unique opportunity to train a kitchen staff and influence thousands of meals daily prior to distribution. Major concerns are that the foods are often purchased pre-portioned and

the cooking equipment is automated in an assembly line. Menu changes must fit into the equipment and production process and the food specifications required of food companies.

In decentralized service, all food is prepared on each school campus under the supervision of a site manager. This type of program creates a sense of ownership by the staff. Training at the site involves identification of the readiness of each employee. Employees may be responsible for only single types of foods, e.g., the baker, the main entree cook. For this type of service, training is directed toward skill development of the different preparation positions.

For either delivery system, point-of-choice nutrition information can be placed adjacent to foods to complement classroom education. For example, a label could read, "Tossed Salad with Flaked Tuna, 1 and 1/2 cup, 144 calories, 241 RE vitamin A, 36 mg vitamin C," or "Hamburger on Whole Wheat Bun: 266 calories, 41% fat, 362 mg sodium." This type of information has been used to guide individuals in making healthy food choices with comparisons and nutrient information (Cinciripini, 1984; Schmitz and Fielding, 1990; Davis-Chervin, Rogers and Clark, 1984; Anderson and Haas, 1990). Color-coding, such as a stop light, has been effective with children (Simons-Morton et al., 1991).

Since school menus are increasingly being evaluated by a nutrient standard, computerized databases are now being used by employees. Increasing the technical skills of child nutrition employees can be accomplished by integrating the computer training into routine procedures. Many programs are available, such as Computrition, Inc., DINE Systems or NutriKids (Computrition, 1992; Dennison, Dennison and Frank, 1992; LunchByte, 1993; Frank, 1985). Each system has unique characteristics, ranging from extensive food production, purchasing and inventory programs on Computrition to evaluation by USDA meal components on NutriKids.

NutriKids is a food database designed specifically for child nutrition programs. It contains more than 3,400 common ingredients and 240 USDA recipes. The DINE System has more than 4,000 foods. It produces a printout with an overall menu score based on consensus dietary recommendations, e.g., less than 30 percent fat and less than 3,300 mg of sodium (Dennison, Dennison and Frank, 1993; Frank, 1985).

Community Partnerships

Developing partnerships with the community is a growing trend for child nutrition directors. A community advisory group of eight to twelve members can consist of a community leader; a local pediatrician; a grocery store owner; a restaurant owne; an American Cancer Society or American Heart Association representative; an elementary school teacher; a newspaper; radio or TV reporter; a clergyperson; a health agency representative; a local nutritionist; and/or a popular personality. The advisory group can respond to the program philosophy, needs, progress and any changes in format. This group can reinforce and publicize positive efforts in child nutrition programs.

Conversely, child nutrition directors and the nutrition education specialists they employ can serve as nutrition resources for the media and community health efforts. For example, Connie Evers, MS, RD, is a specialist with the Portland Public Schools who periodically writes a column focusing on child nutrition for the *Portland Oregonian*. Unfortunately, only 8 percent of child nutrition directors employ such a specialist, often due to lack of funds (Frank and Desai, 1992).

National Directions

The USDA and its regional offices provide the major direction and impetus for school food programs. The nutritional well-being of children is influenced by USDA's acceptance and integration of national nutrition directives into its own programs. USDA oversees the commodity program that provides surplus foods to schools annually. The trend has been to provide healthier commodities to schools that need the price break that commodities offer. For example, in 1970, American cheese, ground beef with fat not to exceed 30 percent, fruit packed in heavy syrup, and hydrogenated vegetable fat were common commodities. These items have been replaced with mozzarella cheese, ground beef with fat not to exceed 22 percent and soybean salad oil. Today, ground turkey, extra-lean frozen beef patties and diced chicken appear on the commodity list, along with processed cheese with reduced sodium, sliced peaches in light syrup, and almond butter. Changes are still needed, but improvements in commodities are evident.

The ASFSA and its state chapters support a 65,000 national membership. The association is the mouthpiece for child nutrition professionals, with active lobbying efforts in Congress. In 1992 and 1993, efforts were directed toward universal feeding and increasing participation in NSLP, breakfast and summer feeding programs.

The ADA and the School Food Services Dietetic Practice Group are major professional organizations of registered dietitians employed in school systems. In addition, many food companies employ registered dietitians who manage complete health care lines and specialty lines for schools, e.g., S. E. Rycoff, Arrow-Sysco and ConAgra. Child nutrition directors and managers work directly with the food companies to achieve lower fat, sodium and sugar products for their menus.

Many nonprofit organizations have programs available to schools. The American Heart Association and the American Cancer Association have each developed excellent nutrition education materials, such as *Changing the Course, Early Start* and *Heart Works*. Working collaboratively with these organizations and professional volunteers can be advantageous to schools with budget restrictions. Continuing education hours can be accrued for teachers and child nutrition employees. Additionally, complete up-to-date and effective curricula from these organizations can link classroom education with the cafeteria and tap parents and community resources.

The Association of State School Nutrition Directors and Supervisors meets annually to update programs on USDA guidelines and pending national legislation affecting school meals, to discuss innovations, and to provide continuing education. These directors oversee all USDA food programs in schools and daycare facilities in their respective states.

Major Nutrition Initiatives

Several objectives in *Healthy People 2000* (U.S. Department of Health and Human Services, 1990) set the nutrition agenda for schools. (See Figure 2.) The Pediatric Panel Report of the National Cholesterol Education Program (NCEP) underscores these objectives for children two years and older by recommending maintenance of a healthy body weight and an eating pattern with less than 30 percent of total energy as fat, 10 percent as saturated fat, and less than 300 mg of cholesterol per day (NCEP, 1991). This pattern requires a high complex-carbohydrate intake, not only to reach the lower fat composition, but also to achieve adequate calories for growth and development of children.

A fiber recommendation for children is needed, yet is only speculative at this time. Fiber intake of ten-year-old children in the Bogalusa Heart Study from 1973 to 1982 averaged 4 to 5 g. A 25/25 standard has been suggested, i.e., 25 percent of the total energy intake for children as fat and 25 grams of fiber per day (Wynder, Weisburger and Ng, 1992). An increase in complex

---

Figure 2
Healthy People 2000 **Objectives Relevant for Child Nutrition in Schools**

2.10 To reduce iron deficiency to less than 3% among children ages 1 through 4 and among women of childbearing age.

2.17 To increase to 90% the proportion of school lunch and breakfast service and child care food services with menus that are consistent with the *Dietary Guidelines for Americans.*

2.19 To increase to at least 75% the proportion of the Nation's schools that provide nutrition education from preschool through 12th grade, preferably as part of quality school health education.

2.3 To reduce overweight to a prevalence of no more than 15% among adolescents ages 12 through 19.

2.5 To reduce dietary fat intake to an average of 30% of calories or less and average saturated fat intake to less than 10% of calories among people age 2 and older.

2.6 To increase complex carbohydrate and fiber-containing foods in the diets of adults to 5 or more daily servings for vegetables (including legumes) and fruits, and to 6 or more daily servings for grain products.

2.7 To increase to at least 50% the proportion of overweight people age 12 and older who have adopted sound dietary practices combined with regular physical activity to attain an appropriate body weight.

2.8 To increase calcium intake so at least 50% of youth ages 12 through 24 and 50% of pregnant and lactating women consume 3 or more servings daily of foods rich in calcium, and at least 50% of people age 25 and older consume 2 or more servings daily.

Source: U.S. Department of Health and Human Services, Public Health Service. *Healthy People 2000.* DHHS Publication No. 91-50212. Washington, DC.

carbohydrate to achieve a 30 percent or lower fat-eating pattern naturally creates a high fiber eating pattern.

The USDA *Pyramid Guide to Eating* (1992) is the visual presentation of the dietary guidelines. Fats, oils and sweets are at the tip of the pyramid, followed by lowfat meat and dairy products. Whole grain starches, breads and cereals, fruits and vegetables form the bottom segments signifying more servings for a healthier food pattern. The Pyramid Guide conveys three important concepts:

1. Balance foods higher in nutrients with those lower in nutrients.
2. Choose a variety of foods each day.
3. Eat moderate portions of foods.

The Pyramid Guide was preceded in 1989 by California's Assembly Bill 2109. This bill mandated the California Department of Education to develop nutrition guidelines for all food and beverages sold on school campuses in California. The *Nutrition Guidelines for California School Foods* (California Department of Education, 1991) presented a three-tiered approach to dietary modification of lunch and breakfast menus. Each level reduces fat content and increases fiber content through an increase in whole-grain foods, fruits and vegetables. (See Figure 3.)

Tier 1 has the least change. At this level, modification occurs primarily in the quality of the food that children receive—for example, fresh fruit rather than canned or whole-grain bread rather than plain white bread. *Tier 2* decreases the quantities of certain foods and replaces them with increased quantities of others to maintain the calories children need for energy and growth. For example, less butter is used on vegetables, and gravies and rich desserts, which add calories primarily in the form of fat, are served less frequently. Lower-fat forms of meat, cheese, milk and desserts are used. Calories are increased by adding servings of bread and bread alternates and fruits and vegetables.

Figure 3

Three-Tiered Approach to Menu Planning in Child Nutrition Programs Following the Nutrition Guidelines for California School Foods.

Component	Tier 1		Tier 2		Tier 3	
	Grade K-3	Grade 4-12	Grade K-3	Grade 4-12	Grade K-3	Grade 4-12
Fruit or Vegetable • offer fresh produce whenever possible	1/2 cup (at least 1/4 cup fresh 3 times/week)	3/4 cup (at least 1/4 cup fresh 3 times/week)	3/4 cup (at least 1/4 cup fresh 5 times/week)	1 cup (at least 1/4 cup fresh 5 times/week)	1 cup (at least 1/4 cup fresh daily)	1-1/4 cup (at least 1/4 cup fresh daily)
Meat/Meat Alternate (M/MA)** • emphasize lean and lower sodium choices • serve beans as meat/meat alternate at least once a week	1-1/2 oz. (at least 1/4 cup beans/week = 1/2 oz. M/MA)	2 oz. (at least 1/4 cup beans/week = 1/2 oz. M/MA)	1-1/2 oz. (at least 1/2 cup beans/week)	2 oz. (at least 1/2 cup beans/week)	1-1/2 oz. (at least 1/2 cup beans/week)	1-1/2 oz.** (at least 1/2 cup beans/week)
Bread/Bread Alternate (B/BA) • emphasize whole grain products	2/day or 10/week (at least 3 servings/week are whole grain or all B/BAs contain at least 25% whole grain)	2/day or 10/week (at least 3 servings/week are whole grain or all B/BAs contain at least 25% whole grain)	2/day or 12/week (at least 5 servings/week are whole grain or all B/BAs contain at least 33% whole grain)	2/day or 12/week (at least 5 servings/week are whole grain or all B/BAs contain at least 33% whole grain)	2/day or 12/week (at least 1 serving/day is whole grain or all B/BAs contain at least 33% whole grain)	3/day or 15/week (at least 1 serving/day is whole grain or all B/BAs contain at least 33% whole grain) (1 serving may be a "healthy" dessert)
Milk • offer lower-fat choices	8 oz.	8 oz.	8 oz.	8 oz.	8 oz.	8 oz.

* Refer to California Daily Food Guide (California Department of Health Services, 1990) for specific food suggestions.
** Requires prior approval from USDA to decrease M/MA.

Source: California Department of Education. 1991. *The Nutrition Guidelines for California School Foods.* Sacramento, CA.

Tier 3 has the greatest change. This is the last step for increasing servings of beans, fruits and vegetables. All high-fat desserts are replaced with fresh fruits; whole-grain breads are served; and minimal fat is added in cooking. Reaching this tier achieves the nutrition guidelines for child nutrition programs. Nutrient content at this level reflects 30 to 35 percent of the total calories as fat and one-third of the RDAs for vitamins and minerals with moderation of sodium and sugar.

The eating pattern identified in California's nutrition guidelines is based on the *California Daily Food Guide* (California Department of Health Services, 1990), currently used by California for all nutrition programs. The guide provides quantitative, lifecycle dietary recommendations with ethnic-, age- and gender-specific food guides. This guide provides continuity for programs and for the public. If the pattern is followed in childhood, transition to adolescence and adulthood is easier and probable. The California guide and the Pyramid Guide are complementary.

Challenges

Many factors provide challenges to child nutrition programs. There are a variety of ways to address these challenges.

Impact of Funding Sources. School districts receive USDA funding for meals that are served according to USDA menu standards. Milk yields an additional reimbursement. Each district should work to increase its reimbursement rate by offering nutritious meals and promoting participation by students through marketing to parents. Schools can choose whether to participate in the School Breakfast Program; however, with hungry and high-risk children slipping through the cracks, schools should ensure that their policies allow all children access to the SBP, the NSLP and the Summer Food Service Program.

Healthy E.D.G.E. The ASFSA offers an initiative called *Healthy E.D.G.E.: Eating, the Dietary Guidelines and Education.* This initiative focuses first on team building in schools and communities to help incorporate the *Dietary Guidelines for Americans* as part of the school policy. It also emphasizes activities that will effectively improve the nutritional health of students (ASFSA, 1991). It is the impetus for child nutrition employees to practice healthy menu planning for school children.

Child Nutrition as a Component of Comprehensive School Health. Comprehensive school health is based on a planned, sequential pre-kindergarten through twelfth grade curriculum that addresses the physical, mental, emotional and social dimensions of the child (Allensworth and Kolbe, 1987). Child nutrition and food service is one of the eight major comprehensive school health components. School cafeterias and campus food sales are a primary prevention arena—a learning laboratory for children, where demonstration and education studies can be conducted to evaluate menu changes and student acceptability (Frank, Vaden and Martin, 1987). With national efforts to legislate comprehensive school health in our schools, support for this initiative strengthens each component, e.g., child nutrition, physical education, and its respective programs.

Professional Development. The ASFSA has a strong commitment to continuing education addressing sanitation, safety, meal planning and health promotion in schools. School districts should support the food service staff and share expenses in training and upgrading this aspect of the school environment. Often child nutrition employees are at the low end of pay scales; their work may be seen as tertiary to education and physical fitness. Such an attitude is demeaning and unnecessary. No hungry or malnourished child can think, concentrate and participate at his or her fullest potential, and well-trained child nutrition employees provide the programs that protect children against hunger and malnutrition.

A statewide census of training needs queried 547 directors and 1,266 managers in California (Frank et al., 1992). "Training programs" was reported as the number one influence on career development. "Food preparation" and "healthy menu planning" were the two future courses respondents felt would be "most helpful" in their daily work. On-the-job training was the most common form of training, and respondents preferred either their school site or their district office for training.

To train child nutrition employees in healthy menu planning, *Shaping Healthy Meals for School Children* was developed as a ten-lesson curriculum to be taught in the train-the-trainer format (Frank and Desai, 1992). This curriculum uses the California Daily Food Guide and has been approved for continued education units by the California School Food Service Association. The curriculum integrates several worksheets from the American Cancer Society's cafeteria training manual, *Changing the Course*. It is only one of several excellent "hands-on" curricula available to schools

Cafeteria intervention in the form of inservice training can follow a population approach and be given to all participating schools in a district or to multiple districts in a county. Training in school districts must be formalized in a consistent, sequential manner, such as monthly or bimonthly, even though it is seldom done. A train-the-trainer format strengthens the likelihood that the school district will sustain the program. This format identifies employees to be trained who then become trainers for their peers.

Applying National Directives
An action plan to adapt child nutrition programs to achieve *Healthy People 2000* objectives should be dominated by the RDAs, the Pyramid Guide and the NCEP recommendations. These

directives, if achieved, could reduce eating disorders, promote healthy weight management, reduce nutrient imbalance, enhance nutrition education in the classroom, and ensure that healthy and acceptable meal planning occurs in schools.

The PRECEDE model for school health intervention (Green et al., 1980) can serve as a blueprint for developing an action plan. It addresses predisposing, enabling and reinforcing factors in schools. Predisposing factors are the demographic and population norms, which are often beyond the scope of a program and are not modifiable. Increasing fruit and vegetable intake in the population would establish a new preferred norm. Enabling factors include availability and accessibility in the school, such as the cafeteria, vending machines and campus stores. Reinforcing factors include attitudes and behaviors of peers, teachers, administrators and media that either support or discourage behavioral change. Child nutrition program directors can structure their action plans on the PRECEDE model and reduce unknowns, thereby focusing their energies and budgets on specific modifiable factors.

The nutrition plight of many children, however, must be addressed. Direct services are essential in some settings to complement meals and education at school. For example, the 1992-1993 "Healthy Start Initiative" in California will ultimately provide immediate care clinics on school grounds for high-risk populations. This approach must be mandated nationally. Nutrition should be visible and incorporated from the start as a direct service, especially when obesity, anorexia nervosa, iron deficiency anemia, lead poisoning, hunger and nutrient imbalances are prevalent.

As changes occur in child nutrition programs, actions must be monitored to identify what works and what does not work. Often child nutrition programs lack sufficient evaluation. Evaluation is crucial if major issues are to be corrected. Implementation and process evaluation can include questionnaire and observational measures to assess the program operation. Outcome evaluation can include questionnaires and observational methods to assess program effects on food consumption and nutrient outcome.

A "Meal Quality Assessment Instrument" developed by the California Department of Education requires fifteen to twenty minutes of direct observation and marking on a Scantron form by an observer (Frank, 1992). It tracks qualitative changes in menus. Pre- and post-tests of five to ten items can be used at each training class and summed to establish baseline knowledge of employees (Frank et al., 1989a).

A Basic Nutrition Knowledge Questionnaire with ten to twenty-five items can be developed for students to identify specific groups and knowledge of the role of foods in chronic disease prevention, food misconceptions and perceptions of nutrition messages in the media. Attitudinal questionnaires can focus on student likes and dislikes, such as fruits and vegetables or high-fat and protein foods. Scales using facial expressions are helpful when assessing attitudes of younger children. Behavior can be measured with food records or specific instruments such as the Fat Avoidance Scale or a Food Frequency chart (Frank et al., 1989b; Frank et al., 1992; Block, 1989).

Students' Nutritional Health

The nutritional health of students is a vital consideration in planning child nutrition programs. A student's health depends on the foods ingested and how the body uses them.

Growth and Development
Growth and development are monitored by two common nutritional indicators, height and weight. Many U.S. students today tend to exist at one of the extremes, either too heavy or too light

for age or height. Children who exceed the recommended weight by 15 percent are considered overweight; those who exceed it by 20 percent are considered obese. Excess weight predisposes children to high blood cholesterol and sets them on a track for chronic disease (Berenson et al., 1980). At the other extreme, underweight and malnourished children present a different mosaic of nutritional problems, many of which begin during infancy and the preschool years.

The most common problems among Head-Start children in Massachusetts were overweight and short stature (13 percent each) and iron deficiency anemia (12 percent). About 20 percent of physically or developmentally disabled children had short stature, compared with 15 percent of the Asian children. Acute undernutrition was not prevalent. Overweight among Hispanic, African-American and White children was 17 percent, 13 percent and 11 percent, respectively (Wiecha et al., 1991).

The Hispanic Health and Nutrition Examination Survey (HHANES) was conducted from 1982 to 1984 and included a probability sample of civilian, noninstitutionalized Hispanics in three areas of the United States: Puerto Ricans in New York City, Mexican Americans in the Southwest and Cuban Americans in Dade County, Florida. The survey found that Hispanic children were shorter than non-Hispanic Whites, but had larger anthropometric measurements and greater weight for height than average American children. Hispanic children in all age groups were heavier than non-Hispanics, and their overweight represented increased fatness in the trunk. Twenty-three percent of the children surveyed had an abnormal weight for their age: 19 percent were overweight and 4 percent were underweight. Ten percent of the Hispanic children had abnormal hemoglobin levels, and this increased to 23 percent if borderline cases were counted. Hemoglobin is the oxygen-carrying protein of the red blood cells and the best indicator of overall nutritional status (Monsen, 1988).

Children of migrant workers may be at increased risk for receiving inadequate nutrition prior to school entrance. These children experience poor housing with limited cooking facilities. They are victims of a lack of prenatal care for their mothers, who also lack sufficient funds to provide nutritious foods for their children. Migrant children exist at a poverty level that has negative effects on their lifestyle and school potential (Good, 1990).

Key findings in a 1991 survey (Food Research and Action Center) of childhood hunger in the United States include:

- About 5.5 million children under 12 years of age are hungry.
- An additional six million children are at risk of hunger.
- Hungry children are two to three times more likely than children from non-hungry, low-income families to have suffered from individual health problems such as unwanted weight loss, fatigue, irritability, headaches and inability to concentrate in the six months prior to the survey.
- Children with a specific health problem are absent from school almost twice as many days as those not reporting specific health problems.

These data alert us to the high-risk children who enter our schools annually. Often we forget that many seemingly healthy children do not have adequate eating environments from the time they are born until they enter the school door.

Recommended Dietary Allowances

For proper growth and development, children need an array of nutrients on a daily basis. RDAs are used to evaluate how sufficient children's total daily food intakes are (National Research Council, 1989). The U.S. Department of Agriculture bases the meal planning guide for school meals on achievement of one-third of the RDAs for school lunch; breakfast is planned to achieve about one-fourth of the RDAs for healthy children (U. S. Department of Agriculture, 1983).

Children generally consume about one-fourth of the day's energy, fat and protein intakes at lunch, but one-third or more of their calcium and sodium levels (Frank, 1980). The 1987/1988 National Food Consumption Survey found that 20 percent of adolescent boys and 40 percent of adolescent girls did not drink milk on the day of the survey (Wotecki, 1992). Although consumption of the total school lunch is the goal, consuming at least the milk is essential for growing children. A study of 164 healthy White children reported that those who consumed more than 1,000 mg of calcium per day had a higher bone mineral content than children who consumed less than 1,000 mg (Chan, 1991). The higher bone mineral content is especially crucial for girls to prevent osteoporosis later in life.

In cross-sectional surveys of ten and fifteen-year-old children in Bogalusa, Louisiana, school lunch analysis reported 22 percent and 29 percent of total energy intake from fat and 20 percent and 29 percent from carbohydrate. Sugar intake represented more than one-half the total carbohydrate intake (Frank et al., 1986). Sodium averaged one-third of the recommended daily range. Parcel analyzed school lunch aliquots as yielding 39 percent of the day's total fat intake (Parcel et al., 1987). There is still room for improvement.

Eating Patterns and Behaviors

The home and leisure-time environment of children may either complement or contradict efforts at school. Parents and teachers serve as role models for children in eating behaviors as well as in other health behaviors. Teachers influence eating patterns via the knowledge they impart and the personal habits they practice.

Elementary students are more susceptible to the teacher role model, whereas peers emerge as an adolescent's major role model.

Kirk and Gillespie (1990) identified two new roles for parents and how they affect children's food choices, i.e., the "meaning creator" and the "family diplomat." Previously, mothers functioned as nutritionists, economists and "managers-organizers," but today preparation time and catering to individual preferences influence food choices as much as nutrition. Children seem to mimic the "all or nothing" attitude of their parents. Many identify foods as "good" or "bad." In fact, 73 percent of fourth to eighth graders surveyed in a national sample worried about fat and cholesterol. About 85 percent felt they should avoid all high-fat foods, while 77 percent felt they should never eat high-sugar foods (National Center for Nutrition and Dietetics and International Food Information Council, 1991c).

About one-half (54 percent) of the children eat with their families every day; 35 percent eat with the family only three to five times per week. Students who give themselves the best nutrition rating eat more frequently with their families. Skipping meals and snacks influences dietary adequacy, yet many children skip meals. In a sample of American students in fourth through eighth grades, more than half the students had skipped breakfast (57 percent). Forty-one percent had skipped lunch, and 17 percent had skipped dinner (National Center for Nutrition and Dietetics and International Food Information Council, 1991b).

Of 639 fourth- and sixth-grade students, 9 percent reported skipping breakfast within the past 24 hours, and 5 percent reported eating nothing the entire morning. The most common reason for missing meals was dislike of particular meals or snacks, lack of time or forgetting to bring food. Thirty percent of the students met the recommended number of servings from the four food groups then being taught, but 44 percent did not eat the recommended fruit and vegetable servings. Students who ate breakfast and had a morning snack were three times more likely to meet all food group recommendations (Bidgood and Cameron, 1992).

A survey of the breakfast habits and behaviors of 382 children in third and fourth grades revealed that children who ate breakfast exhibited other healthful habits such as brushing teeth and taking vitamin/mineral supplements. Students who skipped breakfast were significantly more tired and hungry when they arrived at school, yet no significant social and emotional behavior problems or concerns were noted (Lindeman and Clancy, 1990).

Resnicow (1991) studied the relationship between breakfast habits and plasma cholesterol in schoolchildren nine to nineteen years old. Only 4 percent reported not eating breakfast regularly, but these were also less likely to believe in the benefits of breakfast. Controlling for age, gender and body mass index, those who skipped breakfast had significantly higher total cholesterol levels (172 mg percent) compared with those who ate breakfast, (160 mg percent). Students who ate ready-to-eat fiber cereals had lower cholesterol levels than all other breakfast eaters. Those who skipped breakfast also reported a higher intake of high-fat snacks, while traditional breakfast eaters reported significantly lower intake of high-fiber/low-fat snacks.

Observation of a cross-sectional sample of White and Hispanic preschoolers and their parents indicates the need to educate children from varied cultural backgrounds about important dietary behaviors (Frank et al., 1991). Significantly higher scores for fat-avoiding behaviors were noted for White preschoolers (n=143) than Hispanic preschoolers (n=198).

Preliminary data from the 1987/1988 National Food Consumption Survey report indicate that children one to nineteen years old average 35 to 36 percent of their total calories from fat.

Saturated fat was 14 percent; polyunsaturated fat, 6 percent; monounsaturated fat, 13 to 14 percent; and dietary cholesterol, 193 to 296 mg. This eating pattern has predisposed children to a health-risk behavior that manifests in excess weight and high blood cholesterol levels. At least 25 percent of American children and adolescents exceed the acceptable 170 mg percent serum cholesterol level (Wotecki, 1992).

The low fruit and vegetable intake of children is common. About 90 percent of children participating in a National Heart, Lung and Blood Institute demonstration/education project called "Catch" state that they eat fresh fruit at home most of the time. About three-fourths of White and African-American children appear sure they can eat fresh fruit instead of a candy bar. However, of 407 Los Angeles Hispanic children, only 3 percent consume four servings of fruits and vegetables a day (Palmer and Johnson, 1992).

An analysis of the 1982–1983 HHANES data set composed of 3,356 Hispanic children (Murphy et al., 1990) provides further alarming data. The children surveyed consumed fruits and vegetables less often than the other food groups. Data indicated these children instead chose their calories from the meat, dairy and breads/cereals groups.

These data are alarming because students are responsible for making most of their own food selections by the time they reach the fourth grade. Sixty-five percent choose their own breakfast, 46 percent their lunch, and 74 percent their snacks; although 73 percent report their mothers choose the dinner. Most students (87 percent) are responsible for cooking or preparing some of their own meals. Eighty percent make their own breakfast, and 57 percent are involved in buying food for meals or snacks (National Center for Nutrition and Dietetics and International Food Information Council, 1991b).

Avoidance of certain foods due to intolerances or hypersensitivities may not be well founded. Although many individuals think they have a food allergy, true food allergies affect only 0.3 to 7.5 percent of children and less than 1 percent of adults (Sampson, Buckley and Matcalf, 1987). Food intolerance, which involves an abnormal physiologic response to a food, is more common. Hyperactivity is a different condition, distinguished by signs of developmentally inappropriate inattention occurring in 5 to 10 percent of young school children (American Psychiatric Association, 1980). Food allergies do not cause hyperactivity; however, caffeine and alcohol stimulate the nervous system.

Iron Intake and Lead Exposure

A significant decline in the prevalence of anemia has been observed among healthy children from 1969 to 1986. Credit is given to improved prenatal and infant care for Women, Infants and Children (WIC) Program recipients. Iron deficiency (<3.5 mg percent) remains the most common nutrient deficiency among U.S. children six months to three years of age. Adolescents have an increased demand for iron to compensate for the increased hemoglobin level with growth. Boys need a 350 mg increase per day, while girls need a 455 mg increase because of menses (Johnson, 1990). National surveys report that adolescent girls twelve to nineteen years old have the highest anemia prevalence rates (6 to 14 percent). These adolescents become the mothers of tomorrow (Wotecki, 1992).

Lead exposure has now become the most common environmental disease of childhood (Needleman, 1991). A strong relationship between blood lead level, hematocrit and age has been noted. The higher the blood lead level, the greater the probability of iron-deficiency anemia; a toxic level is between 10 and 25 micrograms/dl (Schwartz et al., 1990). Lead affects nutrition by displacing essential divalent cations (iron, zinc, calcium) in several metabolic functions, and lead toxicity is associated with deficiencies of iron, zinc and calcium (Neggers and Stitt, 1986). Since the body absorbs lead more efficiently during times of growth, children and infants are susceptible to toxicity.

Even at low levels, lead can affect the central nervous system, hearing, blood pressure and physical growth. Initial signs of lead poisoning include diarrhea, irritability and lethargy. The long-term effects of exposure include lower IQ scores, poorer speech and language performance, impaired attention and an increased risk of attention deficit disorder and hyperactivity.

In one study, 55 percent of African-American children living in poverty had blood lead levels greater than 10 micrograms/dl. The blood lead levels of 579 one- to five-year-old children living near a lead smelter ranged from 11 to 164 micrograms/dl. The younger children with higher blood lead levels also had a higher probability of anemia (Schwartz et al., 1990).

Alcohol and Caffeine Excess

Alcohol provides calories and energy, but most adolescents drink it for fun and pleasure. Supplanting nutrient-rich foods with alcohol sets a child in a dangerous nutrition and accident-prone track.

Forty-five percent of White and 48 percent of Native American high school students in Michigan reported using alcohol. Almost half of the White, Native American and Hispanic male users reported heavy alcohol use (Bachman et al., 1991). Prevalence may be higher among dropouts.

The *Youth Risk Behavior Survey* (YBRS) of ninth and twelfth graders in 1990 reported 88 percent had consumed alcohol, with 59 percent drinking at least once during the last thirty days. Males were more likely than females to drink (62 percent to 55 percent), and twelfth graders were more likely than ninth graders to drink. Thirty-seven percent of males had consumed more than five drinks at least once during the last thirty days (Center for Disease Control and Prevention, 1991a).

In an evaluation of drinking habits of rural students in seventh to twelfth grades, it was noted that 39 percent had ridden in a car with a drinking driver in the past six months and 16 percent had driven after drinking. Both activities increased as grade level increased (Sarvela et al., 1990).

Caffeine is a nervous system stimulant. Although not viewed as a negative dietary component, caffeine may be of increasing concern, as it lowers calcium absorption and increases heart rate and respiration. Arbeit and colleagues (1988) reported caffeine intake per kilogram of body weight of White children ten to fifteen years old was comparable to adults, 2.5 versus 2.6 mg/kg. Caffeine sources for children are carbonated beverages, chocolate candy, chocolate pudding and ice cream, and tea.

Inactivity and Obesity

The prevalence of obesity among children six to eleven years has increased 54 percent since 1970; for 12 to 17 year olds, it has increased 39 percent. Hispanic children are among those experiencing as much as a 120 percent increase in the prevalence of obesity during the past twenty years. Excess intake of high-fat and low-complex-carbohydrate foods combined with minimal physical activity is a major potential culprit for this trend. Children need to be conditioned and equipped with skills to shift food intakes toward higher fruit and vegetable consumption. They also need to be encouraged to increase physical activity and reduce TV watching.

In a 1991 study of 4,771 adult females (Tucker and Bagwell, 1991), the amount of TV viewing was inversely correlated with amount of exercise. Women who reported more than four hours of watching television each day had twice the prevalence of obesity as females who watched less than one hour daily. Women who watched three to four hours of television had almost twice the prevalence of obesity as the group that watched less than one hour.

Children who watch more TV than their peers have greater prevalence of obesity and superobesity (Gortmaker, 1987). During prime-time TV programs and commercials, references to food focus on low-nutrient beverages and sweets consumed as snacks. Emphasis is on "good taste" and "fresh and natural" with minimal attention given to foods consistent with healthy guidelines for children (Story, 1990).

The prevalence of obesity among children of military dependents was observed at two major medical centers (Tiwary and Holguin, 1992). The prevalence was greater among adolescents than among young children. The percentage of very obese children increased from 5.5 percent in 1978 to 9.0 percent in both 1986 and 1990. Children of retirees were more likely to be obese (24 percent) than were children of active duty staff (18 percent), irrespective of age and rank of the parents. These data may indicate that lifestyle changes such as retirement have significant effects for children, too.

The relationship between consumption of high-fat foods, low physical activity and obesity was studied using a case-control design and school children with a 30 percent prevalence of obesity. Thirty-five percent of the girls were obese compared with 26 percent of the boys. The children who consumed high-fat foods but had low physical activity had a 38 percent increased risk of obesity compared with children who consumed low-fat foods and had high physical activity (Muecke et al., 1992).

Eating Disorders and Self-Image

Approximately one million adolescents are affected by anorexia nervosa and bulimia. These eating disorders are thought to arise from pressure to be thin, depression, biological errors and poor self-concept. The *Youth Risk Behavior Survey* (CDC, 1991b) reported that 69 percent of male students considered themselves at the right body weight and 17 percent thought they were underweight. Fifty-nine percent of female students considered themselves at the right body weight, and 7 percent thought they were underweight. African-American students considered themselves less overweight than White or Hispanic students. About 44 percent of the girls were trying to lose weight, but only 15 percent of the boys reported this intent. Even 27 percent of girls who considered themselves at the right weight reported currently trying to lose weight. Weight-loss methods included exercise, skipping meals, taking diet pills and inducing vomiting, which girls reported significantly more often than boys.

One survey reported that 454 White girls, 14 to 19 years old, who responded that their guardians "always" lectured them about food, had significantly higher scores on "drive for thinness" and "ineffectiveness" subscales. Girls who responded that their guardians were unaware of their problems also had higher scores on the "ineffectiveness" and "interpersonal distrust" subscales (Larson, 1991).

In another study, 12 percent of African-American, low-income adolescents thought they had an eating disorder. Those 14 years or older were more likely to think about vomiting to lose weight. Females identified more emotional concerns about being overweight or the need to lose weight. The "desire to do everything perfectly" was related to eating disorders among the middle school students, whereas "feeling ineffective as a person" was related to eating disorders among high school students. Students who had a self-perceived eating disorder were more often above the 50th percentile for weight for height, and accurately perceived themselves as such (Balentine, 1991).

A 22-item questionnaire on weight perceptions was administered to inner-city African-American and White adolescent students, 12 to 17 years old. Forty percent of heavy African-American females compared to 100 percent of heavy White females perceived themselves as overweight and the trend was similar for heavy males. African-American males were more likely to believe that emotions affected eating behavior than White males. African-American females felt lack of exercise accounted for their weight, while White females felt eating habits accounted for theirs. Girls obtained their weight control information from television, family, friends and magazines. Boys used television, family and athletic coaches for advice (Desmond et al., 1989).

After a program to educate high school students, staff and teachers about eating disorders, more questions about eating disorders were answered correctly by participants than by controls (Shisslak, Crago and Neal, 1990). Information alone, however, does not change behavior.

Meeting the Challenge

A current school health education challenge is to address the major nutrition issues. Documenting how eating behavior influences health and how eating behavior in childhood initiates adolescent and adult eating patterns is essential. With structured action plans to coordinate important contributors, the major national initiatives and the dominant nutrition issues, we can meet the challenge and improve the nutritional well-being of children.

Acknowledgments

The author thanks Selina Moralis Lai, MS, for technical assistance and review of the manuscript, and Colleen Odlum for typing assistance.

References

Allensworth, D. D., and L. J. Kolbe. 1987. The comprehensive school health program: Exploring an expanded concept. *Journal of School Health* 57 (10): 31.

American Dietetic Association. 1991. *Survey of American dietary habits.* Chicago: The Wirthlin Group.

American Psychiatric Association. 1980. *Diagnostic and Statistical Manual (DSM III).* 3d ed. Washington, DC.

American School Food Service Association. 1985. Educational pathways for growth: A master plan for education. *School Food Service Journal* 39(6): 38-70.

American School Food Service Association. 1988. *Professional development handbook.* Englewood, CO.

American School Food Service Association. 1990. *Youth Advisory Council—At the starting line.* Alexandria, VA.

American School Food Service Association. 1991. *The healthy E.D.G.E. in schools.* Supplement to the *School Food Service Journal* (March).

Anderson, J., and M. H. Haas. 1990. Impact of a nutrition education program on food sales in restaurants. *Journal of Nutrition Education* 22:232-238.

Arbeit, M. L., T. A. Nicklas, G. C. Frank, L. S. Webber, M. H. Miner and G. S. Berenson. 1988. Caffeine intakes of children from a biracial population: The Bogalusa heart study. *Journal of the American Dietetic Association* 88 (4): 466-470.

Bachman, J. G., J. M. Wallace, P. M. O'Malley, L. D. Johnston, C. L. Kurth and H. W. Neighbors. 1991. Racial/ethnic differences in smoking, drinking, and illicit drug use among American high school seniors, 1976-89. *American Journal of Public Health* 81:372-377.

Balentine, M., K. Stitt, J. Bonner and L. Clark. 1991. Self-reported eating disorders of Black, low-income adolescents: Behavior, body weight perceptions, and methods of dieting. *Journal of School Health* 61(9): 392-396.

Berenson, G. S., C. A. McMahan, A. W. Voors, L. S. Webber, S. R. Srinivasan,

G. C. Frank, T. A. Foster and C. V. Blonde. 1980. *Cardiovascular risk factors in children—the early natural history of atherosclerosis and essential hypertension.* New York: Oxford University Press.

Bidgood, B. A., and G. Cameron. 1992. Meal/snack missing and dietary adequacy of primary school children. *Journal of the Canadian Dietetic Association* 53:164-168.

Block G., C. Clifford, M. D. Naughton, M. Henderson and M. A. McAdams. 1989. Brief dietary screen for high fat intake. *Journal of Nutrition Education* 21:199-207.

California Department of Education. 1991. *The Nutrition Guidelines for California School Foods.* Sacramento, CA.

California Department of Health Services. 1990. *California daily food guide.* F-89-559. Sacramento, CA.

Centers for Disease Control and Prevention. 1991a. Alcohol and other drug use among high school students—United States. *Journal of the American Medical Association* 266:3266-3267.

Centers for Disease Control and Prevention. 1991b. Body weight perceptions and selected weight-management goals and practices of high school students—United States. *Journal of the American Medical Association* 266:2811-2812.

Chan, G. M. 1991. Dietary calcium and bone mineral status of children and adolescents. *American Journal of Diseases of Children* 145:631-634.

Cinciripini, P. M. 1984. Changing food selections in a public cafeteria. *Behavior Modification* 8:522-539.

Davis-Chervin, D., T. Rogers and M. Clark. 1985. Influencing food selection with point-of-choice nutrition information. *Journal of Nutrition Education* 17:18-22.

Dennison D., K. F. Dennison, and G. C. Frank. 1993. The DINE evaluation process: Improving food choices of the public. *Journal of Nutrition Education,* in press.

Desmond, S. M., J. H. Price, C. Hallinan and D. Smith. 1989. Black and white adolescents' perceptions of their weight. *Journal of School Health* 59 (8): 353-358.

Dubinsky, L. D., and J. H. Bodner. 1991. Food for thought: Starting a K-3 nutrition education program. *Journal of School Health* 61 (4): 181-183.

Food and Nutrition Board, National Academy of Sciences, National Research Council. 1989. *Recommended dietary allowances.* 9th ed. Washington, DC.

Food Marketing Institute. 1989. *Trends: Consumer attitudes and the supermaket.* Washington, D.C.

Food Research and Action Center. 1991. *Community childhood hunger identification project.* Washington, DC.

Frank, G. C. 1980. Dietary studies of infants and children. In *Cardiovascular risk factors in children—The early natural history of atherosclerosis and essential hypertension,* eds. G. S. Berenson et al., 111-123. New York: Oxford University Press.

Frank, G. C. 1985. Nutrient profile on personal computers—A comparison of DINE with mainframe computers. *Health Education* 16:16-19.

Frank, G. C., 1993. Evaluating meal quality in school food service. *School Food Service Research Review.* (Manuscript.)

Frank, G. C., and S. Desai. 1992. Shaping healthy meals for school children. Long Beach, CA: California State University, Long Beach.

Frank, G. C., R. P. Farris, J. L. Cresanta and T. A. Nicklas. 1986. Dietary intake as a determinant of cardiovascular risk factor variables. Chapter X, Part A: Observations in a pediatric population. In *Causation of Cardiovascular Risk Factors in Children: Perspectives on Causation of Cardiovascular Risk in Early Life,* ed. G. S. Berenson, 254-291. New York: Raven Press.

Frank, G. C., T. Nicklas, J. Forcier, L. Webber and G. S. Berenson. 1989a. Cardiovascular health promotion of children: The Heart Smart School Lunch Program, part I. *School Food Service and Restaurant Review* 13 (2): 130-136.

Frank, G. C., T. Nicklas, J. Forcier, L. Webber and G. S. Berenson. 1989b. Cardiovascular health promotion of children: Student behavior and institutional food service change, part II. *School Food Service Restaurant Review* 13 (2): 137-145.

Frank, G. C., T. A. Nicklas, L. S. Webber, C. Major, J. F. Miller and G. S. Berenson. 1992. A food frequency questionnaire for adolescents: Defining eating patterns. *Journal of the American Dietetic Association* 92:313-318.

Frank, G. C., A. Vaden and J. Martin. 1987. School health promotion: Child nutrition programs. *Journal of School Health* 57 (10): 451-460.

Frank, G. C., M. Zive, J. Nelson, S. Broyles and P. Nader. 1991. Fat and cholesterol avoidance among Mexican-American and Anglo preschool children and parents. *Journal of the American Dietetic Association* 91 (8): 954-961.

Good, M. E. 1990. A needs assessment: The health status of migrant children as they enter kindergarten. San Jose, CA: San Jose State University. (ERIC Document Reproduction Service No. ED 338 460.)

Gortmaker, S. L. 1987. Increasing pediatric obesity in the U.S. *American Journal of Diseases in Children* 141:535-541.

Green, L. W., M. W. Kreuter, S. G. Deeds and K. B. Partridge. 1980. *Health education planning—A diagnostic approach*. Palo Alto, CA: Mayfield Publishing.

Hong, L., G. C. Frank, R. Toma and H. Lee. 1992. The nutrient analysis and sensory evaluation of a new recipe for school lunch—modified Chinese meat bun. Abstract presented at the California Dietetic Association, April 1992.

Johnson, A. A. 1990. Iron deficiency: Pediatric epidemiology. In *Functional Significance of Iron Deficiency. Annual Nutrition Workshop Series, Volume III*, ed. C. Enwonuw, 57-65. Nashville, TN: Meharry Medical College.

Kirk, M. C., and A. H. Gillespie. 1990. Factors affecting food choices of working mothers with young families. *Journal of Nutrition Education* 22:161-168.

Larson, B. 1991. Relationship of family communication patterns to eating disorder inventory scores in adolescent girls. *Journal of the American Dietetic Association* 91 (9): 1065-1067.

Levy, S. R., B. K. Iverson and H. J. Walberg. 1980. Nutrition education research: An interdisciplinary evaluation and review. *Health Education Quarterly* 7 (2): 107-126.

Lindeman, A. K., and K. L. Clancy. 1990. Assessment of breakfast habits and social/emotional behavior of elementary schoolchildren. *Journal of Nutrition Education* 22:226-231.

LunchByte Systems. 1993. NutriKids. Rochester, NY.

May, C. D. 1980. Food allergy: Perspective, principles, practical management. *Nutrition Today* 15 (6): 28-31.

Monsen, E. R. 1988. Iron nutrition and absorption: Dietary factors which affect bioavailability. *Journal of the American Dietetic Association* 88 (7): 786-790.

Muecke, L., B. Morton-Simons, I. W. Huang and G. Parcel. 1992. Is childhood obesity associated with high-fat foods and low physical activity? *Journal of School Health* 62 (1): 19-23.

Murphy, S. P., R. O. Castillo, R. Martorell, and F. S. Mendora. 1990. An evaluation of food group intakes by Mexican-American children. *Journal of the American Dietetic Association* 91 (3): 388-393.

National Center for Nutrition and Dietetics and International Food Information Council. 1991a. *Study of children's eating habits: Families still eat together.* Chicago, IL: American Dietetic Association.

National Center for Nutrition and Dietetics and International Food Information Council. 1991b. *Study of children's eating habits: Kids at the table: Who's placing the orders?* Chicago, IL: American Dietetic Association.

National Center for Nutrition and Dietetics and International Food Information Council. 1991c. *Study of children's eating habits: Kids earn good marks for nutrition knowledge.* Chicago, IL: American Dietetic Association.

National Center for Nutrition and Dietetics and International Food Information Council. 1991d. *Study of children's eating habits: Where do kids get nutrition information?* Chicago, IL: American Dietetic Association.

National Cholesterol Education Program. 1991. Pediatric Panel Report. April.

National Research Council. 1989. *Diet and health: Implications for reducing chronic disease risk.* Washington, DC: National Academy Press.

Needleman, H. 1991. Lead exposure: The commonest environmental disease of childhood. *Bulletin of National Center for Clinical Infant Programs* 11:1-6.

Neggers, Y. H., and K. R. Stitt. 1986. Effects of high lead intakes in children. *Journal of the American Dietetic Association* 86 (7): 938-940.

Palmer, R., and A. Johnson. 1992. Personal communication. Institute for Preventive Research, USC. Los Angeles, CA.

Parcel, G. S., B. G. Simmons-Morton, N. M. O'Hara, T. Baranowski and B. Wilson. 1987. School promotion of healthful diet and exercise behavior: An integration of organizational change and social learning theory interventions. *Journal of School Health* 57 (4): 150-156.

Portland Public Schools. 1989. Fundamental Understanding of Nutrition (F.U.N.) Program. A comprehensive nutrition education program for grades K-3, Nutrition Services.

Resnicow, K. 1991. The relationship between breakfast habits and plasma cholesterol levels in schoolchildren. *Journal of School Health* 61 (2): 81-85.

Sampson, H., R. Buckley and D. Metcalfe. 1987. Food allergy. *Journal of the American Medical Association* 258: 2886-2890.

Sarvela, P. D., D. J. Pape, J. Odulana and S. M. Bajracharya. 1990. Drinking, drug use, and driving among rural midwestern youth. *Journal of School Health* 60 (5): 215-219.

Schmitz, M. F., and J. E. Fielding. 1986. Point-of-choice nutritional labeling: Evaluation in a worksite cafeteria. *Journal of Nutrition Education* 18:S65-S68.

Schwartz, J., P. J. Landrigan, E. L. Baker, W. A. Orenstein and P. E. von Lindern. 1990. Lead-induced anemia: Dose-response relationships and evidence for a threshold. *American Journal of Public Health* 80:165-168.

Shisslak, C. M., M. Crago and M. E. Neal. 1990. Prevention of eating disorders among adolescents. *American Journal of Health Promotion* 5:100-106.

Simons-Morton, B. G., G. S. Parcel, T. Baranowski, R. Forthofer and N. M. O'Hara. 1991. Promoting physical activity and a healthful diet among children: Results of a school-based intervention study. *American Journal of Public Health* 81:986-991.

State of California. 1989. Assembly Bill 2109, Speier.

Story, M., and P. Faulkner. 1990. The prime time diet. A content analysis of eating behavior and food messages in television program content and commercials. *American Journal of Public Health* 80: 738-740.

Tiwary, C. M., and A. H. Holguin. 1992. Prevalence of obesity among children of military dependents at two major medical centers. *American Journal of Public Health* 82 (3): 354-357.

Tucker, L. A., and M. Bagwell. 1991. Television viewing and obesity in adult females. *American Journal of Public Health* 81 (7): 908-911.

U.S. Department of Agriculture. 1983. *Menu planning guide for school food service.* Program Aid 1260. Washington, DC.

U.S. Department of Agriculture. 1992. *Nutrition guidance for the child nutrition programs.* FNS-279. Washington, DC.

U.S. Department of Agriculture. 1992. *The pyramid food guide.* Washington, DC.

U.S. Department of Agriculture and U.S. Department of Health and Human Services. 1988. *Nutrition and your health: Dietary guidelines for Americans.* 2d ed. Home and Garden Bulletin No. 232 and 322-1. Washington, DC.

U.S. Department of Health and Human Services, Public Health Service. 1988. *The Surgeon General's report on nutrition and health.* DHHS Publication No. (PHS) 88-50210. Washington, DC.

U.S. Department of Health and Human Services, Public Health Service. 1990. *Healthy People 2000.* DHHS Publication No. (PHS) 91-50212. Washington, DC.

Wiecha, J. L., C. A. Grandon, P. Fisher-Miller and D. Seder. 1991. *Nutrition counts: Massachusetts nutrition surveillance system, FY90 annual report.* Massachusetts: Department of Public Health. (ERIC Document Reproduction Service No. ED 338 423.)

Wotecki, C. E. 1992. Nutrition in childhood and adolescence—Parts 1 and 2. *Contemporary Nutrition* 17 (2): 1-2.

Wynder, E. L., J. H. Weisburger and S. K. Ng. 1992. Nutrition: the need to define "optimal" intake as a basis for public policy decisions. *American Journal of Public Health* 82 (3): 346-350.

Chapter 16

Educating About HIV/AIDS

Kathleen R. Miner, PhD, MPH, CHES

A IDS is the disease of the twentieth century. It is an infectious viral illness that adversely affects the human immune system. Its history is short and its pathology complex. Both its history and its pathology provide insight into the complexity of the school challenge that AIDS presents.

As we begin understanding the severity of this disease, the tragedy of denial becomes clear. As we study its chronology, the necessity of acceptance becomes obvious. The only question that remains is, Are our schools sufficiently dedicated to the well-being of children to take the actions necessary to safeguard children against the major disease of their time?*

*Comprehensive school health includes policy, as well as environmental and curricular approaches to ensuring a safe and healthy school setting. This description would apply to schools' response to AIDS. Throughout this chapter, discussions of the school response will focus on specifics related to HIV and AIDS. However, many prominent AIDS education agencies recommend that AIDS education fall within the context of a comprehensive school health program (Center for Disease Control and Prevention, 1988).

The History of AIDS
and Its Relation to Schools

Although the term *AIDS* was not yet coined, the Centers for Disease Control and Prevention (CDC) identified the first case of AIDS in 1981. Soon after the first case, physicians in New York and San Francisco began reporting a number of homosexual men with a form of cancer called Kaposi's sarcoma. The incidence of this type of cancer was highly unusual for men in their 30s and 40s. Kaposi's sarcoma is more typically found in older adults, people of Mediterranean ancestry and individuals with severely compromised immune systems.

In addition to seeing this uncommon form of cancer, physicians began seeing homosexual men with other rare conditions, including a bacterial pneumonia, Pneumocystis carinii, and a fungal throat infection, esophageal candidiasis. As is the case with Kaposi's sarcoma, these diseases are often found in individuals whose immune systems are not functioning properly (Centers for Disease Control and Prevention, 1981).

The occurrence of these unexpected diseases in homosexual men caused a number of physicians to speculate that the homosexual community was afflicted with a new form of disease that affected the immune system. This new disease was called Gay Related Immune Disease or G.R.I.D. However, soon after the first cases were identified, physicians began seeing immune-compromising conditions in populations other than homosexual males. The term G.R.I.D. no longer accurately reflected the nature of the disease, so the name was changed to Acquired Immune Deficiency Syndrome (AIDS). As increasing numbers of people were becoming ill in the United States, cases also were showing up in of Africa, Europe and Asia. It is a peculiarity of the epidemic in the United States that the first cases were identified in homosexuals.

In most of the world, a majority of the cases have been identified in heterosexuals.

During the early years of the epidemic, the schools had very little interest in the subject of AIDS. The etiology of the disease was unknown, and the precise mechanism of transmission was unclear. Moreover, the occurrence of the disease seemed to be limited to the gay communities of New York and San Francisco. Even in cities where there were large communities of homosexual adults, there was no compelling justification for large-scale caution or concern. Because AIDS did not appear to infect school-age children and its disease process was so puzzling, there seemed to be no imperative for any form of school response.

The 1980s

During the early 1980s, nearly 80 percent of the AIDS cases in the United States were in six large cities in five states: New York, San Francisco, Los Angeles, Newark, Miami and Houston. By the end of the decade, cases of AIDS had been reported from every state, U. S. territory and most cities. Currently, more than thirty metropolitan areas report a cumulative incidence of more than 1,000 cases (Centers for Disease Control and Prevention, 1992).

Although the vast majority of reported AIDS cases in the 1980s were still from the homosexual community, the number of cases identified in individuals who used injectable drugs was increasing. Soon after the association between needle use and AIDS was described, women began to be diagnosed with similar symptoms. These women were exposed to the infection either because they were injecting drugs themselves or because they were the sexual partners of infected men. In the view of many researchers, infected women added two very serious dimensions to the AIDS epidemic: the confirmation of heterosexual transmission and the possibility of mother to baby (perinatal) transmission. By the mid-1980s, many cases of AIDS were showing up in people who had had transfusions with blood or blood products, especially young men with hemophilia.

Several hemophilia-related AIDS cases reported from central Florida made national news because the young men suffered discrimination both at home and in school. Their community insisted that these young men be removed from direct contact with other children and adults, especially while at school. Under national scrutiny, these students and their families experienced personal violence and social rejection. Media attention forced the local school to contend with a range of AIDS issues, from instructional to environmental.

Soon after the Florida incident, Ryan White, a midwestern youth with hemophilia, became a national figure because of his willingness to fight publicly the school discrimination he was experiencing. His story was so widely publicized that schools everywhere were pressured to develop local AIDS policies. These events, as well as disclosures that prominent public figures had died of the disease, made the subject of AIDS one that the schools could no longer dismiss.

As AIDS began its spread across the geography of the United States and into populations other than gay men, a demand for a better understanding of the disease and of its transmission mechanisms began. Scientists in France and the United States first isolated the human immunodeficiency virus (HIV) in 1983. These same scientists confirmed that HIV causes AIDS in 1984.

An unfortunate legacy of the United States response to AIDS is that it was not until the disease had spread to "safe" populations, such as those with hemophilia, that the American public began demanding that intensive research be initiated and prevention and education programs be started. With this increased pressure, schools began to take action. Many schools initiated policies outlining the procedures necessary to respond to students and personnel who might be infected and began the difficult task of developing an instructional response to the AIDS epidemic.

The 1990s and the Future

By the end of the 1980s, more than 100,000 people in the United States had died of AIDS-related causes. The rate at which people were dying of HIV/AIDS was accelerating. In 1990 alone, approximately 39,000 people died of AIDS-related causes, accounting for nearly one-third of all deaths since the beginning of the epidemic. Currently, about 100 people with AIDS die each day, which equates to one AIDS death every fifteen minutes.

The data indicate that during the 1990s, HIV will continue to spread across this nation with great speed. HIV will continue to penetrate into populations other than homosexual males. The future will include increasing numbers of HIV infection in women, children, adolescents, heterosexuals, injection drug users and people of color. Hispanics and Native Americans in the United States, and Asians, particularly Thais, worldwide, along with the homosexual community, will continue to suffer disproportionately from this disease.

At its current rate of increase, HIV/AIDS will become a leading cause of death among youth and young adults in the United States and will place a substantial burden on the country's social and economic resources. The United States can ill-afford to lose its young productive citizens to a costly disease at a time when the demography has shifted toward an older population (National Commission on AIDS, 1991).

The schools will be expected to take direct leadership in ensuring that young people and their families are aware of the transmission routes and the prevention steps necessary to avoid infection. They will be expected to use culturally appropriate HIV/AIDS education materials targeted toward African Americans, Hispanics, Native Americans and other ethnic minorities. Moreover, the schools will be expected to have clear policies regarding the response to infected individuals, including students, faculty and staff.

Key Points
1. HIV/AIDS is not a gay disease. In most of the world, HIV is transmitted heterosexually.
2. HIV infection is not confined to a few places in the United States. Every state and most cities have reported people infected with HIV.
3. HIV/AIDS is becoming a leading cause of death in young adults in the United States.

Basic AIDS Pathology and Its Effect on the School Environment

HIV is a type of virus called a retrovirus, which means that it has a central nucleic acid core of RNA rather than the more common viral core of DNA. Because of the biochemical differences between RNA and DNA, retroviruses are more difficult to study. They are unstable in their genetic make-up, which makes developing a vaccine or producing medicines against them a greater challenge than against DNA-cored viruses. The basic structure of the virus consists of an outer coat of protein and the inner core of RNA. When infected with HIV, the human body generates antibodies against the protein coat of the virus.

HIV selectively infects certain cells in the human body. The primary cells that are infected are types of white blood cells called T-helper (T4 or CD4) lymphocytes and the macrophages. These white blood cells are responsible for the normal functioning of the human immune system and the production of antibodies. HIV infection results in the destruction of these cells.

Without these cells, individuals can no longer make antibodies against infectious microorganisms. They therefore become ill from diseases that are normally prevented by antibody action. Many of the symptoms associated with AIDS are called opportunistic infections, because they are caused by microorganisms that take the "opportunity" to infect individuals with compromised immune systems. These microorganisms are widespread and are not normally pathogenic. In the presence of a diminished immune system, they cause serious and often life-threatening infections. This explains the curiosity surrounding the rare types of infections seen in the first cases of AIDS.

Even though HIV attacks the white blood cells responsible for making antibodies, not all of the cells are destroyed at once. The human body continues to make more white blood cells, which, in turn, continue to recognize HIV as a pathogen and make antibodies against the virus. However, as the number of viruses increases, the immune system becomes overwhelmed and gradually loses the ability to produce enough white blood cells and the corresponding antibodies. This begins the AIDS disease process.

With the discovery of the virus that causes AIDS, scientists began to make a distinction between being infected and having AIDS. Individuals are considered to have AIDS when they begin to show signs of opportunistic infections or their white blood cell counts are very low. In the absence of low white blood cell counts and opportunistic infections, individuals are considered to be HIV infected. All people with AIDS are HIV infected, but not all people with HIV infection have AIDS.

The average time between the initial infection and the body's inability to produce sufficient white blood cells is from seven to ten years. During the time between infection and illness, infected persons have no apparent disease but are capable of transmitting the infection to others. This duration of time is called the incubation (or latent) period. What makes AIDS unique is the length of the incubation period. It is unlike other infectious diseases, such as measles, tuberculosis or gonorrhea, in which the incubation period allows for an estimation of the conditions of exposure (person, place and time). AIDS' long incubation makes defining the conditions of exposure very difficult.

Children with AIDS are susceptible to opportunistic infections, just as adults with AIDS are. Children with AIDS who attend school are likely to become infected with microorganisms that would not be pathogenic to healthy students. When people are asked what they fear most about having children with AIDS in school, a frequent response is the fear of "spreading the AIDS infection." Yet, in reality, it is the other way around. People with AIDS are more likely to pick up infections from other individuals, pets and the environment than are noninfected people. Because there is no evidence that HIV is spread through casual contact, children with AIDS will not spread the disease to other children who share the same classroom, bathroom or cafeteria (Lifson, 1990).

It is impossible to tell "just by looking" whether individuals are infected with HIV. In fact, the infected individuals themselves may not know their disease status. Therefore, it is essential that school curricula explain the need to be careful with sexual encounters and drug use at all times and not just at times when there is a perception of high risk.

Serological Testing

Advances in the understanding of the composition and behavior of the human immunodeficiency virus allowed scientists to develop procedures for testing blood for evidence that it might be HIV infected. The bases of the HIV testing are procedures that measure the presence or absence of the antibodies made by the white blood cells against the virus. The first tests became available in 1985 and were used to screen the donated blood supply. This same year the use of the tests expanded to include testing the HIV status of individuals.

Two tests are usually used in tandem to determine the HIV status of individuals. These tests are called the Enzyme-Linked Immunoassay (ELA) and the Western Blot (WB). Due to the different biochemical nature of the tests, and to ensure that the results are as accurate as possible, individuals are considered to be positive when their blood samples yield two positive ELA tests and one positive Western Blot.

For babies born to HIV-infected mothers, the testing scenario is somewhat different. The procedure for testing the blood of infants for HIV infection is the same as for adults. However, all babies are born with immature immune systems. They are unable to make antibodies on their own for the first six to nine months of their lives. Nature protects newborns by providing them with doses of their mothers' antibodies until such time as they are capable of making their own.

Therefore, testing the blood of newborns for the presence of HIV antibodies is a test of the presence of their mothers' antibodies. All babies born to HIV-positive mothers will test positive during their first months of life. Although estimates vary, children will have to be approximately 12 months old before confirmatory HIV testing can be done to assess accurately whether they are making their own antibodies against the virus. Children who are not infected will lose their maternally acquired antibodies and will test negative. Children who are infected will begin to produce their own antibodies against HIV and will continue to test positive.

Negative results from the serological tests do *not* prove that individuals are free from HIV. Because the tests measure the presence or absence of antibodies to the virus and not the virus itself, there is a possibility that the titer (amount) of antibody in the blood is insufficient to produce a positive test. This would be the case with newly infected individuals. Even though their tests may be negative, such people could still transmit HIV to others. Generally, it takes from six weeks to several months for the number of antibodies to reach an amount that can be measured.

Scientists continue to explore serological testing procedures that measure the presence or absence of the virus. Confirmation of the virus would allow for the determination of HIV status very early in the infection cycle. The most promising procedures involve analyzing blood for pieces of the protein coat that surrounds the outside of the virus. However, it will be many years before these tests will be widely available.

With the onset of serological testing, a false sense of assurance that infected persons can be identified has developed. As can be seen from the nature of the testing, however, this is not the case. Therefore, large-scale screening programs and required testing associated with obtaining marriage licenses or teaching certificates is an unwise use of resources. These resources could be better used by developing quality HIV/AIDS educational materials for use in community interventions and comprehensive school health programs.

In the absence of a cure, the reality is once positive, always positive. If individuals test positive and their condition becomes known, they may experience discrimination and bigotry through being denied health care benefits, professional advancement and/or access to children.

For the schools, there are several important responses to serological testing. The first has to do with the increasing likelihood that people will become aware of infected yet still healthy students, teachers or other staff. The schools must have policies that describe their response to infected people. These policies should address such things as how to handle the confidentiality of personnel and student records, answer inquiries about the HIV status of these individuals, provide staff development HIV programs, and react to demands from the public to remove HIV-positive individuals from the classroom. (See Appendix F for characteristics of effective policies.)

The second response is in regard to curricula. As society increasingly calls for universal HIV testing, the public might falsely accept the absoluteness of the HIV test. Students must be instructed as to the purpose, reliability and validity of the HIV testing protocols. For example, young people may be fooled into believing that individuals are not subject to infection if they carry an "HIV-free" result from serological tests. An HIV-free designation could provide the illusion of immunity, thereby encouraging them to engage in sexual or needle-sharing activities without precautions. The over-reliance on serological testing procedures is both erroneous and dangerous. The school curriculum must be diligent in dispelling this myth.

Key Points

1. Not all babies born to infected mothers will develop HIV infection.
2. Babies who develop HIV infection during infancy were born to mothers who had the infection.
3. All babies born to HIV-infected mothers will test positive for HIV at birth, but only 20 to 30 percent will actually have HIV infection.

Development of Chemotherapy

Not until the late 1980s were any drugs available to forestall the demise of the immune system associated with HIV. The currently available medications (AZT, ddI, ddC) work by suppressing a key step in the life cycle of the virus. These drugs inhibit the reproduction of the virus in cells that are newly infected, but do not stop production in cells already infected. Because they do not stop the initial infection and do not destroy all of the virus, these drugs are not vaccines or cures. Rather, they are considered treatments that slow down the progression of the disease.

These drugs are life extenders; they can give a greater quality and quantity of life to infected individuals. Nevertheless, they are strong medications with powerful side-effects that many infected people cannot tolerate. Often, even in the presence of advancing disease, people will elect to stop the medications. There is continuing research to find a vaccine and a cure, but progress is slow and the possibility of this happening is unlikely for many years to come.

With the onset of potent therapies has come an increase of two important time durations: (1) the time between initial infection and the onset of AIDS, and (2) the time between the diagnosis of AIDS and death. With each of these extensions, serious issues force schools to examine their approach to HIV/AIDS.

Children who are born infected with HIV can be expected to live longer. As therapies and treatments for children born with HIV become more effective, these children can be expected to live to school age. These children will enter school with their age cohorts and progress with them through the primary, elementary and secondary grades.

Beyond the social problems that could develop because HIV-positive children are attending school, many of these children will require special procedures and medications to be administered at school. To administer some of the therapies, school personnel may require technical skills and access to specialized equipment.

As therapies for adults also become more effective, the schools can expect to see personnel with HIV remain active in the school environment. Individuals who are known to be infected or who are ill will be able to remain productive employees. In order to avoid potential AIDS-associated discrimination, schools need to prepare in advance for the possibility of having HIV-infected children and adults in their setting.

In 1992, the Americans with Disabilities Act prohibited discrimination toward people with HIV infection. In truth, much of the intolerance associated with this disease is difficult to prove and receives tacit, if not overt, support from the public. The schools can expect to have an awkward time balancing the rights of infected persons, be they students or employees, and the expectations of their voting constituents.

Transmission Routes and Their Role in the School Curriculum

From the earliest days of the AIDS epidemic, many scientists believed that AIDS was an infectious disease. This led them to search for the causative agent, the human immunodeficiency virus (HIV). The identification of the virus was not discovery enough to provide an understanding of the entire infection process. It was important to detail the means by which infected individuals transmit the virus to noninfected individuals.

Exposure to Body Fluids
HIV has been isolated from a variety of body fluids, including blood, semen, vaginal secretions, breast milk, urine, tears and saliva. Clearly, any body substance that contains white blood cells has the potential of transmitting the virus.

Although the virus has been found in the listed substances, often the concentration of the virus is so low that these fluids are not considered to be very infectious. This is true for tears, urine and saliva. Casual contact with these fluids is not likely to transmit the infection.

However, blood, blood products, semen, vaginal secretions and breast milk have high concentrations of the virus and are considered to be very infectious. Activities that result in contact with these fluids are classified as high-risk behaviors and should be conducted with precaution. It is very common for blood and blood products to carry pathogens. Hepatitis B is a prevalent and notable example of a bloodborne disease.

Activities that prevent the transmission of HIV will also prevent other forms of serious infections. Therefore, the protocols for HIV/AIDS prevention are recommended as responsible precautions for a wide range of potentially harmful conditions.

In a school environment, many events, such as sports and recreation activities, increase the possibility that people will be exposed to body fluids. For the safety of everyone, schools must have procedures and supplies available that will protect individuals from exposure to blood. These procedures should include access to latex gloves when handling cuts, changing bandages or dressing wounds.

Another common concern is the care of younger or disabled children who are still in diapers, have toilet accidents, vomit or display other behaviors that could result in body fluid contact. Beyond sound sanitation and hygiene procedures, little is necessary to prevent the spread of HIV should any of these children be infected. To prevent the spread of all sorts of infections, personnel should always use latex gloves when handling diapers and other soiled materials. Only in the presence of blood would there be any risk of HIV transmission. In the event of blood, the use of latex gloves would be sufficient. Disposal of diapers should follow standard hygienic procedures (Grossman, 1988).

Some children with behavioral disorders will act out by biting other children. There is no evidence that AIDS is transmitted by biting (Lifson, 1990).

Sexual Behavior

The transmission of the virus through sexual contact occurs in both homosexual and heterosexual activities. These activities include sexual contact between men, between women and men, and possibly between women. The potential for transmission exists with different forms of sexual intercourse, including penile/anal, penile/vaginal and oral/genital sex. There is no form of intimate sexual activity that is completely risk free.

The relationship between the risk of transmission and the various types of intercourse is not known precisely. Evidence does suggest that the sexual partner who is the recipient of the semen has a greater risk of becoming infected than the donating partner. This evidence appears to hold true for both homosexual and heterosexual couples. Additional data suggest that individuals who have genital lesions or ulcers are more likely to transmit or receive the virus. Likewise, sexual activities that cause tissues to rupture or produce blood would also increase the risk of HIV transmission (Osmond, 1990).

The proper use of latex condoms with nonoxynol-9 is an effective means of inhibiting the transmission of HIV (Wofsy, 1988). Although the risk of transmission during unprotected sexual activity is not known, studies suggest that the risk of transmitting the virus from an infected person to a noninfected person with one sexual encounter while using a condom is one in 500 (Cohen, 1990).

Candid discussions about sexual behavior are a tricky proposition for the schools. Sexual expressions are deeply rooted in moral, social and cultural beliefs. Yet, HIV/AIDS is a disease for which candid discussions are necessary if people are going to understand both the severity of the disease and the precautions required to protect themselves from possible exposure.

Many people would like to deny the sexual behavior of adolescents or blame it on curiosity aroused by sexuality education. Developmentally, adolescence is the time for sexual discovery and experimentation. According to the Report of the National Commission on AIDS (1991):

> Recent studies revealed that by age 15, 27% of the girls and 33% of the boys were sexually active. Half of the girls had sex by age 17 and half of the boys by age 16; three out of every four unmarried 19-year-old women and five out of six unmarried 19-year-old men had had sexual intercourse.

Teenage pregnancy rates testify to the level of sexual activity in this population. In spite of protests to the contrary, teenagers are a sexually active population, at risk for HIV infection. In 1988, AIDS was the sixth leading cause of death in 15 to 24 year olds. During the years of the 1990s, AIDS cases in adolescents have increased by 77 percent (AIDS Clinical Care, 1992). These data suggest that teenagers in the United States are sexually active in ways that place them at risk for HIV.

This same group of young people are exposed to the open display of condoms and other contraceptive measures in grocery and convenience stores. Condom jokes and references are on television news and entertainment shows. Specialty condom stores have opened. Condom ads now appear in magazines, newspapers and on television. Yet, school teachers and counselors cannot describe how to use condoms effectively for the prevention of HIV and other sexually transmitted disease (STD). Without question, adolescents live in an ambiguous society—one where they can buy condoms by the dozen but cannot be instructed on how to use them.

Regardless of the social pressures not to act, the schools, along with other social systems, must assume their role of instructing youth on the steps necessary to prevent exposure to HIV. It is unconscionable that sexually active teenagers are permitted to remain ignorant and vulnerable to a deadly disease. Unlike the stigma of getting a "social disease" or the trauma of an unplanned pregnancy, HIV/AIDS is fatal. At a minimum, teachers should be permitted to discuss anything that can be purchased at a grocery store.

Injection Transmission

Transmission of the virus through injection is one of the most certain methods of infection. The sharing of needles between an infected person and a noninfected person amounts to a direct inoculation of the virus. The actual risk of transmission is related to the number of exposures and the concentration of the virus in the contaminated syringe. In some injection-drug-using communities, the prevalence of HIV infection exceeds 67 percent of the population (Chaisson, 1990).

Schools must be relentless in their inclusion of substance use and abuse content in the curriculum. There is little room for a soft response to this problem. Few people object to the schools taking a strong instructional stand in the prevention of drug use. However, the role of the schools in the treatment side of the drug-use equation is less agreed upon.

Young people who are already using injection drugs progressively increase their risk of infection with every shared needle. Moreover, adolescent HIV-infected drug users can be the sexual partners of noninfected, non-drug-using adolescents, further increasing the likelihood of heterosexual transmission of HIV. To reduce the risk of HIV transmission, schools need to take leader-ship roles in advocating for increased numbers of treatment pro-grams for adolescents.

Although in principle few people object to providing drug treatment programs, most do not want schools to pay for these programs. They see the drug problem as a criminal justice one, not an educational one. Even those who want to support a school role in providing drug treatment for adolescents face the dilemma of allocating revenues to either education interventions or to treatment programs.

Of greater controversy is the call by the National Commission on AIDS to instruct individuals about "safe" needle use. By using bleach to clean the paraphernalia between each injection, the risk of transmission is greatly lowered. Another more contentious recommendation is to develop needle exchange programs, which would allow intravenous drug users to exchange used needles for clean ones.

Beyond the legality issues, this recommendation raises some of the same concerns as those associated with sex education. Many people believe that teaching individuals how to engage in "safer" drug use is tantamount to endorsing the behavior. The appropriate role of the schools in these controversial recommendations will vary according to the prevalence of substance use in their commu-nities and the availability of other drug intervention programs.

Blood Transfusions

Prior to the universal testing of the United States blood supply in 1984, a blood transfusion that contained HIV was a significant inoculation of the virus. People receiving such transfusions almost certainly developed HIV infection with the corresponding pro-gression toward AIDS. A special subpopulation that received enormous numbers of transfusions was people with hemophilia.

When hemophiliacs experience bleeding, they need to infuse themselves with concentrated blood products to stop the bleeding and prevent permanent damage to their joints. As a result of their multiple blood transfusions, many hemophiliacs developed AIDS. Since the beginning of the universal testing program, people with hemophilia are able to take care of their disease without risk of contracting HIV.

Young men with hemophilia became infected with HIV in the early 1980s. They will be a part of the school environment for many years to come. This accentuates the necessity for school policies that outline the procedures for managing HIV-infected students.

Perinatal Transmission

Transmission from infected mothers to their children can occur during fetal development, during delivery and during breastfeeding. The risk of transmission was once considered to be very high, in the range of 60 to 75 percent. Recent studies have lowered the risk of transmitting HIV between mothers and their children to a more modest estimate of 20 to 30 percent (Wofsy, 1990). The precise risk of transmission of the virus by breastfeeding is unknown. However, due to the large number of white blood cells in breast milk, most protocols for HIV prevention recommend that HIV-positive mothers not breastfeed their infants. Due to the biology of the immune system, all babies born to infected mothers will test positive for HIV at birth. This positive test is not confirmatory for the HIV status of the child, but is confirmatory for the status of the mother.

Although there is little direct connection between the perinatal transmission characteristics of HIV and the role of the school curriculum, beyond what might be included in a parenting class or early childhood class, there remains a need for the schools to be knowledgeable of the conditions associated with perinatal transmission. As more women become infected, the numbers of children born exposed to HIV will increase. With the currently available treatments, these children will be healthy enough to enter preschool and early intervention programs such as Head Start. As the treatments improve, HIV-infected children will remain healthy for longer periods and will be entering regular school programs. Soon it will be commonplace for HIV-infected children to participate fully in the entire range of school activities. Once again, this speaks to the need for comprehensive school HIV/AIDS policies.

Casual Spread

Even more controversial than discussing the sexual transmission of the virus is the discussion of contracting HIV infection through casual contact. Although there is no evidence that HIV is spread through such activities as hugging, sharing eating utensils, using the same shower or soap, breathing the same air, or sleeping in the same room, people are reluctant to believe it.

HIV/AIDS seems so mysterious that people expect a more complex and unfamiliar mechanism of transmission. For some people, sexual behavior and drug use are too ordinary to explain away the noxiousness of this disease. Therefore, they doubt the accuracy of the reports from the Centers for Disease Control and Prevention.

In spite of this skepticism, no documentation supports a conspiracy of germ warfare or medical experiments gone awry. Likewise, there is no evidence that HIV is spread through bites of mosquitoes or other insects. HIV is not spread through the air. HIV is not spread by hugging infected people or touching their belongings. After studying more than 200,000 cases of AIDS, there are no known cases linked to any of these behaviors or events.

Regardless of this overwhelming evidence, many people still believe that casual transmission is possible. In the presence of HIV/AIDS, this belief can turn to fear. This fear results in the hostility many schools experience after admitting HIV-infected children or employing HIV-infected personnel.

Key Points

1. There are several very definite ways in which HIV can spread from one person to another:
   - unprotected sexual activity with infected persons
   - sharing contaminated needles with infected persons
   - transfusion or major contact with infected blood
   - transmission between mother and child during fetal development, delivery or breastfeeding
2. These are the only ways HIV is spread.
3. HIV is not spread through casual contact.

Cofactors for Transmission and Their Role in the School Program

Transmission cofactors are those conditions that do not directly transmit the virus but do increase the likelihood that HIV-transmitting behaviors will occur.

Substance Use

The first cofactor is substance use other than injection drugs. Drugs tend to impair judgment, lower inhibitions and increase the thrill of risk taking. After several alcoholic drinks, a snort of cocaine or a few pills, individuals can feel more immune from harm. This feeling increases the chances of unprotected intercourse occurring or the chances that injection drugs will be tried.

Moreover, the continued use of substances can result in a

dependency that is costly to maintain. Many young people resort to participating in "sex for drugs" in order to sustain their dependency. Those who perform sex for drugs place themselves in double jeopardy, because they are engaging in numerous sexual encounters and are unlikely to take prevention action to avoid infection with HIV or other STD.

As schools develop programs and adopt curricula directed toward the reduction of substance use, they need to be mindful of the relationship between intoxication and exposure to risk. Classroom discussions about substance use can be used as opportunities to reinforce the HIV/AIDS prevention messages. Likewise, discussions about HIV/AIDS are opportunities to expand the content to include substance use prevention messages.

Sexually Transmitted Disease

The second cofactor of concern is the presence of STD. Many STDs cause genital lesions that can facilitate the viral transmission from one person to another. STD may also increase the likelihood of transmission by expanding the numbers of white blood cells that can come into contact with infected body fluids. STDs that have been associated with increased transmission include syphilis, herpes simplex and chancroid.

Non-lesion-producing STD may also increase the risk of transmission because many of these STDs attract the HIV target cells to the infected areas (oral, anal or genital). For people infected with HIV, having an STD increases the likelihood of spreading the infected cells to noninfected partners. For noninfected people, having an STD increases the likelihood that receptor cells will come into contact with body fluids containing HIV (Osmond, 1990).

In addition to the risk of transmitting HIV, STD is a measure of unprotected sexual activity in a population. Since World War II, and until recently, syphilis has been on the decline in the United States. During the last years of the 1980s, however, many urban and rural communities began experiencing a dramatic rise in the number of syphilis cases, especially in the younger populations in which sex for drugs is a factor.

Left untreated, syphilis can be a debilitating disease, with major social and health consequences to the infected persons and to the children born to syphilitic mothers. The symptoms of syphilis come in four stages that extend over a lifetime if the disease is untreated. The most noticeable symptom is a sore called a chancre which appears from a week to three months after exposure. If individuals have both syphilis and HIV, the virus is present in very high concentration in chancres, and these sores make the transmission of HIV more likely.

Many STDs, most notably syphilis and gonorrhea, are treatable with penicillin and other antibiotics. Strains of gonorrhea within the United States have become resistant to antibiotics, resulting in an increased spread of the penicillin-resistant strains. In women, the inability or failure to treat STD can result in serious infections that penetrate the reproductive system, causing pelvic inflammatory disease and sterility. Untreated oral gonorrhea can result in a disseminated infection that spreads throughout the entire body. The symptoms associated with gonorrhea usually appear from several days to a couple of weeks after exposure. They can be very mild in women and are often overlooked.

Gonorrhea is often accompanied by chlamydia, which is the most common bacterial STD in the United States. In women, chlamydia can cause very serious problems, such as pelvic inflammatory disease, sterility, urinary tract infections and possible complications during pregnancy. In men, chlamydia usually causes an inflammation of the urethra, prostate and/or rectum. Anal chlamydia has also been associated with the sexual abuse of children.

Chlamydia is treated with large doses of antibiotics. Although the symptoms associated with chlamydia are so mild that they may go unnoticed, when they do appear it will be from one to two weeks following exposure. Characteristics of chlamydia that increase the risk of HIV transmission are unusual vaginal bleeding and bleeding after intercourse.

The condition called herpes is caused by viruses and comes in two varieties: herpes simplex virus Type I (HSV I) and herpes simplex virus Type II (HSV II). In general, HSV I occurs around the face and mouth and causes fever blisters or cold sores. HSV I does not appear to be transmitted from one person to another.

HSV II occurs in the genital area and causes blisters similar in appearance to the cold sores associated with HSV I. These painful blisters break and ooze fluid full of the virus. HSV II can be transmitted through direct contact with the virus found in the blisters. A greater acceptance of oral sex practices has led to HSV II blisters also occurring near the mouth and oral cavity.

Herpes infection has active stages when the blisters are present and remission periods when there is no sign of the disease. Although transmission is more likely during the active stage, it can occur during times of remission as well. Once infected with HSV II, there can be periods of remission followed by reoccurrences throughout life. There is no cure for herpes infection. Symptoms of the disease occur between two days and three weeks after exposure. People with active HSV II are at greater risk for HIV transmission.

Another common viral STD, genital warts, is caused by Human papillomavirus (HPV). There are more than twenty types of HPV that cause warts or flat lesions in the human genital area. There is some evidence that HPV is associated with increased risk of cervical cancer. The cures for HPV are similar to those used in treating warts on other parts of the body: they are burned off chemically or removed surgically. Symptoms of HPV infection occur from three weeks to eight months after exposure. The relationship between presence of genital warts and the transmission of HIV is not known.

Just as with HIV, viral STD infections are neither easily treatable nor curable. Antibiotics, although effective against many bacterial STDs, are not efficacious in treating viral infections. Untreated STDs are very serious, but they rarely result in death.

HIV, which is transmitted in a similar fashion, is both untreatable and fatal. Another striking difference between STD and HIV is the length of time from exposure to symptoms. With most STDs, the time between infection and symptoms can be from a few days to many months; with HIV, the time ranges from seven to ten years. Regardless of the comparisons between HIV and STD, one fact is indisputable: people who place themselves at risk for STD are simultaneously placing themselves at risk for HIV.

Many school health curricula include the discussion of HIV/ AIDS in the subject area of sexually transmitted disease. This fits comfortably with the sexual transmission of the virus. HIV/AIDS and other STDs are prevented through similar means: abstinence, mutual monogomy, and condom use. The inclusion of HIV/ AIDS with STD provides a larger conceptual frame from which to describe the harmful social and economic consequences that result from infectious diseases that are left unchecked.

This relationship provides an opportunity to highlight the public health approach to curbing the spread of disease, which includes an analysis of the circumstances that surround exposure to the infectious agent. The public health approach concentrates on behaviors that place people at risk for the infection rather than emphasizing the nature of the persons who are infected. By embedding HIV/AIDS discussions in the larger topic of STD, these discussions are less vulnerable to attack from groups who oppose the inclusion of HIV/AIDS in school health programs in stand-alone HIV/AIDS units. Additionally, linking STD and HIV/AIDS can strengthen young people's sense of vulnerability about becoming infected through unprotected sexual intercourse. However, it is important not to lose sight of the other routes of HIV transmission, most specifically injection drug use.

Tuberculosis

Although not a true cofactor, tuberculosis (TB) is emerging as a serious consequence of the HIV epidemic. During the early 1900s, tuberculosis was a leading cause of death in the United States. TB is a very infectious, contagious and debilitating disease. The bacterium that causes TB, *Mycobacterium tuberculosis,* is spread from infected people to noninfected people through the air. People who are infected can easily spread the disease to others through coughing, sneezing and spitting. However, with improved diagnosis and treatment, the disease had been on the decline until the middle 1980s. Most states closed their TB sanitariums and the former American Tuberculosis Association changed its name to the American Lung Association.

Now the incidence of TB is on the rise in populations whose immune systems are compromised by HIV, poor nutrition, alcoholism, drug use and other degenerating illnesses. It is now quite common to find active TB in people with HIV/AIDS, the homeless, alcoholics and drug users. There is a serious correlation between the risk factors for TB and the risk factors for HIV. Many populations who are infected with HIV are also infected with TB. Unlike HIV, where the virus is not transmitted through casual contact, TB is spread very easily by breathing the TB bacillus.

Coincidental to the rise of TB cases, there has been an increasing incidence of drug-resistant TB strains. These strains persist in an infectious and contagious state even after several rounds of treatment protocols. The fear of drug-resistant TB can result in many people with HIV/AIDS, or those who engage in risk behaviors associated with HIV/AIDS transmission, being denied medical or social services.

Because historically the schools were often associated with TB epidemics, in many states school teachers were required to have annual chest X-rays or tuberculin skin tests prior to the beginning of the school year. With the decline of TB, many schools dropped these requirements during the 1970s. In the event of an epidemic of drug resistant strains of TB, the public could demand the return of X-rays and skin tests for school personnel.

In early school health curricula, the prevention of TB was included as part of the content. With the advances of modern medicine, most school health curricula deleted any references to TB. A parallel deletion occurred in the curricula of medical and health professional schools. Many practicing physicians, nurses and public health officials have never treated patients with TB.

If the TB problem continues to grow, schools might be asked to include TB education as part of the comprehensive school health program. Additionally, public health officials might require school health personnel to obtain continuing education about the diagnosis and treatment of tuberculosis.

Ignorance Is *Not* Bliss

AIDS jolted the American people. It has awakened us to the scary reality that a disease anywhere is a possibility of a disease everywhere. The decade of debate over the propriety of including discussions about homosexuality, sexual practices, STD and condoms in school curricula wasted valuable time. The failure to take swift, direct and persistent action to alert the public about the pathology of HIV/AIDS has placed entire populations at risk for contracting it.

AIDS has reminded us that the adage "Ignorance is bliss" was incorrect. While the nation was engaging in fruitless arguments about the vulgarity of the disease and the worthiness of the people it infected, AIDS was becoming a leading cause of death in the country. If AIDS has taught us anything, it has taught us that denial, fear and condemnation do not prevent epidemics. The question remains, Do the schools have the courage to take their rightful place in protecting America's children against the major disease of their time?

If we do have the courage to prepare our children to handle today's realities of HIV/AIDS, we will be investing in our future. Not only will we be preparing them to avoid a mortal disease, we will be modeling for them the type of valor they will need to respond to the disease realities of tomorrow. There is no assurance that AIDS is the last "new" disease that will test our sensibilities and require bold action. And what happened with the HIV/AIDS epidemic should never happen again.

References

AIDS Clinical Care. 1992. Medical care of HIV-infected adolescents. 4 (12): 95-98.

Centers for Disease Control and Prevention. 1981. Kaposi's sarcoma and pneumocystis pneumonia among homosexual men—New York City and California. *Morbidity and Mortality Weekly Report* 30:305-308.

Centers for Disease Control and Prevention. 1988. Guidelines for effective school health education to prevent the spread of AIDS. *Morbidity and Mortality Weekly Report.* 37 (suppl. no. S-2): 1-14.

Centers for Disease Control and Prevention. 1992. *HIV/AIDS Surveillance.* Atlanta, GA. (Single copies are available free from National AIDS Clearinghouse, P. O. Box 6003, Rockville, MD 20849-6003.)

Chaisson, R. E. 1990. Transmission of HIV in intravenous drug users. In *The AIDS knowledge base,* ed. P. T. Cohen, M. A. Sande and P. A. Volberding,

1.2.6-1.2.6-4. Waltham, MA: The Medical Publishing Corp.

Cohen, P. T. 1990. Safe sex, safer sex, and prevention of HIV infection. In *The AIDS knowledge base,* ed. P. T. Cohen, M. A. Sande and P. A. Volverding, 11.1.4-11.1.4-10. Waltham, MA: The Medical Publishing Corp.

Grossman, M. 1988. Children with AIDS. In *The Medical Management of AIDS,* ed. M. A. Sande and P. A. Volberding, 319-329. Philadelphia, PA: W. B. Saunders.

Lifson, A. 1990. Transmission of HIV in households. In *The AIDS Knowledge Base,* ed. P. T. Cohen, M. A. Sande and P. A. Volberding, 1.2.11-1.2.11-3. Waltham, MA: The Medical Publishing Corp.

National Commission on AIDS. 1991. *Americans living with AIDS.* (Available from National Commission on AIDS, 1730 K Street NW, Suite 815, Washington, DC 20402.)

Osmond, D. 1990. Heterosexual transmission of HIV. In *The AIDS knowledge base,* ed. P. T. Cohen, M. A. Sande, and P. A. Volberding, 1.2.4-1.2.4-9. Waltham, MA: The Medical Publishing Corp.

Osmond, D. 1990. Homosexual transmission of HIV. In *The AIDS knowledge base,* ed. P. T. Cohen, M. A. Sande, and P. A. Volberding, 1.2.3-1.2.3-3. Waltham, MA: The Medical Publishing Corp.

Wofsy, C. 1988. Prevention of HIV transmission. In *The medical management of AIDS,* ed. M. A. Sande and P. A. Volberding, 29-43. Philadelphia, PA: W. B. Saunders.

Chapter 17

Injury Prevention

David A. Sleet, PhD

The health status of American children has changed significantly in the last forty years. Widespread immunization programs have virtually eliminated the threat of infectious diseases such as polio, diphtheria and pneumonia. However, one health problem continues to threaten the life and health of school-age children and youth—injuries. Childhood injury is the major cause of excess child mortality in the United States; it causes more deaths to school-age children than all childhood diseases combined (Rosenberg, Rodriquez and Chorba, 1990). In fact, injury is today's primary public health problem for Americans under the age of 44.

In contrast to the reductions in infectious disease rates, the number of injury deaths has shown only a slight decline in the last twenty years. From 1975 to 1986, while deaths from collisions between motor vehicles and pedestrians declined by 16 percent, injury deaths from homicide declined by only 7 percent; and suicide deaths increased by 2 percent (Baker et al., 1992). Recent data suggest that injuries to American children and youth could be dramatically reduced by improving programs for injury prevention and control.

The school plays an important role in encouraging injury prevention. Behavioral, environmental and social control measures can be implemented in the school to ensure the safety of children and youth. The school's role as a community resource also provides an opportunity for school administrators and teachers to play a more active part in advocating state and federal injury prevention legislation, local and community regulation, and district and school policy reform. Parents and teachers need training in effective injury prevention education programs at school, at home and in the community. Children need the foundation of decision-making skills regarding injury-risk behaviors and injury-avoidance strategies.

Injury as a Public Health Problem

According to the National Academy of Sciences (1988), "Injury is probably the most underrecognized major public health problem facing the nation today." Injuries, both unintentional and intentional, are a major public health problem in America. In fact, each year, injury is the number one cause of death among school-age children and youth in virtually every country in the world (Egger, Sleet, Harrison et al., 1993). Why then hasn't injury prevention been given a more prominent place in health promotion and disease prevention efforts?

One reason injury prevention traditionally has not been embraced within public health is that injuries have been considered the result of "accidents." *The Oxford English Dictionary* defines the term *accident* as "an event without apparent cause...unexpected

...happening by chance." In geology, an accident is "an irregularity on a surface, the explanation of which is not readily known."

Accidents have been viewed as random and uncontrollable "acts of fate," unpredictable and unavoidable. But this is not true. We know from the science of injury prevention that the events that cause injury are not accidents or random events—they are predictable and many are preventable.

The modern public health approach recognizes injury as a public health problem that can be understood and controlled with the same measures we have directed against disease. Injury results from the interactions among an injury-producing agent (such as kinetic energy), the environment (such as a playground) and a susceptible host (such as a young, curious child).

Injury can be controlled by preventing its occurrence or minimizing its severity. In the case of a sports injury, damage to the host—the person harmed—is brought about through a rapid transfer of kinetic energy (from movement). Changing this pattern of energy transfer, either by making the host more resistant to it or by separating the host from the energy exchange in the environment, is part of the science of injury prevention.

Research and practice in injury control indicate who is at risk for particular injuries and what works to prevent such injuries. A "systems approach" in the schools, one that combines structural, environmental and educational elements, is likely to yield the best results. This approach requires the involvement of school districts, teachers, social workers, police, principals, engineers, playground designers, sports medicine experts, coaches, road safety professionals and health professionals. Prevention will pay off only through multidisciplinary collaboration. This collaboration is especially important in the area of violence prevention.

What Is Injury?

The word *injury* has its root in the Latin term *in juris,* which literally means "not right." The dictionary defines injury as "harm of any kind, done or sustained." Injury, as used in public health, is defined as "unintentional or intentional damage to the body resulting from acute exposure to thermal, mechanical, electrical, or chemical energy or from the absence of such essentials as heat or oxygen" (National Committee for Injury Prevention and Control, 1989). The terms *injury* and *trauma* are often used interchangeably.

Although there are many kinds and causes of injury, two main categories have been defined. *Acute exposure to energy* includes injuries resulting from falls, motor vehicle crashes, firearms, violence and many sports injuries (kinetic); fires and burns (thermal); poisonings (chemical); electrocution (electricity); and radiation. *Absence of essentials* includes lack of oxygen (as in asphyxiation or drowning) and lack of heat (as in hypothermia or frostbite). Injury may be *intentional* (deliberate), as in murder or suicide, or *unintentional* ("accidental") as in a fall or poisoning.

Since the term *accident* implies an unavoidable event, it should not be used when referring to injury—the medical consequence of an event that may be largely preventable. Using terms such as *injury control* and *injury prevention* rather than *accident prevention* helps make clear the potential for preventing such events. As former U.S. Surgeon General C. Everett Koop put it:

> We must accept that the injuries associated with motor vehicles are not "accidents" and that much can be done to reduce them. We must realize that violence in the forms of abuse, assault or suicide is...within the purview of...the health system. An informed and aroused public can change the behavior

of each of us, but more importantly, it must lead to community outrage and action in regard to unsafe playgrounds, automobiles, highways, work places, toys, homes and use of handguns." (National Committee for Injury Prevention and Control, 1989)

The Magnitude of the Problem

While you read this chapter, approximately nine Americans will be killed and about 765 others will suffer a disability from injury. On an average day in the United States, more than four hundred people die and 170,000 seek medical care as a result of injuries (National Committee for Injury Prevention and Control, 1989). On average, there are ten unintentional injury deaths and about one thousand disabling injuries every hour (National Safety Council, 1992).

From a few months of age through age 44, injuries are the leading cause of death in the United States. One source estimated that for children ages five to nine, the risk of dying from injuries during the next 15 years is 2.6 times greater than the risk of dying from all other causes combined (Budnick and Chaiken, 1985).

About 75 percent of children's injury mortality is caused by unintentional injury, with motor-vehicle-related injury deaths responsible for the greatest proportion. The remaining 25 percent is caused by violence, principally homicide and suicide. In 1988 in the United States, injury claimed the lives of more than 22,000 children under age 19; it accounted for 80 percent of the deaths from all causes in the 15- to 19-year-old age group (Children's Safety Network, 1991). As C. Everett Koop once noted: "If a disease were killing our children in the proportions that injuries are, people would be outraged and demand that this killer be stopped" (Koop, 1989).

Figures 1, 2 and 3 present childhood injury deaths by cause and age. When viewed together, motor-vehicle-related injuries are the major cause of death in school-age children and youth.

Figure 1 shows that the four leading causes of injury death to elementary-school-age children (ages 5-9) in 1988 were pedestrian, motor vehicle occupant, fire/burns and drowning. Pedestrian and motor vehicle occupant injuries accounted for nearly 40 percent of all deaths in this age group.

For middle-school-age children (ages 10-14), the leading causes of injury death are motor vehicle occupant, pedestrian, homicide, suicide and drowning. Intentional injuries account for nearly 20 percent of the injury deaths of these children. (See Figure 2.)

For high-school-age youth (ages 15-19), motor vehicle occupant injuries are the leading cause of injury-related death. Twice as many 15 to 19 year olds die as occupants of motor vehicles than from any other cause. After motor vehicle occupant deaths, homicide and suicide are the major causes of mortality in this age group. (See Figure 3.)

Costs

Overall, estimated total lifetime costs of all injuries in 1985 exceeded $158 billion, with unintentional injuries accounting for two-thirds of these costs. Injury costs include emergency medical treatment and rehabilitation costs, as well as costs due to lost productivity and the value of goods and services not produced because of injury. One study found that among children ages zero to 19, three causes of injuries account for 60.5 percent of the total initial medical costs: transportation injuries, falls and sports injuries (Malek et al., 1991).

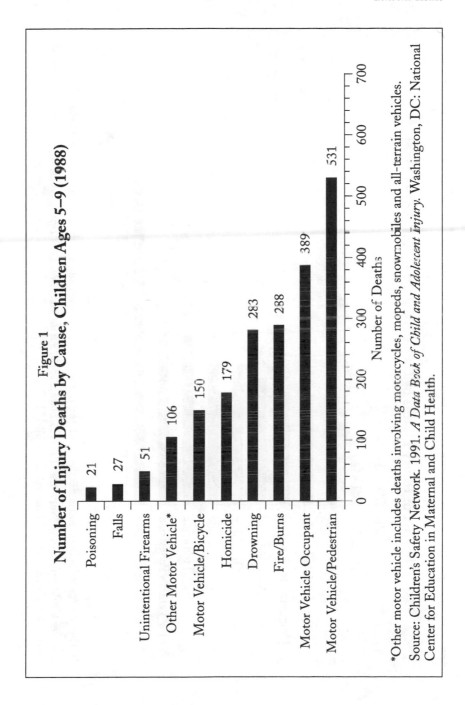

Figure 1
Number of Injury Deaths by Cause, Children Ages 5–9 (1988)

*Other motor vehicle includes deaths involving motorcycles, mopeds, snowmobiles and all-terrain vehicles.

Source: Children's Safety Network. 1991. *A Data Book of Child and Adolecent Injury.* Washington, DC: National Center for Education in Maternal and Child Health.

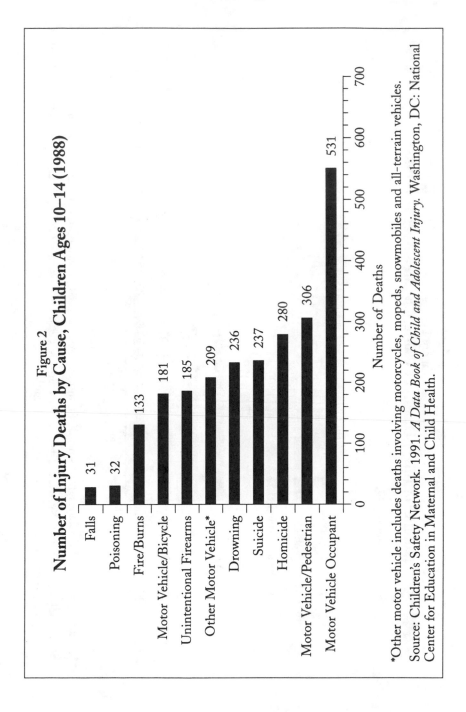

Figure 2

Number of Injury Deaths by Cause, Children Ages 10–14 (1988)

*Other motor vehicle includes deaths involving motorcycles, mopeds, snowmobiles and all-terrain vehicles.

Source: Children's Safety Network. 1991. *A Data Book of Child and Adolescent Injury.* Washington, DC: National Center for Education in Maternal and Child Health.

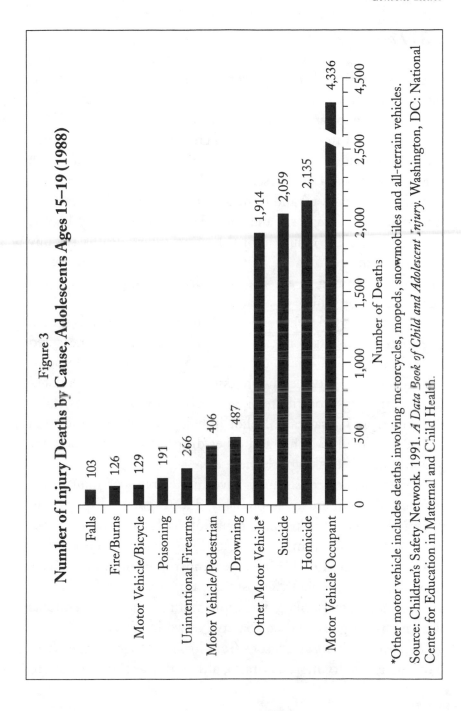

Figure 3
Number of Injury Deaths by Cause, Adolescents Ages 15–19 (1988)

Cause	Number of Deaths
Falls	103
Fire/Burns	126
Motor Vehicle/Bicycle	129
Poisoning	191
Unintentional Firearms	266
Motor Vehicle/Pedestrian	406
Drowning	487
Other Motor Vehicle*	1,914
Suicide	2,059
Homicide	2,135
Motor Vehicle Occupant	4,336

Number of Deaths

*Other motor vehicle includes deaths involving motorcycles, mopeds, snowmobiles and all-terrain vehicles.
Source: Children's Safety Network. 1991. *A Data Book of Child and Adolescent Injury.* Washington, DC: National Center for Education in Maternal and Child Health.

Risk Factors

Injury types and rates vary according to demographics, age, sex, stages of growth and development, and environmental risks. Consequently, injury prevention strategies must be tailored to individual risk groups and developmental stages.

Age. Deaths from aspiration and choking are high in infancy. Deaths from drownings peak at around age three, as do burn deaths from house fires. Preschoolers die from falls, as pedestrians (usually in a driveway) and from poisonings. Pedestrian deaths in traffic increase to age six and then decline, replaced by bicycle injuries to age 14. Unintentional firearm injury deaths steadily increase from ages 5 to 19. Homicide and suicide show dramatic increases beginning at age 15, as do drownings, poisonings and deaths as motor vehicle occupants.

Alcohol/Drugs. Alcohol and its role in injury commands special attention as a risk factor. The effects of alcohol can be measured across virtually all injury categories. About half of all motor vehicle and homicide deaths are associated with alcohol. Alcohol and other drugs contribute significantly to suicide, fires, falls, drownings and assaults. Alcohol impairs physical abilities and affects judgment. Alcohol and other drugs can also increase aggression and risk-taking behavior.

Gender. Males consistently have higher rates of injury than females. This difference is probably due to greater exposure to risks and increased risk-taking behavior. Males are also 2.5 times more likely to die from injury (U.S. Department of Health and Human Services, 1991). Males are almost four times more likely to be victims of homicide, almost three times more likely to drown and 6.5 times more likely to be the victim of an unintentional firearm discharge (Children's Safety Network, 1991).

Socioeconomic status. Persons from lower socioeconomic status have higher injury mortality rates, although there are exceptions for certain types of injuries. Families in lower-income areas are also less likely to have safety devices on hand, such as child safety restraints, fire extinguishers and smoke detectors.

Geography/Residence. Rural populations have higher injury death rates than urban residents, probably due to greater hazards, higher road speeds, and delays in obtaining emergency assistance. Climate, seasonal changes and access to quality medical care are also characteristics of geography that affect injury rates and injury outcomes. Fire-related deaths are more common in areas with poor housing standards and crowding; drowning in hot climates, in summer, and among residents with backyard pools; homicides and poisonings in large metropolitan cities; unintentional and intentional shooting deaths in homes with easy access to guns; and motor vehicle deaths among residents in less densely populated areas.

Ethnicity. Higher death rates from unintentional injury occur among African Americans than among Whites over the entire age range (Gulaid et al., 1988), with African-American males generally having the highest death rates. Native Americans and Native Alaskans have disproportionately higher death rates from motor vehicle crashes, residential fires and drowning (Indian Health Service, 1989), especially in reservation states in the western United States. Suicides are also prevalent among some tribes (Smith et al., 1992). These differences may reflect important socio-economic, environmental or lifestyle factors.

Nonfatal Injuries

Injury deaths are only a small part of the problem. Millions are incapacitated by injuries; many suffer lifelong disabilities. Nonfatal injuries account for one in every six hospital days and one in every ten hospital discharges (U.S. Department of Health and Human Services, 1991). A population-based study in Massachu-

setts found that for each injury death, there were 42 hospitalizations and 1,121 emergency room visits (Gallagher, 1991). More
than 25 percent of all emergency room or hospital visits are for the
treatment of injuries (Rivara and Mueller, 1987). In addition,
injuries are the leading cause of physician contacts. One out of
four Americans seek medical care for an injury each year. At the
current rate, one in nine children born today will be hospitalized
for an injury during the first 15 years of life.

Childhood injury mortality figures are shocking. However,
mortality is only a small part of the total injury picture. Interventions targeted solely at injury deaths may neglect nonfatal injuries
that require hospitalization and may leave children permanently
disabled. Interventions targeted only at preventing injury deaths
may neglect the potential for preventing more frequent and costly
disabling and nonfatal injuries.

Controlling Injuries

Advances in injury prevention have been dominated by one of
two, frequently conflicting, approaches: "active" or behavioral approaches and "passive" or environmental approaches. Although
both have an important role to play, neither approach presents a
complete solution to the injury problem. Health promotion approaches provide an alternative that allows for both behavioral and
environmental intervention to control injuries (Sleet, Wagenaar
and Waller, 1989).

Active Versus Passive Approaches

Active approaches require some human effort or behavioral change
to be effective. Active approaches can be simple, relying on one-
time behavior (placing dangerous equipment out of reach of children) or more complex frequent behavior (putting on a bicycle

helmet). Active interventions place the emphasis for prevention almost entirely on the individual. They emphasize behavioral change and modification of lifestyle. The approach is epitomized in the view that the great majority of controllable risk factors associated with injuries are behavioral in nature and that injury prevention can be realized through individuals taking greater responsibility for their own health (Roberts, Fanurik and Layfield, 1987).

Passive approaches require little or no human effort to be effective, relying instead on changes in the environment or in technology. Passive approaches (such as smoke detectors, air bags, break-away goal posts) work automatically to protect people from injury. Automatic protection places emphasis on modifications in the physical environment (playing fields and surfaces, protective equipment) and the psychosocial environment (modified rules, social norms and expectations), as well as in products that cause injury (chemicals, machine tools, pools, guns). These modifications require little or no individual action on the part of those being protected. This approach stresses the importance of the role of the social, political, economic and physical environments in determining injury behavior (Wilson and Baker, 1987).

Although active and passive approaches overlap considerably, they have important differences. Passive approaches, when applied to large populations, have the greatest potential for effectiveness, but they are not available for all injury risks and are frequently difficult to implement. For example, the passive approach to sliding injuries in baseball through the use of detachable bases requires individual action in replacing the bases correctly.

Active approaches, such as putting on a helmet or driving within the speed limit, require frequent, repeated action and high motivation. Active approaches often don't influence those at greatest risk, such as teenagers, who may not be motivated to take protective action frequently.

Health Promotion Approaches

Health promotion is the "combination of educational and environmental supports for actions and conditions of living conducive to health" (Green and Kreuter, 1991). Health promotion seeks to change social and environmental factors that influence injury risk behavior. Individual and community actions, fostered by education, stimulated by social and organizational change, and encouraged through public policy, legislation and enforcement, are the immediate objects of health promotion approaches to injury prevention (Sleet, Egger and Albany, 1991).

Schools have placed increasing emphasis on health promotion approaches in programs for changing diet, exercise and substance use behaviors in school-age children and youth. These same approaches must now be used to prevent injuries (Sleet, 1984). As stated by Mason and Tolsma (1984):

> Persons can hardly be expected to avoid the health risks imposed by personal choices when they do not know or understand these risks, when they lack the knowledge or skills needed to choose a healthier lifestyle, or worst of all, when they seek guidance or support from their community and it is unavailable to them.

Effective injury prevention programs in schools must incorporate passive protection where feasible (automatic guards on dangerous equipment, soft playground surfaces) and promote individual behavior change when possible (incentives for bicycle helmet use, education on safe pedestrian practices). Most injuries have both environmental and behavioral determinants, and the solution to reducing injury rests in using both approaches simultaneously.

Selecting Appropriate Strategies

There are three generally accepted strategies for injury prevention and control.

- Education/Behavior Change
- Legislation (Policy)/Enforcement
- Engineering/Technology

Strategies are often selected in combination after an analysis of the situation. Identifying strategies that may be effectively implemented over the long term and those that may be used for more immediate results is helpful. Such identification can lead to interventions designed to change school policies to create safer environments, legislative actions such as passage of more stringent regulations or enforcement of existing laws, efforts to change children's behaviors at school to reduce individual risk of injury, or fundamental changes in the design or use of products to make them safer for use at school.

The three types of strategies each target different causative factors in injury. The education/behavior change strategies primarily target changes in host or individual risk behavior. Legislation/ enforcement strategies primarily target the environment through changes in laws, regulations, policy and compliance. Engineering/ technology strategies primarily target the agent (vehicle or vector) of injury and reduce the amount or release of energy through changes in design.

However, the strategies do overlap and may affect more than one segment of the problem simultaneously. For example: An education/behavior change directed toward decreasing individual drinking and driving behavior may also have an effect on strengthening existing drinking/driving laws or enforcement. It may also lead to the development of better technology for testing the blood-alcohol content of drinking drivers (Geller et al., 1991). An example of the targeted use of these three types of strategies in the prevention of sports injuries at school and how these strategies may overlap is presented in Figure 4.

Since most sports injuries result from human contact, there is great potential for improving injury rates by education/behavior change strategies. Some of the means for reducing individual risk in sports include:

- increased screening for age/developmental appropriateness of participation
- improved individual and game supervision
- training for coaches
- player education and improved conditioning
- more effective practice sessions and competency
- parent education
- safety and injury prevention incentives and rewards

Legislation/enforcement strategies can contribute to injury reduction through changes in the environment, both the physical and the sociocultural environment. Changes in the physical environment can be encouraged by passing regulations or guidelines on the proper use of protective gear, surface and equipment requirements, enforcing rules and policies on first-aid training, emergency-care access and transport and suitable practice conditions. Changes in the sociocultural environment can be encouraged through requiring minimal insurance, mandating parental involvement, establishing minimal accreditation standards for coaches and trainers, and altering and enforcing the rules of the game to minimize injury.

Improvements in engineering/technology can affect the agents of injury and thus affect the nature and chances of injury. Protective equipment, such as mouthguards, shoulder pads, headgear, shin pads, footwear, helmets and leg padding all result from

Figure 4

Causative Factors and Interaction Between Intervention Strategies
in Prevention of Sports Injuries at School

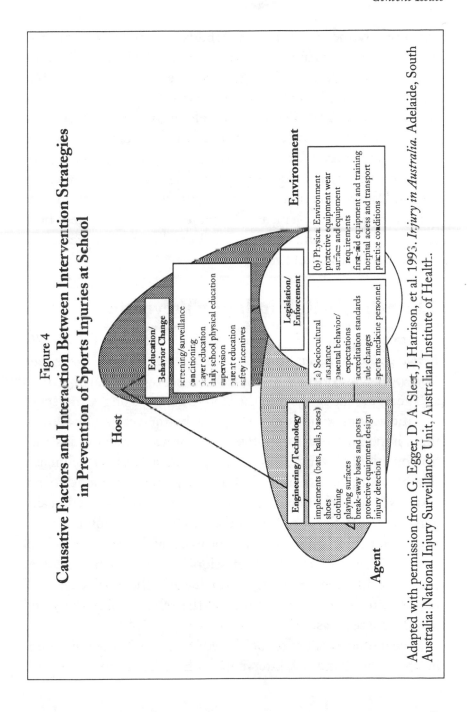

Adapted with permission from G. Egger, D. A. Sleet, J. Harrison, et al. 1993. *Injury in Australia*. Adelaide, South
Australia: National Injury Surveillance Unit, Australian Institute of Health.

advances in the design and suitability of products to protect against injury. Similarly, agents of injury such as bats, balls, bases, cleats, goal posts and playing surfaces should be modified to further minimize injuries during contact.

In some cases, as with football helmets, technology has been combined with regulation and education to guarantee maximum benefit to the player. Unfortunately, helmets, while protecting the host from injury, are frequently themselves the source of injury to others. Using a multiple causation approach to prevention provides a basis for implementing interventions that address both behavioral factors and environmental conditions that predispose school-age children and youth to injuries.

The School's Role in Injury Prevention

In late 1990, the U.S. Public Health Service released *Healthy People 2000: National Health Promotion and Disease Prevention Objectives*. This document establishes a set of national objectives and goals to reduce injury in the United States, along with a set of specific actions to achieve these goals by the year 2000. One of these important health objectives is to "provide academic instruction on injury prevention and control, preferably as part of quality school health education, in at least 50 percent of public school systems (grades K through 12)" (Objective 9.18). A related health personnel objective is to "include academic instruction on injury prevention in schools that train primary and secondary school educators and recreational professionals" (U.S. Department of Health and Human Services, 1991). Clearly, these objectives will require effort and cooperation from the school, community and health care settings.

The development of school-based injury prevention programs has been slow, and few interventions have been properly evaluated. Since injury prevention has recently become a major public health issue, reexamination of the role of the schools in providing injury prevention has begun (Wojtowicz, Macrina and Bolton, 1990).

Educators see students almost every day, so are in a unique position to identify injury problems and potential solutions. An injury prevention program in the schools should be integrated with a comprehensive school health education program. As in school health, many opportunities and resources for improving injury prevention at school already exist (Nelson, 1986). These include policies and procedures, staff training, curriculum development, facilities and environment, and health services.

Policies and Procedures

Administrative rules and regulations can help keep children safe at school. School policies can promote positive behaviors conducive to injury prevention (such as wearing bicycle helmets) and restrict undesirable injury risk-taking behavior such as carrying weapons to school. Every school should develop written policies and procedures for the prevention and treatment of injuries.

School policies may cover first aid and emergency care, record keeping, disaster preparedness, traffic control, personal protection, inservice and school security. A school policy might provide teachers with inservice time for injury prevention training or specify curriculum development and integration. It might prescribe procedures to be followed in sports/recreation programs to improve safety, prescribe specific injury prevention methods to be followed for students with special needs and handicapping conditions, or identify the hours of instruction devoted to injury prevention within the school curriculum. School injury prevention policies and procedures need to be developed, communicated and systematically followed by teachers, administrators and students.

Staff Training

Most teachers will have had little formal training in the problems of injury and injury prevention. Teachers, coaches, administrators and other staff (including bus drivers, nurses, student teachers, aides and custodial staff) must be oriented to school policies and procedures designed to prevent injuries. Teacher training may occur through workshops, preservice seminars, inservice training or formal coursework. Group-oriented curricular development and team teaching, independent study, and community education opportunities (extended studies, open university, training seminars) can also be used to improve teacher competence in injury prevention. Administrators may need to work out efficient means for more careful supervision of students at school.

In addition to helping teachers use new materials in the classroom, many of these activities will also help reduce injury potential for staff by increasing awareness and personal protective action against injury. As new school curricular developments in injury prevention emerge (such as violence prevention), teachers will require further inservice education and training.

Curriculum Development

Few comprehensive curricula exist for teaching about injury prevention. The instructional philosophy driving health education in schools should also influence the development of injury prevention modules and materials.

An injury prevention curriculum or module should be designed to reduce the frequency and severity of injuries—both at school, at home, on the road and in the community—from the early grades through high school. It should enable students to acquire new knowledge about injury risks and improve attitudes about reducing risks. It should also provide skills in personal decision making and behavioral change to modify personal and environmental risks for injury (Sleet, 1992). The curriculum may focus on specific risks, such as violence, by promoting the use of appropriate conflict resolution methods, or provide for a wide range of objectives and activities in injury control.

Elementary Curricula

One formal curriculum available to elementary teachers is *Preventing Injury: A Safety Curriculum* (ETR Associates, 1991). The curriculum is offered in four volumes, for preschool/kindergarten, grades one and two, grades three and four, and grades five and six. *Actions for Health* (ETR Associates, 1992), a comprehensive health curriculum for kindergarten through grade six, includes lessons on injury prevention at each grade level.

ETR Associates also offers *Safety Is No Accident: Children's Activities in Injury Prevention* (Kane, 1992) and an accompanying poster, *Safety Power!* for children in kindergarten through third grade. Many community groups and agencies are also good sources for school programs and materials covering a variety of injury prevention topics.

Secondary Curricula

The *Teenage Health Teaching Modules* (Education Development Center, 1991) include an injury prevention module for secondary teachers. This comprehensive instructional curriculum covers both intentional and unintentional injury prevention and includes classroom and follow-up activities for grades nine and ten.

Part of ETR Associates' Contemporary Health Series, *Entering Adulthood: Skills for Injury Prevention* (Hunter and Lloyd-Kolkin, 1991) is an injury prevention curriculum for grades nine through twelve. *Into Adolescence: Stopping Violence* (Post, 1991) is an injury prevention curriculum for middle school students, grades five through eight.

Prothrow-Stith (1987) has developed a curriculum that focuses on violence prevention among adolescents, intended to supplement the *Teenage Health Teaching Modules.* This ten-session curriculum addresses violence prevention between peers and tries to show high school students the extent to which they are at risk for homicide, and positive ways to deal with anger and aggression.

A health professionals' training package of four modules (Introduction, Firearm Injuries, Burn Injuries to Children, Falls Among the Elderly) is also available (EDC, 1990). The package includes both slides and scripts in each module.

Facilities and Environment

Injury is determined by a complex interaction between environmental and individual factors. Interventions in schools that focus only on the individual factors may be limited in effectiveness because they ignore hazards in the physical facilities and school environment. Yet merely pointing out hazards to persons responsible for school environments may be insufficient to abate the hazards (Sacks et al., 1992).

A safe school environment includes not only the physical buildings and playgrounds, but also instructional areas such as laboratories; wood, metal, auto and electrical shops; and physical education/locker facilities. One study in Italy found that 50 percent of the cases of injuries to school children in Milan occurred in the gymnasium (Pagano et al., 1987). Changing the physical environment to reduce risk of injury may include controlling or removing hazards such as wet flooring, unsafe stairs, spilled chemicals, cracked or broken glassware, inadequate lighting, poor ventilation, insufficient space and unsafe playgrounds.

Many hazards can exist in school design, such as hard surfaces, equipment at excessive heights, and equipment made from unyielding materials such as iron and cement. Supervision in playground activity and constant surveillance for playground hazards by all teachers and administrators is necessary. Many studies favor a "child-centered playground safety curriculum approach," combining developmental capabilities of children with education, skill development, and use of safe and appropriate equipment (King and Ball, 1989).

Opportunities for injury prevention may also extend to factors in the psychosocial environment. Family stress, alcohol and drug abuse, and violence create an environment where injuries are more likely (Molloy, 1987). Many studies have found a relationship between injuries and adverse sociocultural environments such as neighborhood crowding and family dysfunction, and there is a strong relationship between injuries and socioeconomic conditions such as poverty, financial problems in the home and substandard housing (Berger, 1985; Mare, 1982). Reconsidering the influence of environments at school, such as parking lots, restrooms, common grounds and hallways, may result in interventions that help curb violence at school.

Health Services

Health professionals working in schools are in a unique position to observe and record injuries and intervene in controlling them. Most schools have established procedures for at least two health services related to injuries: emergency treatment and care of injuries for both students and staff, and injury reporting and record keeping.

Emergency Treatment

Every school should have procedures for handling medical problems and emergencies, including injuries to students and staff. Medical personnel on site (school nurse or physician) usually attend to the treatment of minor injuries, but should be alert to the need for more comprehensive care in particular instances. School personnel also need to be aware of signs of child abuse and follow standard reporting procedures and referral to appropriate follow-up care.

All school personnel should be properly trained in basic first-aid procedures to manage common injuries such as cuts, nose-bleeds, sprains, etc., and more advanced first-aid and CPR to manage life-threatening circumstances until more qualified help can be obtained. Some states (e.g., California) now require all teachers to be certified in CPR.

Injury Reporting

Any injury that causes a student or staff member to miss or leave school (or miss or leave work) or involves property damage should be reported on a standard injury report form. Such forms vary, but in general contain information related to the nature of the injury, part of the body injured, days lost from school or work, treatment given, witnesses, location and description of the circumstances of the injury.

Accurate injury-reporting tools and methods to identify and monitor the number and kinds of injuries at school are essential to an examination of injury trends and the identification of opportunities for intervention. A consistent injury-reporting system may also help identify particularly high-risk individuals, groups or unsafe environments at the school. Record keeping also serves an important function in cases of liability and in lawsuits. One study (Bremberg, 1989) found substantial underreporting of injuries at school when reporting was done by the school nurse. When other staff were involved in reporting injuries, a two-fold increase in the number of injuries reported was found (Wojtowicz, Macrina and Bolton, 1990).

Data should be collected on *all* injuries occurring at school, those treated by school personnel and those referred out for care. This information should become part of the official school health records.

Recommendations for Specific Injury Problems Affecting Schools

There are many areas in which schools can work to reduce injuries. Some suggestions for a variety of these areas follow.

Traffic Injuries

Traffic injuries include injuries to occupants of cars, vans, motorcycles and buses, to pedestrians, and to bicyclists. This category is the largest single source of injury deaths to children and youth. A school injury prevention program should strive to reduce specific traffic-related injuries. Efforts can be coordinated with the state department of transportation, the department of education and local public works and road departments.

Motor vehicle occupant death rates peak at ages 16 to 19, with males at higher risk. Alcohol consumption is a leading factor in traffic crashes that result in serious injuries and fatalities. Nearly 40 percent of all fatally injured drivers have sufficient alcohol in their systems to be legally intoxicated (National Highway Traffic Safety Administration, 1988).

Safety belts are 40 to 55 percent effective in reducing serious injury and death in a crash. The risk of death in a crash for an unrestrained child is 11 times that of a restrained child. While all states require child safety seat use, only about two-thirds of the states have mandatory safety belt use laws for older children, adolescents and adults. Estimates of safety belt use rates are only about 60 percent nationwide, and parents who do not use safety belts themselves are less likely to use restraints for their children

(Russell, 1993). Strong law enforcement is a key to increasing safety belt use.

Schools should require that children being dropped off at school in private vehicles be properly restrained—either by the use of a child safety seat or a safety belt. Children who are transported on school outings should be properly restrained at all times.

Pedestrians

Pedestrian injuries to children and youth are generally an urban problem. Among school-age children, pedestrian injury deaths are highest among five to nine year olds. Peaks in pedestrian injuries occur in the fall and winter. Two-thirds of fatalities occur between sunset and dawn; most occur to males and away from intersections (National Highway Traffic Safety Administration, 1988). Fatalities to older children are usually the result of "darting out" into traffic while playing (Rivara and Barber, 1985; Brison, Wicklund and Mueller, 1988) and inadequate perceptual motor development to judge speed and distance of oncoming traffic (Arnold, 1990).

Some argue that young children should not be taught how to cross the street safely, but instead should be taught *not* to cross streets without supervision (Modena et al., p. 63). Older children can be successfully taught to watch for oncoming traffic and not to dart into the street. One school education program, "Willie Whistle," demonstrated dramatic success in reducing child pedestrian injuries in the local setting (Preusser and Lund, 1988). Other ways to reduce child pedestrian injuries include (National Committee for Injury Prevention and Control, 1989):

- one-way streets
- pedestrian lights in high-risk areas
- "talking" or audio signals at pedestrian intersections
- changing bus stop locations

- use of sidewalks, roadway barriers, crossing signs and signals
- use of crossing guards and escorts for young children

Motorcycles

Motorcycle crashes kill about one hundred children each year (Modena et al., 1991). Among 15 to 34 year olds, one out of every ten traffic fatalities involves a motorcycle driver or passenger (National Highway Traffic Safety Administration, 1988). As a group, motorcyclists have a fatality rate 19 times that of car drivers. Death rates are highest between ages 18 and 24 and are ten times higher for males than females. The two factors that most affect death rates are amount of travel (exposure to hazards) and use of a protective helmet.

Helmet laws have reduced motorcyclist deaths dramatically by reducing head injuries, although only a handful of states have passed (and enforce) such laws. Experience and training appear to influence crash rates, as does increased visibility (Cercarelli et al., 1990). Motorcyclists increase their risk by ignoring road rules related to proper signaling, lane changing, speed, following distance and alcohol use. Schools can regulate the use of motorcycles on school grounds by requiring speed limits, daytime running lights, helmet use and reflective/protective clothing.

Mopeds

Mopeds and minibikes pose additional risks to young adolescents, since some licensing laws allow youth as young as age 13 to operate these vehicles on public roads (U.S. Department of Transportation, 1988). Each year, more than 13,000 children and youth are treated in emergency rooms for injuries sustained in crashes on these vehicles (Modena et al., 1991).

Vehicle instability at speeds above 25 miles per hour, coupled with young and inexperienced drivers and riders and lack of conspicuity on the road, result in a high collision probability. High speed and lack of a helmet and protective clothing increase the severity of injury in the event of a crash.

Schools can regulate the use of these vehicles on school grounds, mandate driver and rider education, require and enforce the use of helmets and protective/reflective clothing, prohibit passenger travel and consider changes in the school road environment to minimize vehicle/moped mix.

Bicycles

Preadolescent bicyclists are at highest risk for bicycle injuries. About 90 percent of bicyclist deaths result from collisions with motor vehicles, and four out of five deaths result from head injury (Modena et al., 1991). Most nonfatal injuries occur from bicycle falls. Bicycle death rates rise rapidly after age four and peak among males at age 13. The peak times for bicycle injuries are after-school hours, from 3:00 to 7:00 p.m.

Although bicycle helmets are the most effective intervention against head injuries, helmet use among children and youth remains low. Howard County in Maryland became the first U. S. jurisdiction to mandate use of helmets by cyclists under 16 years of age (Scheidt, Wilson and Stern, 1992). Australian studies clearly show the effectiveness of locally organized helmet incentive and rebate programs (Bikewest, 1990) and statewide bicycle helmet legislation (Centers for Disease Control and Prevention, 1993a.).

Schools can require helmet use by children who ride bikes to school, initiate regular bicycle safety checks, organize a bicycle helmet rebate scheme (some schools in Australia purchased helmets at cost and provided them at a discount to parents and students), and initiate school and community bike education programs. These activities will increase community acceptance of safe bicycle travel and encourage community action for more effective mandatory legislation.

Bicycle paths and lanes on roads in and around school can reduce the potential for collisions with vehicles. Reflective clothing, helmets, and lights and reflectors (on the bicycle or on the rider) should be encouraged. Changes in the roadway, such as barriers separating bicyclists from traffic and ensuring safe cycling surfaces, will help reduce collisions.

Children should not be encouraged to ride a bike before they are developmentally ready (both physically and perceptually). Children should be taught traffic rules, be provided with bicycle riding training and testing, and use only bikes with safety features such as chain guards, spoke covers, safe handlebars, effective brakes, reflectors and lights. The bicycle should be the right size for the child. Bikes that are too big for the child are most dangerous.

School Buses

Each school day, about 22 million children are transported more than 18 million miles in school buses, yet school bus passenger fatalities are remarkably low—fewer than twenty children per year. Most school bus fatalities occur to pedestrians or students who are getting on or off the bus or as they cross the street in front of a bus (Insurance Institute for Highway Safety, 1985).

Schools can help improve passenger safety by taking an active part in monitoring driver fitness, passenger behavior and vehicle safety, as well as periodically reviewing policies and procedures for school bus use. Increasing the safety of school bus travel, the focus of a National Academy of Sciences study (Transportation Research Board, 1989), includes the following strategies:

* installing and using swing-out stop arms and strobe lights on the bus to prevent drivers from passing stopped school buses
* use of escorts for children exiting the bus and crossing the street
* school bus driver training

- route and stopping location reviews to minimize risk to children
- speed limit posting
- safe loading/unloading zones at school

Recreation/Sports Injuries

The risks of injury from recreational activities and sports is greatest during adolescence. For the 13 to 19 year old, sports are the most frequent cause of nonfatal injuries requiring medical treatment among both males and females. A Massachusetts study of childhood injuries found that one in every fourteen adolescents will be seen in an emergency room or be hospitalized for a sports-related injury every year (Guyer and Gallagher, 1988).

Although the majority of injuries are minor, twice as many males as females are injured in sports and recreational activities. Injury rates vary markedly between sports, as illustrated in Figure 5.

Football is especially hazardous to boys. The National Athletic Trainers' Association found that 37 percent of all high school football players were injured at least once during 1987. The highest sports injury rates for secondary school girls occurs in basketball, the woman's sport with the most contact (National Committee for Injury Prevention and Control, 1989).

Trauma to the face, head, eyes and mouth account for the largest proportion of sports injuries. Mouth protectors and face guards have greatly reduced these injuries in football, but are not required in baseball and ice hockey, where injuries to the face and mouth are also frequent (McGinnis and Degraw, 1991).

While injuries from team sports are more frequent, injuries resulting from recreation and individual sports are more severe. "Track and field, bicycling, horseback riding and ice skating entail higher risks for head injuries than contact team sports such as football" (Children's Safety Network, 1991).

Figure 5
Sports Injury Rates per 100,000 Participants

Sport	Rate per 100,000 Participants
football	2171
ice hockey	2089
baseball	2089
basketball	1858
soccer	910
bicycling	905
skate boarding	878
horseback riding	465
volleyball	370
roller skating	349
ice skating	335
water skiing	199
racquetball	168
tennis	118
golf	104
swimming	93
archery	66

Adapted with permission from the C. V. Mosby Company, a subsidiary of Times Mirror. W. H. Creswell and I. M. Newman. 1993. *School Health Practice*. 10th ed. St. Louis, MO: Times Mirror/Mosby.

It is estimated that about 54 percent of sports injuries are due to physical contact, 30 percent to terrain and surfaces and 15 percent to equipment hazards. Prevention of sports injuries is a major element in coaching, training and sports medicine practice. Major preventive initiatives include:
• increasing the number and quality of trained coaches
• educating students to avoid sports injuries
• changing the environment to reduce hazards (e.g., break-away baseball bases to prevent sliding injuries)
• the use of protective clothing and padding

- rule changes
- improved maintenance of playing fields
- improved response and quality of after-injury care

Schools with recreational and sports programs can do much to reduce the incidence of injuries. One important requirement is the mandatory use of appropriate protective gear. Although mouth guards are mandatory for high school football, few organized leagues and intramural sports require protective gear.

School policies requiring accurate reporting of sports and recreational injuries are essential to prevention. Well-organized and supervised recreation and sports programs are also necessary, as are trained personnel, enforcement of rules and regulations and safe equipment.

The school environment can also be modified to reduce injuries. For example, injuries from sliding into fixed-post bases in baseball (costing an average of $1,223 per sliding injury) could be reduced by 95 percent through the use of break-away bases, which cost about $48 per base to install (Robertson, 1990). Other environmental hazards such as exposed sprinklers, potholes, broken glass, dangerous playing surfaces and inadequately fenced playing fields often contribute to playground injuries. Modifications in rules or requirements for special footwear in certain activities (as in indoor aerobic dance training) to accommodate different playing surfaces and environments are also actions the school can take.

Suicide

Suicide among young people ages 15 to 24 has increased nearly 300 percent over the past thirty years, with the major increase occurring among youth ages 15 to 19. Suicide is the second leading cause of death in this age group and the eighth leading cause of death in the United States overall. Approximately 30,000

Americans commit suicide each year. Although the rate for male adolescents is comparatively low, there has been a steady increase in suicide among all youth ages 15 to 19 since the mid-1950s (U.S. Department of Health and Human Services, 1991). Reports of suicide-like behavior (thoughts or actions) have been documented among children as young as age three (Trad, 1990).

In addition to completed suicides, attempted suicide is also a serious problem among adolescents. It is estimated that for every completed suicide, there are twenty suicide attempts among young people ages 15 to 19 (Alcohol, Drug Abuse and Mental Health Administration, 1989). In several surveys of adolescents in the general population, as many as 10 percent reported having at- tempted suicide at least once (U.S. Department of Health and Human Services, 1990). Students whose suicide attempts resulted in medical injuries are at higher risk of repeated (and completed) suicide attempts in the future.

Studies of suicidal behavior (defined as thoughts or actions that might lead to self-inflicted death or serious injury) among school children indicate that rates are increasing. The studies indicate that suicidal behavior is infrequent among elementary school children (12 percent) but increases progressively among junior high (35 percent), high school (65 percent) and college students (50-65 percent). Actual attempts ranged from a low of 3 percent for elementary school students to 11 percent for high school students and 15 to 18 percent for college students (Garrison, 1989). The most commonly identified correlates include depres- sive symptoms, social and personal problems, family disorganiza- tion and life stress.

School teachers, administrators and other personnel working with adolescents should be trained to recognize the warning signs of suicide and take appropriate actions (Cole and Siegel, 1987). Some professionals recommend the use of schoolwide screening instruments for signs of suicidal behaviors (Reynolds, 1991). Some of the warning signs school personnel may be able to recognize include:

- previous suicide attempts
- suicide threats or statements about a desire to die
- depression
- sudden changes in behavior
- substance use
- loss of a parent or loved one
- child abuse
- runaway behavior

Schools should give special attention to children and youth who have attempted suicide or who were close friends with suicide victims. School counseling programs can be developed to assist children and adolescents to manage grief and stress more appropriately and to help in cases of personal crisis. Some school curricula are available to help students understand more about suicide, increase awareness of depression, and improve coping skills and personal resources (California Department of Education, 1987; Burton, 1990). However, more evaluation research on these programs is needed to determine their impact.

Schools need to review and adopt specific guidelines for crisis management in cases of student suicide to prevent "suicide clusters" at school and to help manage the publicity and media attention (Centers for Disease Control and Prevention, 1988). School administrators should work closely with mental health professionals in the community to coordinate services and referrals. Resources exist in every community, through public health departments, social service agencies and mental health centers, to assist schools in managing this growing problem.

Schools should also do what they can to control the possession of lethal means for suicide at school, such as carrying a firearm. Firearms are both the most common and most lethal methods used in suicide and homicide.

In 1992, the Centers for Disease Control and Prevention reviewed the rationale and evidence for the effectiveness of various suicide prevention strategies. CDC made the following recommendations, which may be relevant for school-based programs:

- Ensure that new and existing suicide prevention programs are linked as closely as possible with professional mental health resources in the community. Many strategies are designed to increase referrals of at-risk youth; this approach can be successful only to the extent that there are appropriate, trained counselors to whom referrals can be made.
- Avoid reliance on any one prevention strategy. Most good programs incorporate several strategies at once.
- Incorporate promising but underused strategies with current programs where possible. The restriction of lethal means by which to commit suicide may be the most important candidate strategy here. Peer support groups for those who have felt suicidal or have attempted suicide also appear promising.
- Expand suicide prevention efforts for young adults ages 20 to 24, among whom the suicide rate is twice as high as for adolescents.
- Incorporate evaluation efforts into all new and existing suicide prevention programs, preferably efforts based on measures such as the incidence of suicidal behavior or ideation. Be aware that suicide prevention efforts, like all health interventions, may have unforeseen negative consequences. Evaluation measures should be designed to identify such consequences, should they occur.

Interpersonal Violence

Each year, more than 20,000 people die and more than 2 million are victims of interpersonal violence in the United States. Homicide and assault are an especially important public health problem among school-age adolescents and young adults. Since 1984, the homicide rate among adolescents 15 to 19 years old has risen 53 percent, and among young people ages 15 to 24, homicide is the second most common cause of death (Roper, 1991). Homicide is the most common cause of death for both African-American females and African-American males ages 15 to 34 (Hammett et al., 1992). Nearly two-thirds of homicide victims are killed with firearms, and 75 percent of these victims are killed with a handgun.

The United States ranks first among industrialized countries in violent death rates. Some have called firearm deaths "a uniquely American epidemic." In the United States, gun deaths occur at a rate more than 90 times greater than in any other country (Rice, MacKenzie and Associates, 1989). During 1986 and 1987, a two-year period, the number of people who died from firearm injuries in the United States was even greater than the number of U.S. casualties during the entire Vietnam War (Kellerman et al., 1991).

Violence is frequently the first response for many adolescents in cases of emotional and mental stress. It is often used as a mechanism for coping with conflict. More than ever, the problems of violence are penetrating the schools—gang recruitment and activity, weapon carrying, and in-school and after-school altercations and fighting behavior. Among the instruments of violent death, firearms and knives rank ahead of all other means.

One-half million assaults are believed to occur on school campuses every year. According to a 1987 school survey, 135,000 boys carry a handgun to school daily in the United States (Calhoun, 1991). Among eighth and tenth graders, almost 7 percent of boys and 2 percent of girls reported carrying knives to school nearly every day (ASHA, AAHE and SOPHE, 1989).

It is estimated that more than 2,000 students and forty teachers are physically attacked on school grounds *each school hour.* Another 900 teachers are threatened (National Education Association, 1993). In 1990, school buildings were the site of 5.3 percent of all nonfatal violent victimizations of persons ages 12 and older. Another 4.5 percent of such assaults occurred on school property (Bureau of Justice Statistics, 1992).

Violence rates in secondary schools are highest in school districts marked by higher crime rates and more street gangs (National Research Council, 1993). A victimization survey by the National Institute of Education (1978) reported higher rates of student violence in schools in which students perceive signs of ineffective social control, such as undisciplined classrooms, lax enforcement of school rules and a weak principal. It is not clear whether lack of school control gives permission that encourages violent behavior or whether high violence levels in the school create fear among administrators and teachers that undermines discipline.

There is evidence that violence levels are related to students' attachments to the values schools seek to promote. In secondary schools, violence rates increased with the percentages of students who did not aspire to good grades, who did not view their curricula as relevant, and who did not believe that their school experience could positively influence their lives (National Research Council, 1993).

Youth gangs are another important problem for schools. Youth gangs exist in nearly every state and in small towns as well as large urban centers (Lazaroff, 1992). Gang activity increases in communities with little social organization, few jobs, poor schools, high poverty and high substance use rates. Schools can help by offering early intervention programs, including after-school activities, drug prevention programs and expanded social opportunities (School Social Services Administration, 1990).

Much remains to be learned about effective means of reducing violence at school, at home and in the community (Mercy and Fenley, 1991). There are large gaps in our understanding of the causes and best preventive strategies for violence in schools and communities, since the underlying causes of violence tend to vary from community to community (Prothrow-Stith and Weissman, 1991). Each school must assess its own needs and adopt a framework for violence prevention that addresses those needs. Schools can take important steps, however, in their efforts to reduce or discourage violence.

Many schools use conflict resolution skill training to help students manage their anger and hostile feelings in nonviolent ways. Some of these strategies include planning ahead and having a strategy for conflict, setting the right tone for discussion, using good communication skills and working toward compromise and acceptable solutions without violence (Hunter and Lloyd-Kolkin, 1991). Other schools train students in teams to mediate arguments before they escalate into fights.

Curricula have been developed for various grade levels that seek to change attitudes toward violence and improve interpersonal skills as ways to curb violence, such as ETR Associates' *Into Adolescence: Stopping Violence*, a curriculum for students in grades five through eight (Post, 1991). Violence curricula that focus on developing peer mediation and conflict resolution skills are most widespread in schools but need further evaluation (Prothrow-Stith, 1989; Selman and Glidden, 1987).

The recent work of the Virginia Association of School Superintendents (1992) and the National Education Association (NEA, 1993; NEA, n.d.) provides encouraging signs that schools are taking an active part in violence prevention and control. Helping adolescents deal with anger in productive, nonviolent ways is one step toward diffusing the enormous injury burden resulting from the increasing incidence of violence in society. National health objectives for the year 2000 include specific violence prevention objectives, many of which cannot be fully met without the help of schools (Iverson and Kolbe, 1983).

While studies of the effectiveness of various curricula in reducing violent and abusive behavior are inconclusive, there is some evidence that they can help improve social problem-solving abilities in adolescents (Guerra and Slaby, 1990). One program in Hawaii trained students in a two-day course to mediate conflicts. In one school, 135 disputes were mediated by students, and 104 agreements were reached. In another school, the number of fights dropped from 83 to 19 during the first two years of the program (Mason, 1993).

Modifying the school environment also has promise as a violence prevention strategy. Barring weapons from school grounds and enforcing the Gun-Free School Zone Act of 1990, which makes it a federal crime to bring firearms onto school property (U.S. Code of Federal Regulations, 1991), are helpful steps schools can take. It is estimated that one-fourth of major urban school districts now use metal detectors. Other schools are employing school security personnel and school surveillance methods to "disarm" potential violence at school.

Spatial characteristics of schools can influence the probability of violence by increasing crowding and opportunities for confrontations. Implementing architectural and social planning principles can create a safer school environment. The impersonality of school routines, conformity and school failure may contribute to feelings of anger, frustration and resentment that may predispose students to violence. Poorly designed school grounds and space may also facilitate crime and violence. These features of school life may be open to possible, as yet untried, interventions.

A multifaceted community-based approach to violence prevention among youth is recommended in the CDC document *Prevention of Youth Violence: A Framework for Community Action* (1993b). This document identifies many promising approaches to preventing youth violence in the community, including educational strategies, legal and regulatory change, and environmental modifications. Many of the recommended strategies are relevant to schools but need to be properly evaluated for their effectiveness.

The recommended education strategies include:
- adult mentoring
- early childhood education
- social-skills training
- peer education
- parenting education
- conflict resolution

Legal and regulatory changes relate to limiting the access to and carrying of weapons and controlling the use of and access to alcohol and other drugs. Environmental changes relate to the social, work, recreational, academic and physical environments.

In one of the most comprehensive approaches to preventing school violence produced by a school system, the Virginia Association of School Superintendents (1992) held a Summit on School Violence, attended by leaders of seven educational organizations. The summit produced a set of recommendations directed at all levels, from the home, school and community to legislators. They include:
- outreach programs to the homes of disruptive youths
- emergency communications systems in the schools
- development of strong and consistent discipline policies

- policies blocking expelled students from reenrolling in neighboring schools
- gun control legislation
- expanded access for at-risk students to early intervention efforts (such as Head Start and Chapter 1) known to improve school success

Schools and communities are close partners in the Virginia plan for resolving the problem of school violence. What has begun in Virginia may be a useful model for progress in other states. In fact, all injury prevention efforts need partnerships. While educators have an important role to play in injury prevention, other facets of society—parents and other family members, community members and government at all levels—must contribute to the solutions.

References

Alcohol, Drug Abuse and Mental Health Administration. 1989. *Report of the secretary's task force on youth suicide, Vol. 1*. DHHS Publication No. (ADM) 89-1621. Washington, DC.

Arnold, P. 1990. Pedestrians in traffic. *Proceedings of Roadwatch*. Perth, Australia: University of Western Australia.

American School Health Association, Association for the Advancement of Health Education and Society for Public Health Education. 1989. *National adolescent student health survey: A report on the health of America's youth*. Oakland, CA: Third Party Press.

Baker, S. P., B. O'Neill, M. Ginsburg and G. Li. 1992. *The injury fact book*. New York: Oxford University Press.

Berger, L. R. 1985. Childhood injuries. *Public Health Reports* 100:572-574.

Bikewest. 1990. *Bicycle helmet rebate scheme—Evaluation*. Perth, Australia: State of Western Australia Department of Transportation.

Bremberg, S. 1989. Is school-based reporting of injuries at school reliable? A literature review and an empirical study. *Accident Analysis and Prevention* 21 (2): 183-189.

Brison, R. J., K. Wicklund and B. A. Mueller. 1988. Fatal pedestrian injuries to young children: A different pattern of injury. *American Journal of Public Health* 78:793-5.

Budnick, L. D., and B. P. Chaiken. 1985. The probability of dying of injuries by the year 2000. *Journal of the American Medical Association* 254 (23): 3350-52.

Bureau of Justice Statistics. 1992. *Criminal victimization in the United States, 1990.* Washington, DC.

Burton, N. D. 1990. *Entering adulthood: Understanding depression and suicide.* Santa Cruz, CA: ETR Associates.

Calhoun, D. 1991. *Teens on target: Teens as resources in violence prevention.* Paper presented at Fifth California Conference on Injury Control for Children and Youth. Costa Mesa, California.

California Department of Education. 1987. *Suicide prevention program for California public schools: Implementation and resource guide.* Sacramento, CA.

Centers for Disease Control and Prevention. 1988. CDC recommendations for a community plan for the prevention and containment of suicide clusters. *Morbidity and Mortality Weekly Report* 37 (Suppl. S-6): 1-12.

Centers for Disease Control and Prevention. 1992a. *Position papers from the Third National Injury Control Conference.* Atlanta, GA: U.S. Public Health Service, National Center for Injury Prevention and Control.

Centers for Disease Control and Prevention. 1992b. *Youth suicide prevention programs: A resource guide.* Atlanta, GA.

Centers for Disease Control and Prevention. 1993a. Mandatory bicycle helmet use in Victoria, Australia. *Morbidity and Mortality Weekly Report* 42 (18): 359-363.

Centers for Disease Control and Prevention. 1993b. *Prevention of youth violence: A framework for community action.* Atlanta, GA: Public Health Service, Center for Injury Prevention and Control.

Cercarelli, L. R., P. K. Arnold, D. L. Rosman, D. Sleet and M. L. Thornett. 1992. Traffic exposure and choice of comparison crashes for examining motorcycle conspicuity by analysis of crash data. *Accident Analysis and Prevention* 24: 363-368.

Children's Safety Network. 1991. *A data book of child and adolescent injury.* Washington, DC: National Center for Education in Maternal and Child Health.

Cole, E., and J. A. Siegel. 1987. Alleviating hopelessness—suicide prevention in the schools. *Public Health Review* 15:241-255.

Creswell, W. H., and I. M. Newman. 1993. *School health practice,* 10th ed. St. Louis: Times Mirror/Mosby.

Dunne-Maxim, K. 1991. Can a suicide prevention curriculum harm students' health? *The School Administrator* 48 (5): 25.

Education Development Center. 1990. *Educating professionals in injury control* (EPIC). Boston.

Education Development Center. 1991. *Teenage health teaching modules (THTM): Preventing injuries.* Newton, MA.

Egger, G., D. A. Sleet, J. Harrison et al. 1993. *Injury in Australia.* Adelaide, South Australia: National Injury Surveillance Unit, Australian Institute of Health.

ETR Associates. 1991. *Preventing injury: A safety curriculum.* Santa Cruz, CA.

ETR Associates. 1992. *Actions for Health.* Santa Cruz, CA.

Fingerhut, L., and National Center for Health Statistics. 1988. Vital statistics, mortality statistics for ages 0-19.

Gallagher, S. 1991. Personal communication with author.

Garrison, C. Z. 1989. The study of suicidal behavior in the schools. *Suicide and Life-Threatening Behavior* 19 (1): 120-130.

Garrison, C. Z., R. E. McKeown, R. F. Valois and M. L. Vincent. 1993. Aggression, substance use and suicidal behaviors in high school students. *American Journal of Public Health* 83 (2): 179-184.

Geller, E. S., J. Elder, M. Hovell and D. Sleet. 1991. Behavioral approaches to drinking-driving interventions. In *Advances in health education and promotion*, vol. 3, ed. W. Ward and F. M. Lewis, 45-68. United Kingdon: Jessica-Kingsley Press.

Green, L. W., and M. Kreuter. 1991. *Health promotion planning: An educational and environmental approach.* Mountain View, CA: Mayfield Publishers.

Guerra, G., and R. G. Slaby. 1990. Cognitive mediators of aggression in adolescent offenders: Intervention. *Developmental Psychology* 26:269-77.

Gulaid, J. A., E. C. Onwuachi-Saunders, J. J. Sacks and D. R. Roberts. 1988. Differences in death rates due to injury among Blacks and Whites, 1984. *Morbidity and Mortality Weekly Report* 37 (Suppl. S-3): 25-32.

Guyer, B., and S. Gallagher. 1988. Childhood injuries and their prevention. In *Maternal and Child Health Practices*, 3d ed., ed. H. Wallace, G. Ryan and A. Oglesby. Oakland, CA: Third Party Publishing.

Hammett, M., K. E. Powell, P. W. O'Carroll and S. T. Clanton. 1992. Homicide surveillance—United States, 1979-1988. *Morbidity and Mortality Weekly Report* 41 (SS-3): 1-34.

Hunter, L. K., and D. Lloyd-Kolkin. 1991. *Entering adulthood: Skills for injury prevention.* Santa Cruz, CA: ETR Associates.

Indian Health Service. 1989. *Trends in Indian health.* Washington, DC: Department of Health and Human Services.

Insurance Institute for Highway Safety. 1985. School buses and seat belts (special issue). *Status Report* 20:1-12.

Iverson, D. C., and L. J. Kolbe. 1983. Evolution of the national disease prevention and health promotion strategy: Establishing a role for the schools. *Journal of School Health* 53 (5): 294-302.

Kane, W. M. 1993. *Safety is no accident: Children's activities in injury prevention.* Santa Cruz, CA: ETR Associates.

Kellerman, A. L., R. K. Lee, J. A. Mercy and J. Banton. 1991. The epidemiologic basis for the prevention of firearm injuries. *Annual Review of Public Health* 12:17-40.

King, K., and D. Ball. 1989. *A holistic approach to accident and injury prevention in children's playgrounds.* London: Great Guildford House.

Koop, C. E. 1989. Testimony before Senate Subcommittee on Children, Family, Drugs and Alcoholism. U.S. Congress, 9 February.

Lawson, D., D. Sleet and M. Amoni, eds. 1984. Automobile occupant protection: An issue for health educators. *Health Education* 15 (5): 25-66.

Lazaroff, S. 1992. Youth gangs: Not new but more violent. *Family Life Educator* 11 (1): 13-15.

Malek, M., B. Chang, S. Gallagher and B. Guyer. 1991. The cost of medical care for injuries to children. *Annals of Emergency Medicine* 20 (9): 997-1005.

Mare, R. 1982. Socioeconomic effects on child mortality in the United States. *American Journal of Public Health* 72:539-547.

Mason, J. O. 1993. The dimensions of an epidemic of violence. *Public Health Reports* 108 (1): 1-3.

Mason, J. O., and D. Tolsma. 1984. Personal health promotion. *Western Journal of Medicine* 141 (6): 772-776.

McGinnis, J., and C. Degraw. 1991. Special issue on Healthy People 2000: National Health Promotion and Disease Prevention Objectives and healthy schools. *Journal of School Health* 61 (7): 292-328.

Modena, H. W., S. P. Baker, S. P. Teret, S. Shock and J. Garbarino. 1991. *Saving children: A guide to injury prevention.* New York: Oxford University Press.

Molloy, P. J. 1987. Childhood injuries. *Public Health Currents* 27 (4): 23-28.

National Academy of Sciences, National Research Council. 1988. *Injury control.* Washington, DC.

National Committee for Injury Prevention and Control. 1989. *Injury prevention: Meeting the challenge.* New York: Oxford University Press.

National Education Association. (n.d.) *School violence: A survival guide for school staff.* Washington, DC: NEA Professional Library.

National Education Association. 1993. A safe haven for children: Curbing violence in schools (advertisement). *Washington Post Weekly,* 21 February 1993.

National Highway Traffic Safety Administration. 1988. *Fatal accident reporting system*. Washington, DC.

National Institute of Education. 1978. Violent schools—safe schools: The Safe School Study report to the Congress. Washington, DC.

National Research Council. 1993. *Understanding and preventing violence*. Washington, DC: National Academy Press.

National Safety Council. 1992. *Accident facts*. Chicago, IL.

Nelson, S. 1986. *How healthy is your school?* New York: National Center for Health Education Press.

Pagano, A., E. Babini, M. Anelli, S. Bernuzzi, S. Lopiccoli and P. Fisher. 1987. Accidents in the school environment in Milan: A five-year study. *European Journal of Epidemiology* 3 (2): 196-201.

Post, J. 1991. *Into adolescence: Stopping violence*. Santa Cruz, CA: ETR Associates.

Preusser, D. F., and A. K. Lund. 1988. And keep on looking: A film to reduce pedestrian crashes among 9-12 year olds. *Journal of Safety Research* 19: 177-185.

Prothrow-Stith, D. 1987. *Violence prevention curriculum for adolescents*. Newton, MA: Education Development Center.

Prothrow-Stith, D., and M. Weissmann. 1991. *Deadly consequences*. New York: HarperCollins.

Reynolds, W. M. 1991. A school-based procedure for the identification of adolescents at risk for suicidal behaviors. *Family and Community Health* 14 (3): 64-75.

Rice, D. P., E. J. MacKenzie and Associates. 1989. *Cost of injury in the United States: A report to Congress*. San Francisco, CA: Institute for Health and Aging, University of California, San Francisco, and Johns Hopkins University.

Rivara, F. P., and M. Barber. 1985. Demographic analysis of childhood pedestrian injuries. *Pediatrics* 76:375-381.

Rivara, F. P., and B. A. Mueller. 1987. The epidemiology and causes of childhood injuries. *Journal of Social Issues* 43 (2): 13-32.

Roberts, M. L., D. Fanurik and D. Layfield. 1987. Behavioral approaches to prevention of childhood injuries. *Journal of Social Issues* 43 (2): 105-118.

Robertson, L. S. 1990. Injury prevention: Environmental approaches. *Critical Reviews in Environmental Control* 20 (1): 1-20.

Roper, W. L. 1991. The prevention of minority youth violence must begin despite risks and imperfect understanding. *Public Health Reports* 106 (3): 229-231.

Rosenberg, M. L., and M. A. Fenley. 1991. *Violence in America: A public health approach*. New York: Oxford University Press.

Rosenberg, M. L., J. G. Rodriquez and T. L. Chorba. 1990. Childhood injuries: Where we are. *Pediatrics* (Suppl.) 86 (6): 1084-1091.

Russell, J. 1993. Impact of adult safety-belt use on restraint use among children <11 years of age–selected states, 1988 and 1989. *Morbidity and Motality Weekly Report* 42 (14): 275-278.

Sacks, J. J., M. D. Brnatley, P. Holmgreen and R. W. Rochat. 1992. Evaluation of an intervention to reduce playground hazards in Atlanta child-care centers. *American Journal of Public Health* 82 (3): 429-431.

Scheidt, P. C., M. H. Wilson and M. S. Stern. 1992. Bicycle helmet law for children: A case study of activism in injury control. *Pediatrics* 89 (6): 1248-1250.

School Social Service Administration. 1990. *Youth gangs: Problem and response.* Chicago: University of Chicago National Youth Gang Suppression and Intervention Project, U. S. Department of Justice.

Selman, R. L., and M. Glidden. 1987. Negotiation strategies for youth. *School Safety* (Fall): 18-21.

Sleet, D A. 1984. Reducing motor vehicle trauma through health promotion programming. *Health Education Quarterly* 11 (2): 113-125.

Sleet, D. A. 1992. *Master the road...safely.* An injury prevention module for Live for Life. Santa Monica, CA: Johnson and Johnson Health Management.

Sleet, D. A., G. Egger and P. A. Albany. 1991. Injury as a public health problem. *Health Promotion Journal of Australia* 1 (2): 4-9.

Sleet, D. A., A. Wagenaar and P. Waller, eds. 1989. Drinking, driving and health promotion. *Health Education Quarterly* 16 (3).

Smith, S. M., B. K. Molloy, H. J. Winick and P. L. Graiter. 1992. Rural American Indian injury patterns. *Journal of Environmental Health* 54 (60): 22-25.

Trad, P. V. 1990. *Treating suicide-like behavior in a preschooler.* Madison, CT: International Universities Press.

Transportation Research Board. 1989. *Improving school bus safety.* Special Report 222. Washington, DC: National Academy of Sciences.

U.S. Code of Federal Regulations. 1991. Gun-Free School Zones Act of 1990 (P.L. 101-647, Section 1702). Amendment to Section 922 of Title 18 of U.S. Code. *United States Code Annotated.* 6 C Statutory Supplement, 1990 Public Laws 101-625 to 101-650. 101st Congress, 2nd Session, February.

U.S. Department of Health and Human Services, Public Health Service. 1991. *Healthy people 2000: National health promotion and disease prevention objectives.* DHHS Publication No. (PHS) 91-50212. Washington, DC.

U.S. Department of Transportation. 1988. *Driver license administration requirements and fees—1988.* Publication FHWA-PL-88-016. Washington, DC: Federal Highway Administration.

Virginia Association of School Superintendents. 1992. *Violence in schools: Recommendations for action by the Education Summit*. Charlottesville, VA.

Wilson, M., and S. Baker. 1987. Structural approach to injury control. *Journal of Social Issues* 43 (2): 73-86.

Wilson, M. H., S. P. Baker, S. P. Teret, S. Shock and J. Garbarino. 1991. *Saving children: A guide to injury prevention*. New York: Oxford University Press.

Wojtowicz, G., D. Macrina and A. Bolton. 1990. Reexamining the role of schools in injury prevention. *Wellness Perspectives: Research, Theory and Practice* 7 (1): 41-49.

Chapter 18

Physical Fitness: A Vital Component for Total Health and High-Level Wellness

Richard L. Papenfuss, PhD

The benefits of physical fitness have become increasingly clear during the past few years. The literature reveals not only the benefits of physical fitness, but how they may be achieved.

> There is now little doubt that regular physical activity of the appropriate frequency, intensity, and duration produces significant health benefits. Most important is the achievement of those specific fitness components which help reduce the risk of hypokinetic conditions including heart disease, back pain, diabetes, osteoporosis, and obesity. (Corbin, 1987)

Physical fitness is an important component in the total health and wellness of children and adults. Physical health and wellness is as important as social, emotional, intellectual and spiritual health. The effective balance of these five dimensions contributes to total health and high-level wellness.

Figure 1 illustrates the five dimensions of total health. The five dimensions represent the spokes of a wheel. When the spokes are of equal length, the wheel turns smoothly (life is balanced). However, when one dimension is extended or reduced in length, the wheel becomes unbalanced and all other dimensions are affected (life becomes difficult).

The physical dimension seeks its own balance in such healthy behaviors as proper diet, stress management, adequate rest and regular exercise. This type of physical fitness contributes to overall

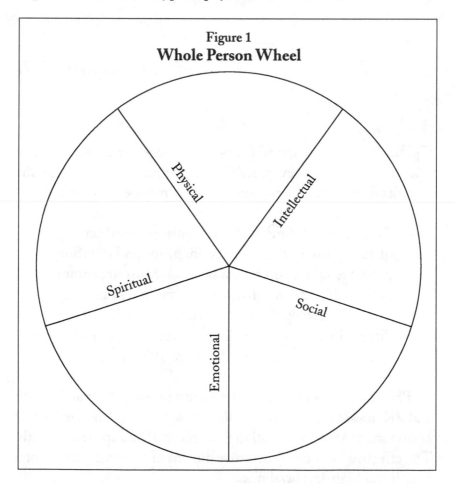

Figure 1
Whole Person Wheel

balance for total health and high-level wellness.

Physical fitness is but one of several important components that comprise the health and wellness of individuals. Ardell, in his book *Planning for Wellness*, suggested that high-level wellness has several components. His model for wellness has been expanded to include a myriad of factors that contribute to high-level wellness. Figure 2 depicts this Wellness Model.

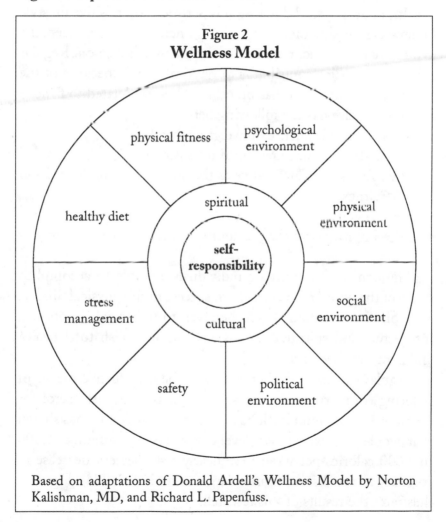

Figure 2
Wellness Model

Based on adaptations of Donald Ardell's Wellness Model by Norton Kalishman, MD, and Richard L. Papenfuss.

The Wellness Model focuses on the need for individuals to assume "self-responsibility" for their own wellness. It also suggests that several external factors must be addressed in order to achieve high-level wellness.

Why Is Physical Fitness Important?

Health in the physical dimension is derived from positive lifestyle behaviors related to diet, stress management, relaxation, sleep, the avoidance of tobacco, responsible alcohol use, and so on. Regular exercise is a major contributor to physical health, because of the synergistic effect that it has on other behaviors related to fitness. Regular exercise has the following benefits:

- has a positive influence on weight control
- aids in stress management and relaxation
- often serves as an alternative to the use of tobacco, alcohol and other drugs
- improves energy level
- helps improve strength, flexibility and endurance

Through regular exercise, individuals are able to accomplish many of the outcomes necessary to success in the physical dimension. Similar attention should be given to the social, emotional, intellectual and spiritual dimensions to accomplish total health and high-level wellness.

Regular exercise has been proven to be an effective means of reducing coronary artery disease, the number one risk factor for premature death among adults in our society. Research has shown that people who exercise at a level that burns a minimum of 2,000 to 3,000 calories per week have nearly a 40 percent decrease in coronary artery disease (Paffenbarger and Hyde, 1984). Figure 3 illustrates the results of this research.

When individuals walk, they tend to burn approximately six to eight calories per minute; when they jog, they burn eight to ten calories per minute. Therefore, someone who implements a walking program of fifty minutes per day, six days per week, would be exercising for three hundred minutes. If this individual burned seven calories per minute, she or he would burn a total of 2,100 calories for the week, which is within the desirable calorie consumption range of 2,000 to 3,000 calories per week.

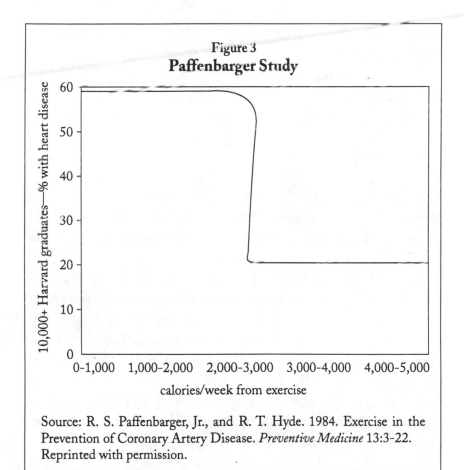

Figure 3
Paffenbarger Study

Source: R. S. Paffenbarger, Jr., and R. T. Hyde. 1984. Exercise in the Prevention of Coronary Artery Disease. *Preventive Medicine* 13:3-22. Reprinted with permission.

Other exercise schedules may be implemented, depending on time available and interests. The encouraging message in Paffenbarger's work is that we do not have to be marathon runners to obtain the positive benefits of exercise in reducing coronary artery disease.

The American Heart Association has identified the following ten risk factors for heart disease:

1. age
2. sex
3. heredity
4. lack of exercise
5. elevated cholesterol
6. high blood pressure
7. smoking
8. stress and tension
9. diabetes
10. overweight and obesity

The first three risk factors (age, sex and heredity) have been called the "uncontrollables." The other seven risk factors can be controlled. The effects of exercise positively influence six of the remaining seven (all except smoking).

Research by the Institute for Aerobic Research also supports the case for regular exercise in the reduction of cancer, the number-two risk factor for American adults. An eight-year study of approximately 13,000 people showed that physical activity reduces the risk of death from virtually all causes, but especially from heart disease and cancer (Blair et al., 1989). Figure 4 illustrates the results of this research. Regular exercise has the potential to dramatically reduce the risk of heart disease, cancer and other causes of death in both men and women.

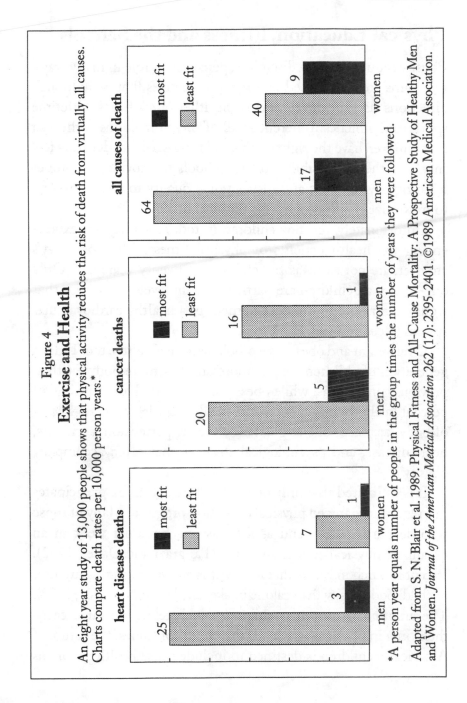

Figure 4
Exercise and Health

An eight year study of 13,000 people shows that physical activity reduces the risk of death from virtually all causes. Charts compare death rates per 10,000 person years.*

all causes of death

cancer deaths

heart disease deaths

*A person year equals number of people in the group times the number of years they were followed.

Adapted from S. N. Blair et al. 1989. Physical Fitness and All-Cause Mortality: A Prospective Study of Healthy Men and Women. *Journal of the American Medical Association* 262 (17): 2395–2401. ©1989 American Medical Association.

Physical Education, Fitness and the Schools

Physical education, as a discipline, perceives its role in many ways. Programs are often based on varying objectives that include such directions as skill development, health-related fitness, lifetime sports and athletics. Inherent in all of these directions is the fact that children have the right to physical fitness. Most educators feel that it is the responsibility of the schools to provide the proper learning environment and instructional quality to allow children to maximize their potential for physical fitness.

Unfortunately, too few children in today's society are experiencing the health benefits of physical fitness. Most of today's children are not as fit as the children of twenty years ago. Only one-half of all children are participating in levels of exercise that would contribute to the development of a healthy cardiovascular system (Ross and Gilbert, 1985).

Overweight and obesity are problematic in children, too. Today's generation of children weighs more and has more body fat than previous generations, while obesity has increased an alarming 54 percent in children ages six to eleven (Bar-Or, 1987). A high level of body fat places one at greater risk for hypertension, accidents, heart disease, and psychological stressors that often accompany obesity.

It is estimated that only one out of three children participates in a regular, organized physical education program. Many of those who do participate spend as little as one hour per week in an organized physical education lesson (Pangrazi and Dauer, 1992). Recent research indicates that inactivity is an even bigger contributor to childhood obesity than calorie intake (Ikeda and Naworski, 1992). The amount of time that children watch television far exceeds their time in physical activity. If this trend continues, the future of American's children is destined to include those health problems related to sedentary living—hypertension, obesity, heart disease, strokes and cancer, to name several (Blair et al., 1989).

National Objectives for Physical Activity and Fitness

The United States has identified specific objectives for physical activity and fitness in *Healthy People 2000: National Health Promotion and Disease Prevention Objectives* (U.S. Department of Health and Human Services, 1991).

A summary list of objectives related to physical activity and fitness follows:

- Reduce coronary artery disease deaths to no more than 100 per 100,000 people (Objective 1.1).
- Reduce overweight to a prevalence of no more than 20 percent among people age 20 and older and no more than 15 percent among adolescents ages 12 to 19 (Objective 1.2).
- Increase to at least 30 percent the proportion of people age 6 and older who engage regularly, preferably daily, in light to moderate physical activity for at least thirty minutes per day (Objective 1.3).
- Increase to at least 20 percent the proportion of people age 18 and older and to at least 75 percent the proportion of children and adolescents ages 6 to 17 who engage in vigorous physical activity that promotes the development and maintenance of cardiorespiratory fitness three or more days per week for twenty or more minutes per occasion (Objective 1.4).
- Reduce to no more than 15 percent the proportion of people age 6 and older who engage in no leisure-time activity (Objective 1.5).
- Increase to at least 40 percent the proportion of people age 6 and older who regularly perform physical activities that enhance and maintain muscular strength, muscular endurance and flexibility (Objective 1.6).

- Increase to at least 50 percent the proportion of overweight people age 12 and older who have adopted sound dietary practices combined with regular physical activity to attain an appropriate body weight (Objective 1.7).

These objectives provide an excellent foundation upon which to develop a comprehensive school health promotion program, which would include:
- physical education
- health education
- home economics/nutrition
- biology
- social sciences
- school food service/cafeteria
- nursing
- counseling

Components of a Physical Fitness Program

Most experts agree on the components necessary for a successful physical fitness program. The American Alliance for Health, Physical Education, Recreation and Dance (AAHPERD) designed assessment strategies utilized in the measurement of each of the components during physical education classes. The common components follow (Pangrazi and Dauer, 1992):

Cardiovascular Fitness. The goal in this component is to develop the heart, blood and respiratory system in order to increase cardiovascular capabilities while simultaneously reducing the risks of morbidity and mortality. Aerobic activities, those requiring the heart to deliver a continuous supply of oxygen to the cells, are necessary for the achievement of a "training effect" on the cardiovascular system. Activities such as walking, jogging, biking, swimming, dance aerobics, basketball, soccer, rope jumping, and cross-country skiing are examples of aerobic activity.

Body Composition. Body composition is an important part of physical fitness. Body composition refers to the amount of body fat an individual has in proportion to lean body mass. It can be determined by several different types of measurement. The most common method of measurement features the use of a skinfold caliper. A series of measurements are applied to a formula that calculates body composition. Achieving a healthy level of body composition is significant in maximizing one's potential for wellness. It is also vital to the reduction of risk factors related to accidents and chronic diseases.

Flexibility. Flexibility contributes to overall physical fitness because it improves the range of movement in which a single joint or series of joints is able to move. This range of movement is important to fitness because it reduces the frequency of injury in exercise and sport, usually improves posture, and may decrease problems with low-back pain.

The recommended type of stretching is static, controlled activity (as opposed to ballistic stretching that uses bouncing movements). Static stretching is safer and less likely to cause injury. It encourages one to slowly stretch the muscles, tendons and ligaments to a point of discomfort, then ease off and hold the stretch for a period of time. Static stretching is recommended both as a warmup in preparation for strenuous activity and for a cool-down following vigorous exercise. Cool-down stretching is extremely helpful in reducing muscle stiffness and soreness from exercise.

Muscular Strength and Endurance. Muscular strength is the ability of a muscle to exert force; muscular endurance is the ability to exert that force over a period of time. To achieve adequate levels of physical fitness, a person must be capable of muscular strength to fulfill the skills necessary for an activity. Muscular endurance is necessary for the activity to be repeated over and over again so improved fitness can occur.

To improve muscular strength, the muscle must be moved while under resistance. To improve muscular endurance, the muscle must be moved repeatedly while under a low-level work load. It is recommended that individuals participate in regular exercise sessions three to four times per week as a means of increasing muscular strength and endurance.

In summary, to achieve a healthy level of physical fitness, emphasis should be placed upon each of the four vital components of fitness: (1) cardiovascular fitness, (2) body composition, (3) flexibility, and (4) muscular strength and endurance.

Student-Based Physical Fitness Programs

Because our students are so unfit, new strategies must be developed to reach this target audience. History seems to indicate that physical education programs alone cannot accomplish the national physical fitness goals established by *Healthy People 2000*. What can we do to improve the health of our children?

Form a physical fitness advisory group consisting of members from the school and community. Membership should be broad-based, including physicians, nurses, clergy, exercise scientists, parents, students, teachers, administrators, etc.

Conduct a study of the existing school policies as they pertain to student physical education requirements. Seek to support school policies that will allow physical fitness opportunities for all students at least three times per week.

Analyze the current physical education curriculum to determine if instruction is designed to achieve healthy levels of physical fitness for all children. Try to positively influence curricula that place a high priority on sports to include a greater emphasis on health-related fitness assessment and supportive activities.

Obtain interdisciplinary support for physical fitness and total health. Encourage disciplines other than physical education to teach toward the building of knowledge, attitudes, skills and behaviors that enhance physical fitness. Use *Healthy People 2000* as a foundation for your objectives.

Network with the community to develop broad-based support for physical fitness objectives within and outside the school. Plan assignments that will encourage students and parents to participate together in fitness activities and assist the community in designing fitness events that will attract wide participation.

Develop reinforcement strategies for those who are achieving personal physical fitness goals. Identify a system that will allow for verbal compliments, written commendations and/or specific awards to those who are accomplishing their physical fitness objectives.

Comprehensive School Health Promotion and Physical Fitness

The responsibility for physical fitness within the total person concept and the wellness model is far too encompassing for any one discipline. Traditionally, physical fitness goals were identified as the sole responsibility of physical education. Today, however, health promotion advocates in North America are recommending an interdisciplinary approach to fitness and the total health of the individual and the community. This comprehensive school health promotion model is still in its developmental stages, but momentum is gathering for the acceptance and integration of this model in numerous school and community settings.

In essence, the school health promotion model suggests that if the health of the school (organization) is to improve significantly a comprehensive approach to health promotion is necessary. This comprehensive approach should not be limited to health education and physical education, but should include home economics, psychology, biology, social sciences and other interested disciplines. It should also incorporate student services and service personnel such as nursing, counseling, administration, food service, bus drivers and custodians. In this process, health promotion becomes integrated within the entire school setting for the benefit of students, teachers, administrators and all other school personnel.

School health educators can play an important role in the promotion of fitness within the school and community settings. Health educators should support all the goals and objectives of *Healthy People 2000*, especially those related to physical fitness, because of the contributions fitness makes toward total health. There are many ways in which school health education may contribute:

- Health educators should be positive role models for students, staff and the community by exemplifying healthy lifestyles, including behaviors related to physical fitness.
- Whenever possible, collegial support should be provided to those who are aspiring to promote physical fitness with the school and community environments.
- The health educator should assist those responsible for curriculum development of physical education to support the goals and objectives of *Healthy People 2000*.
- The school health education program should lend support for physical fitness by planning teaching strategies that reinforce the goals and objectives of physical education's health-related fitness component.
- The school health education program should seek ways to reinforce positive health behaviors of students, staff and the community—especially those behaviors related to improved physical fitness.

- Health educators should seek ways to involve parents and children in the mutual attainment of physical fitness goals and objectives both at home and in the school.
- Community networking should be pursued by the health educator so that opportunities for health-related fitness may be enhanced for children and adults.
- Health educators should assist in the development of special projects designed within the school and community to promote physical fitness activities for children and adults.
- School health educators should be willing to provide leadership in the development of health promotion programs for employees within the school setting.

The challenge for school health educators seems never-ending. But to significantly improve the health of people in our schools and communities, all avenues must be considered.

Health Promotion for School Employees

Traditional thinking in physical fitness has been skewed toward the importance of fitness for students. Recent developments have been more sensitive to the benefits of physical fitness for teachers and all other school personnel. School health promotion can be designed for both school employees and students within the school environment.

The success stories offered here provide evidence to support the concept of school health promotion. These examples are just the beginning of a movement that has the potential to spread across the schools of our nation.

Oregon's Seaside Conference

The Oregon Department of Education, under the leadership of Len Tritsch, developed an annual summer conference in school health promotion. Now in its fifteenth year, the conference attracts more than a thousand school and community leaders to a week-long Seaside Conference. Conference participants are asked to develop a plan of action that they will be able to implement in their respective school and community settings.

This approach has met with so much success that the National Association of School Administrators has financially supported the diffusion of this model throughout other states in the United States. The Seaside Conference has created a ripple effect across the nation. It is increasing the opportunities for schools and communities to become involved in comprehensive school health promotion at the local levels.

Dallas Independent School District

The Dallas Independent School District initiated one of the first attempts in school-based health promotion designed to evaluate the cost-effectiveness of their efforts. The Dallas school health promotion project provided opportunities for school personnel to participate in an employee wellness program that featured such components as exercise, stress management, smoking cessation and weight control. A comparison of absenteeism rates of those who participated with those who didn't indicated that the participants were absent 2.5 fewer days. Because the district had to hire substitute teachers for absent teachers, the savings were significant enough (nearly $500,000) to offset the cost of the school health promotion program (Blair et al., 1984).

Albuquerque Public Schools

In a dissertation study conducted by Beier (1984), the results of a school-based health promotion program showed that teacher and staff absenteeism and self-concept could be significantly improved. Teachers and staff who participated in a regular wellness program offered at the school decreased their absenteeism by two days. The cost savings on substitute teachers more than offset the cost of the health promotion program.

Why Health Promotion in the Schools?

There are several important reasons for health promotion in the schools. Schools collectively represent one of the largest employee groups in the United States. The problems encountered by school employees parallel those problems of any large corporation. As Mark Tager, MD, stated (1985):

> Chances are, your school district is not unlike the national average:
> * One in six of your employees has hypertension;
> * One in ten has problems with alcohol or drugs;
> * Half are obese;
> * Almost a quarter of your male employees will die of cardiovascular disease before age 65.

Given these lifestyle conditions for illness and premature death, it is easy to understand why schools are a necessary focal point for health promotion and wellness.

The economic factors surrounding these conditions also provide an excellent rationale. School districts, like business and industry, have been experiencing escalating costs for employee health insurance coverage. Health insurance rates have sometimes increased by 25 percent or more from one year to the next. Health care costs have been steadily increasing for the past two decades to a point where the United States in now spending more than $600 billion per year on health care costs. This represents about 11 percent of our Gross National Product (GNP). The health care budget is second only to our national defense budget in total dollars spent.

The major costs for health care from illness or disability seem to be related to heart disease, hypertension and low-back pain. Similarly, the major cause of illness and death in the United States continues to be coronary heart disease. The American Heart Association states that cardiovascular disease accounts for more than $64 billion of our annual medical costs. And, yet, when we examine the risk factors of heart disease, it is easy to see that many of the risk factors can be controlled through physical fitness.

The research also supports the conclusion that a successful health promotion program can positively affect absenteeism, disability, job turnover, productivity and morale. Each of these benefits saves money for the employer. Thus, the question is not "Should we start a health promotion program?" but rather, "How do we get started?"

The Need for Health Promotion

One way to attempt to solve the problem of escalating health care costs is to focus more energy on prevention rather than treatment. Many authorities agree that this strategy has tremendous potential for the future of the United States:

> ...any future advances made in improving the nation's health will not result from spectacular bio-medical breakthroughs. Rather, advances will result from personally initiated actions that are directly influenced by the person's health-related activities, values, belief, and knowledge. (Wisconsin Department of Public Instruction, 1985)

Evidence suggests that even a modest health promotion program can have a positive impact on health care costs of employees. A study in Ontario, Canada, correlated physical fitness with medical care. It recorded the frequency of hospital and doctor visits, number of days absent due to illness, and the number of physician claims made under the Ontario Health Insurance Plan. The study concluded that:

- People with higher levels of physical fitness tend to have lower medical claims.
- An estimated reduction of 31 million medical claims could be expected if all adults ages 20 to 69 attained at least average physical fitness.
- People with higher levels of fitness tend to have reduced incidence of coronary artery disease.

The Control Data Corporation studied 5,000 of its employees who participated in their "Stay Well" health promotion program. The results indicated that regular exercisers had a 36 percent decrease in health care expenditures and a significant decrease in hospital stays. These studies offer excellent support for physical fitness as an integral part of the school health promotion program.

Planning a School Health Promotion Program for Employees

The process for planning a school health promotion program for employees does not have to be very difficult or time consuming. Some of the preplanning considerations might include:

- an inventory of available resources within the school and community
- a philosophy upon which the program may be built
- some general goals

For example, goals developed by school staff members from Fairfax County, Virginia, schools included (Tager, 1985):

- greater cohesiveness
- improved communication
- improved self-esteem
- improved morale
- more supportive staff
- reduced absenteeism
- more energy
- greater productivity
- less draw on sick leave bank
- less draw on medical insurance
- reduced job burnout
- greater commitment to the school mission
- greater motivation
- more positive attitudes

The actual implementation phase of such a plan might include the following steps:

Step 1: Screening. In this step, individuals are asked to complete a medical history form designed to screen for serious medical problems that would be deterrents to program participation. A sample medical form is provided in Figure 5.

Step 2: Assessment. A wellness profile could be used as an assessment instrument to determine the strengths and weaknesses of an individual's present lifestyle. See the Healthstyle sample wellness profile in Figure 6.

Step 3: Setting Personal Goals. Based on the wellness profile, individuals are asked to establish some personal health-related goals for themselves. Common choices might include lifestyle changes in such areas as nutritional habits, weight control, exercise, stress management, smoking or safety.

Step 4: Scheduling Activities. Program coordinators assist the participants in scheduling activities that will help them attain their goals. The use of school facilities and school personnel to accommodate the activity sessions requires time and coordination, but also provides ownership, pride and staff cohesiveness when conducted properly. Potential program activities are listed in Figure 7.

Step 5: Reinforcement and Feedback. Planners need to devise methods of reinforcement so participants remain motivated to continue their positive behavior change. Feedback from participants (both positive and negative) to the planners helps improve the quality of the program.

Step 6: Reassessment of Personal Goals. After a designated period of time, individuals are encouraged to assess their progress by re-examining their wellness profile and goal statements.

Step 7: Repeat the Cycle. Individuals may want to continue their present programs or may choose to set new goals for themselves in new areas of lifestyle improvement.

Can School Health Promotion Be Cost Effective?

Education continues to struggle with funding levels that make it difficult to finance all the programs necessary for student and staff growth. In addition, an era of strict accountability forces school administrators to maximize the effects of their budgets. Given the tenor of the times, doesn't it seem appropriate for decision makers in education to support school health promotion programs that are cost-effective? The impact of staff school health promotion programs on absenteeism in both Dallas and Albuquerque has already been discussed. In both cases, absenteeism savings were significant enough to offset the cost of the health promotion program.

Figure 5
Medical History Form

Name _____

School _____

Date _____

1. Age _____   2. Sex _____   3. Race _____

4. Medical Background
Please check if you have had any of the following:

diseases of the heart or arteries _____

diabetes or abnormal blood sugar _____

stroke _____

epilepsy _____

anemia _____

abnormal chest x-ray _____

asthma _____

other lung disease _____

orthopedic or muscular problems _____

If you checked any of the above, please explain in more detail:

_____

_____

_____

5. Present Health Status
Please note if any of the following apply to you:

diseases of the heart or arteries

doctor said blood pressure too high or too low _____

doctor said EKG (electrocardiogram) abnormal _____

diabetes _____

epilepsy _____

stroke _____

chest x-ray abnormal _____

asthma _____

other lung disease _____

orthopedic or muscular problems _____

Please explain in more detail the items you checked:

_____

_____

_____

Figure 5 (continued)

6. Physical Activity

Are you taking part in a regular exercise program? Yes _____
No _____

Do you regularly walk or run one or more miles
without stopping? Yes _____
No _____

If you answered "yes," how many miles do you
average per day or in a typical workout? Miles _____
How long does it take you to cover a mile? Time (Min:sec) _____
Do you lift weights or do calisthenics? Yes _____
No _____

Do you take part in competitive sports? Yes _____
No _____

If "yes," list them: _____
How often? (times per month) _____
If not exercising at present, how long has it been since
you last exercised regularly? _____

7. Cardiovascular Disease in Family

Has anyone in your family suffered from cardiovascular disease (myocardial infarction, hypertension, hyperlipidemia)

Who (What relation to you)	Nature of problem	Age at onset or death
_____	_____	_____
_____	_____	_____
_____	_____	_____
_____	_____	_____
_____	_____	_____

8. Smoking

Do you smoke? Yes _____ No _____
If "yes," how many packs a day? _____
If you're a former smoker, how long ago did you quit? _____

9. Stress and Tension Level

How would you describe yourself?
1. relaxed, not at all tense _____
2. somewhat tense _____
3. moderately tense _____
4. very tense _____

Figure 5 (continued)

10. Medications Used

Please list any medications you are taking:

Medication	Dosage		Taken since:
(Name)	Strength	How often	
_____	_____	_____	_____
_____	_____	_____	_____
_____	_____	_____	_____

Do not write below this line

---

11. Risk Analysis

[To be filled out by program coordinator or consultant]

Risk Factors	Current Level	At Risk (check)
personal history	_____	_____
ECG	_____	_____ (positive)
blood pressure	_____	_____ (>140/90)
inactivity	_____	_____
obesity	_____% fat	_____ (>22-19%)
	_____ height	
	_____ weight	
hyperlipidemia:		
cholesterol	_____ mg%	_____ (>250mg)
triglycerides	_____ mg%	_____ (>150mg)
glucose	_____ mg%	_____ (>110mg)
HDL ratio (total cholesterol divided by HDL)	_____	_____ (>4.5)
family history	_____	_____
smoking	_____	_____
tension	_____	_____ (>level 3)
diabetes	_____	_____
age	_____	_____ (>40)
resting heart rate	_____	_____ (>90)

Adapted with permission from the American Council of Life Insurance and Health Insurance Association of America. M. J. Tager. 1985. *Wellness at the School Worksite: A Manual.* Washington, DC.

Figure 6
Healthstyle: A Self-Test

All of us want good health. But many of us do not know how to be as healthy as possible. Health experts describe *lifestyle* as one of the most important factors affecting health. If fact, it is estimated that as many as seven of the ten leading causes of death could be reduced through common-sense changes in lifestyle. That's what this brief test, developed by the Public Health Service, is all about. Its purpose is simply to tell you how well you are doing to stay healthy. The behaviors covered in the test are recommended for most Americans. Some of them may not apply to persons with certain chronic diseases or handicaps, or to pregnant women. Such persons may require special instructions from their physicians.

	Almost Always	Sometimes	Almost Never
Cigarette Smoking			
If you *never smoke,* enter a score of 10 for this section and go to the next section on *Alcohol and Drugs.*			
1. I avoid smoking cigarettes	2	1	0
2. I smoke only low tar and nicotine cigarettes *or* I smoke a pipe or cigars.	2	1	0

Smoking Score:_____

	Almost Always	Sometimes	Almost Never
Alcohol and Drugs			
1. I avoid drinking alcoholic beverages *or* I drink no more than 1 or 2 drinks a day.	4	1	0
2. I avoid using alcohol or other drugs (especially illegal drugs) as a way of handling stressful situations or the problems in my life.	2	1	0
3. I am careful not to drink alcohol when taking certain medicines (for example, medicine for sleeping, pain, colds and allergies) or when pregnant.	2	1	0
4. I read and follow the label directions when using prescribed and over-the-counter drugs.	2	1	0

Alcohol and Drugs Score:_____

Figure 6 (continued)

Eating Habits	Almost Always	Sometimes	Almost Never
1. I eat a variety of foods each day, such as fruits and vegetables, whole grain breads and cereals, lean meats, dairy products, dry peas and beans, and nuts and seeds.	4	1	0
2. I limit the amount of fat, saturated fat, and cholesterol I eat (including fat on meats, eggs, butter, cream, shortenings, and organ meats such as liver).	2	1	0
3. I limit the amount of salt I eat by cooking with only small amounts, not adding salt at the table, and avoiding salty snacks.	2	1	0
4. I avoid eating too much sugar (especially frequent snacks of sticky candy or soft drinks).	2	1	0

Eating Habits Score:_____

Exercise/Fitness			
1. I maintain a desired weight, avoiding overweight and underweight.	3	1	0
2. I do vigorous exercises for 15-30 minutes at least 3 times a week (examples include running, swimming, brisk walking).	3	1	0
3. I do exercises that enhance my muscle tone for 15-30 minutes at least 3 times a week (examples include yoga and calisthenics).	2	1	0
4. I use part of my leisure time participating in individual, family or team activities that increase my level of fitness (such as gardening, bowling, golf and baseball).	2	1	0

Exercise/Fitness Score:_____

Figure 6 (continued)

	Almost Always	Sometimes	Almost Never
Stress Control			
1. I have a job or do other work that I enjoy.	2	1	0
2. I find it easy to relax and express my feelings freely.	2	1	0
3. I recognize early, and prepare for, events or situations likely to be stressful for me.	2	1	0
4. I have close friends, relatives or others to whom I can talk about personal matters and call on for help when needed.	2	1	0
5. I participate in group activities (such as church and community organizations) or hobbies that I enjoy.	2	1	0

Stress Control Score:_____

	Almost Always	Sometimes	Almost Never
Safety			
1. I wear a safety belt while riding in a car.	2	1	0
2. I avoid driving while under the influence of alcohol and other drugs.	2	1	0
3. I obey traffic rules and the speed limit when driving.	2	1	0
4. I am careful when using potentially harmful products or substances (such as household cleaners, poisons and electrical devices).	2	1	0
5. I avoid smoking in bed.	2	1	0

Safety Score:_____

What Your Scores Mean to You
Scores of 9 and 10
Excellent! Your answers show that you are aware of the importance of this area to your health. More important, you are putting your knowledge to work for you by practicing good health habits. As long as you continue to do so, this area should not pose a serious health risk. It's likely that you are setting an example for your family and friends to follow. Since you got a very high test score on this part of the test, you may want to consider other areas where your scores indicate room for improvement.

Scores of 6 to 8
Your health practices in this area are good, but there is room for improvement. Look again at the items you answered with a "Sometimes" or "Almost Never." What changes can you make to improve your score? Even a small change can often help you achieve better health.

Scores of 3 to 5
Your health risks are showing! Would you like more information about the risks you are facing and why it is important for you to change these behaviors? Perhaps you need help in deciding how to successfully make the changes you desire. In either case, help is available.

Scores of 0 to 2
Obviously, you were concerned enough about your health to take the test, but your answers show that you may be taking serious and unnecessary risks with your health. Perhaps you are not aware of the risks and what to do about them. You can easily get the information and help you need to improve, if you wish. The next step is up to you.

Figure 7
Activities for Health Promotion

exercise/fitness	wellness cooking	low-back pain prevention
smoking cessation	safety education	CPR
nutrition	cholesterol control	alcohol/drug use prevention
weight control	self-care	hypertension control
stress management	parenting skills	retirement

But what about other variables? Wouldn't it also be possible to save money by reducing the high cost of health care? The Ottawa Health Insurance Plan documented the reduction in medical claims by those involved in physical fitness programs. Control Data Corporation showed a 36 percent decrease in health-care costs for those who participated in the "Stay Well" employee health promotion program (Tager, 1985).

Researchers have suggested that the dollars spent on employee health promotion produce savings to the organization of more than one dollar to almost six dollars. Obviously, the costs of an employee health promotion program can have a very positive impact on the financial conditions of an organization.

However, some researchers have warned against evaluating health promotion programs solely on the merits of cost-effectiveness. These experts suggest that considerations should be made on the broader perspective and understanding that health promotion can have a positive impact on the lives of the participants in the physical, mental and social dimensions. These improvements are part of a much larger goal for our population as a society (Breslow, 1990; Warner, 1987). Others have noted that the influence of health promotion on the development of healthful environmental surroundings that contribute to positive lifestyle behaviors is a higher priority than cost-effectiveness (Warner, 1990).

Much could also be said in support of the responsibility of school staff members as role models for the students within their environments. By setting healthy examples in their lifestyle choices to help themselves, they can deliver a strong message to the students with whom they come in contact on a daily basis. This indirect method of teaching may be more powerful than any of us care to imagine.

References

Ardell, D. B., and M. J. Tager. 1982. *Planning for wellness* 2d ed. Dubuque, IA: Kendall/Hunt Publishing.

Bar-Or, O. 1987. A commentary to children and fitness: A public health perspective. *Research Quarterly* 58 (4): 304-307.

Beier, B. J. 1984. A study of the effectiveness of a school-based health promotion program on absenteeism, self-concept, and lifestyle of middle school faculty, staff, and students. PhD diss., University of New Mexico, Albuquerque.

Blair, N., T. Collingwood, R. Reynolds, M. Smith, D. Hagan and C. Sterling. 1984. Health promotion for educators: Impact on health behaviors, satisfaction, and general well-being. *American Journal of Public Health* 74:147-149.

Blair, S. N., H. W. Kohl III, R. S. Paffenbarger, Jr., D. G. Clark, K. H. Cooper and L. W. Gibbons. 1989. Physical fitness and all-cause mortality: A prospective study of healthy men and women. *Journal of the American Medical Association* 262 (17): 2395-2401.

Breslow, L. 1990. A health promotion primer for the 1990s. *Health Affairs* 9 (2): 6-21.

Corbin, C. 1987. Physical fitness in the K-12 curriculum: Some defensive solutions to perennial problems. *Journal of Physical Education, Recreation, and Dance* 58 (7): 49-54.

Curtis, J. D., and R. L. Papenfuss. 1980. *Health instruction: A task approach.* Minneapolis, MN: Burgess Publishing.

Ikeda, J., and P. Naworski. 1992. *Am I fat? Helping young children accept differences in body size.* Santa Cruz, CA: ETR Associates.

Paffenbarger, R. S., Jr., and R. T. Hyde. 1984. Exercise in the prevention of coronary artery disease. *Preventive Medicine* 13: 3-22.

Paffenbarger, R. S., Jr., R. T. Hyde, A. L. Wing and C. C. Hsieh. 1986. Physical activity, all-cause mortality and longevity of college alumni. *New England Journal of Medicine* 314:605-613.

Pangrazi, R. P., and V. P. Dauer. 1992. *Dynamic physical education for elementary school children.* 10th ed. New York: Macmillan.

Ross, J. G., and G. G. Gilbert. 1985. The national children and youth fitness study: A summary of findings. *Journal of Physical Education, Recreation, and Dance* 56 (1): 45-50.

Tager, M. J. 1985. *Wellness at the school worksite: A manual.* Washington, DC: American Council of Life Insurance and Health Insurance Association of America.

United States Department of Health and Human Services, Public Health Service. 1991. *Healthy people 2000: National health promotion and disease prevention objectives.* DHHS Publication No. 91 50212. Washington, DC.

Warner, K. E. 1987. Selling health promotion to corporate America: Uses and abuses of the economic argument. *Health Education Quarterly* 14 (1): 39-55.

Warner, K. E. 1990. Wellness at the worksite. *Health Affairs* 9 (2): 63-79.

Wisconsin Department of Public Instruction. 1985. *A guide to curriculum planning in health education.* Madison, WI.

Contributors to
Volume One

Diane D. Allensworth, RN, PhD, CHES, has served as a faculty member of the Kent State University since 1976. She is an associate professor in the Department of Adult Counseling, Health and Vocational Education. She has also worked with the American School Health Association as the associate executive director for programs. Her responsibilities in the association include directing the Department of Sponsored Programs. In this capacity, she has directed federal grants from the Centers for Disease Control and Prevention, Department of Education, and the Office of Disease Prevention and Health Promotion. Her interest in school health began when she served as the school nurse for seven schools in Northwest Ohio.

Evelyn E. Ames, PhD, CHES, is professor and coordinator of health education at Western Washington University in Bellingham, Washington. She has been involved in health education at the university level for more than 30 years. She also serves as a consultant for various public school health education projects and organizes inservice programs for public school teachers. She has completed a two-year federally funded grant project for inservicing and mentoring elementary teachers in comprehensive school health education. She actively contributes to state and national professional health education organizations.

She is the coauthor of two books: *Designing School Health Curricula: Planning for Good Health* and *Becoming Male and Female* (an adolescent teenage sexuality text).

Judy C. Berryman, MA, is the executive director of the Greater Battle Creek Healthy Lifestyles Project, Battle Creek, Michigan. The project is a school-based health promotion and education project for school staff, students and parents. She has eight years experience as an educator, trainer, lecturer and consultant in the areas of school worksite wellness, community collaboration for healthy children, and comprehensive health education. She has also served as president of the Michigan School Health Association.

Peter A. Cortese, DrPH, CHES, holds a master's and a doctoral degree in public health with an emphasis in school health. He began his professional work as a high school teacher in Keewatin, Minnesota. Following graduate studies at UCLA, he taught in the Los Angeles secondary schools and community colleges and then at the university level. He has been a professor and chair of the Health Science Department at California State University, Long Beach, and is associate dean emeritus of the university's College of Health and Human Services.

He has also served as associate director of the School Health Education Study; director of the Office of Comprehensive School Health, U.S. Department of Education; vice-chair and chair of the National Commission for Health Education Credentialing; chair of the Coalition of National Health Education Organizations; cochair of the Terminology in Health Education Committee; chair of the writing committee that produced "Comprehensive School Health Education—As Defined by the Major National Health Organizations"; and chair of the Implementation Committee for California State Department of Education's "Framework for Health Instruction in California Schools."

In addition, he has been the chair of the School Health Education and Services Section of the American Public Health Association, president of the American Association for the Advancement of Health Education, and president of the Southern California Chapter of the Society for Public Health Education. He has received honor awards from all of the above groups.

He has been actively involved in the work of many voluntary and other public health agencies, has written several juried journal articles and is listed as one of 27 "Key Leaders in Health Education" in the Eta Sigma Gamma Monograph Series.

M. Joycelyn Elders, MD, was director of the Arkansas Department of Health prior to her appointment to the post of Surgeon General. She has served as president of the Association of State and Territorial Health Officers and on the boards of many service organizations. She is a graduate of the University of Arkansas Medical School, where she served as professor of pediatrics. She has also received an honorary doctorate of medical sciences from Yale University. She has appeared on nationwide television and has written more than 150 articles for medical research publications.

Joyce V. Fetro, PhD, CHES, is health education specialist for the San Francisco Unified School District. In that role, she is responsible for inservice training and curriculum development for comprehensive school health education in kindergarten through grade 12. She received her doctoral degree in health education from Southern Illinois University, with an emphasis on evaluation, instrument development and research methods. Her experience in health education spans more than twenty years, including three years as a curriculum specialist, thirteen years as a middle school teacher, two years as a university instructor, and three years conducting research and evaluation studies about the effectiveness of substance use, pregnancy and HIV/AIDS prevention programs. She is the author of *Step by Step to Substance Use Prevention: The Planning Guide for School-Based Programs* (ETR Associates, 1991) and *Personal and Social Skills: Understanding and Integrating Competencies Across Health Content* (ETR Associates, 1992) and is coauthor of *Are You Sad Too? Helping Children Deal with Loss and Death* (ETR Associates, 1993).

Gail C. Frank, DrPH, RD, CHES, is professor of nutrition and director of the Child Nutrition Program Management Center at California State University, Long Beach. Trained as a nutritional epidemiologist, she has more than sixty publications focusing on various aspects of dietary methodology for child respondents, comprehensive school health, nutrient intakes of children and primary prevention programs in schools. She is a national spokesperson for the American Dietetic Association and works directly with print and electronic media at the local, national and international level. In 1990, she was the recipient of the ADA Award for Excellence in the Practice of Dietetic Education and Research. She directs an ADA AP4 Dietetic Internship at California State University and was the recipient of the first ADA grant to incorporate school nutrition training into an ADA internship.

Brian F. Geiger, MS, is a graduate research assistant for the University of South Carolina, School of Public Health School-Community Sexual Risk

Reduction Project for Teens. He has worked as a program director for an outpatient treatment program for adults with chronic mental illness and as a vocational rehabilitation consultant. He has presented papers and workshops on comprehensive health education instruction at statewide conferences and has developed materials for health professionals on Alzheimer's disease and independent-living-skills training. He has served on city and state task forces to plan new housing and services for homeless adults and was a volunteer announcer and member of the planning committee for WRBH-FM Radio for the Blind and Print Handicapped in New Orleans.

Marian V. Hamburg, EdD, CHES, is professor emeritus, New York University, where she established the Department of Health Education and engaged in the professional preparation of school and community health educators for 25 years. Her experience in school health also includes teaching at the secondary level and serving as national school health consultant for the American Heart Association and the March of Dimes. She has held leadership positions in the Association for the Advancement of Health Education, the American School Health Association, the American Public Health Association and the Society for Public Health Education. She has also served on the board of the National Commission for Health Education Credentialing.

Alan C. Henderson, DrPH, CHES, is professor of health science at California State University, Long Beach. He has been involved in professional preparation of health educators for many years. He served as director of the Role Delineation Project for Health Education at the National Center for Health Education. He has worked with numerous professional and community organizations to improve preparation of health educators and meet the health education needs of the public. He is the author of *Healthy Schools, Healthy Futures: The Case for Improving School Environment* (ETR Associates, 1993).

William M. Kane, PhD, CHES, is associate professor of health education at the University of New Mexico in Albuquerque. He is a former public school teacher and coordinator of health education and an author of health education textbooks. He has served as executive director of two national health organizations, the Association for the Advancement of Health Education and the American College of Preventive Medicine, and has been active in the establishment of many national health education initiatives. He is the author of *Step by Step to Comprehensive School Health: The Program Planning Guide* (ETR Associates, 1993).

Nathan Matza, MA, CHES, is a full-time high school teacher, health science mentor teacher and lecturer in the Department of Health Science at California State University, Long Beach. He is a contributing author of the California Health Instructional Framework and a curriculum guide for university health instructors. He is recognized as an expert in health education teaching and has served as mentor teacher for high school students, health teachers and college students. He has written a district health education course of study for Huntington Beach Union High School District and has been selected as a teacher of the year and a finalist for the President's Award for Excellence in Teaching. He has taught for more than 23 years.

Kathleen Middleton, MS, CHES, is editor-in-chief at ETR Associates. She is a nationally recognized expert in the field of school health education and has been involved at local, state and national levels. She taught middle school health education for ten years before entering full-time into educational curricula and materials development. She is the editor of the *Contemporary Health Series* and has been primary author or editor for more than thirty health education curricula. She directed the development, scope and sequence, evaluation and dissemination of *Growing Healthy* for the National Center for Health Education and is coauthor, with Dr. Marion Pollock, of a widely used college textbook, *Elementary School Health Instruction*. She is also the author of *Into Adolescence: Communicating Emotions* (ETR Associates, 1990).

Nancy S. Miller, PhD, was director of external resources for the American Association of School Administrators for ten years. She developed millions of dollars in successful proposals to improve the health of children and youth, including projects to introduce the National Health Objectives, provide HIV prevention training to school leaders, and prevent teen pregnancy through school-based early intervention. In addition to providing technical assistance to these and other school-related programs, she has been a special education teacher, has worked in residential treatment, and assisted in the management of a university-based school service center.

Kathleen R. Miner, PhD, MPH, CHES, has been involved in education since 1968 and health education since 1979. She has authored numerous articles about education and public health, as well as many curricula now being used throughout the state of Georgia. She has also worked as a Health Educator in Egypt, Trinidad and Thailand. She is now an associate professor at the Emory University School of Public Health, where she has been involved in many public health projects, such as the Adolescent Health Concerns Projects of Georgia, the Ryan White Title II AIDS Intervention, the Emory AIDS Training Network and the DeKalb County Teenage Pregnancy Task Force.

Priscilla Naworski, MS, CHES, is the director of the California Healthy Kids Resource Center. She also serves as chair of the Nutrition and Food Services Council for the American School Health Association. She has been active in nutrition education and comprehensive school health programs for more than 15 years. She has published curriculum guides and reviews of materials in these fields and has presented sessions at national and state nutrition and comprehensive health conferences. She has served on the California Children and Weight Task Force, which developed a position paper and training modules for health professionals who deal with children, including children who are overweight. She is coauthor of *Am I Fat? Helping Young Children Accept Differences in Body Size* (ETR Associates, 1992).

Ann E. Nolte, PhD, is distinguished professor emeritus in the Department of Health Sciences at Illinois State University at Normal. She has taught in the public schools of Arlington, Virginia, as well as at universities in Ohio, New York and Illinois. She was also the associate director of the nationwide School Health Education Study (SHES). During her tenure with SHES, she helped develop a curriculum framework for school health education that was conceptually based. She worked actively with administrators and classroom teachers in the development and refinement of classroom materials. At the university level, she has been active in the professional preparation of teachers and as a consultant both locally and nationally in public schools.

Richard L. Papenfuss, PhD, earned his bachelor's and master's degrees at Winona State University in Winona, Minnesota. He earned his doctorate in health sciences from the University of Utah in Salt Lake City. He began his career in school health education in Iowa and Wisconsin and has been actively involved in health promotion as it pertained to adult populations in the areas of cardiac rehabilitation, employee health promotion, patient education and drug education for children, parents and their communities.

He served as president of the Association for the Advancement of Health Education and has published several professional papers and a book. He also coauthored a $1 million grant, funded by the Kellogg Foundation, for the purpose of initiating a health promotion project for students and employees at the University of New Mexico. He also served as chief consultant to the Agency for Instructional Technology in Bloomington, Indiana, for the development of an international drug abuse prevention project. He is currently associate professor and head of the Division of Community and Environmental Health in the School of Health-Related Professions at the University of Arizona.

Nancy S. Perry, MSEd, NCC, NCSC, is the guidance consultant for the Maine Department of Education. In this position, she has worked with health education consultants to develop a coordinated approach to the delivery of health education and school counseling programs to the schools of Maine. She has previously served as a teacher and school counselor at the middle and secondary levels. In 1991-92, she served as president of the American School Counselor Association. During her tenure, she traveled throughout the United States advocating for comprehensive programs based on developmental principles for all students. She has been a presenter at numerous national conferences and has contributed to several books and journals concerning the role and function of school counseling programs.

B. E. "Buzz" Pruitt, EdD, CHES, is an associate professor of health at Texas A&M University, where he teaches and conducts research related to substance use prevention. He began his career in health education as a high school teacher in Lewisville, Texas. A graduate of the University of Texas, he holds a master's in counseling and guidance and a doctorate in education. He has served as executive director of the Association for the Advancement of Health Education and editor of the *Journal of Health Education*. He has received numerous honors for his work as a health educator, including recognition from the U.S. Public Health Service, the ERIC Clearinghouse on Teacher Education, and the Association for the Advancement of Health Education. He has published widely in the field of substance use prevention and was project director for the development of *Education for Self-Responsibility II: Prevention of Drug Use*, a multi-level curriculum for the state of Texas that has been adopted throughout the nation and in several foreign countries.

David A. Sleet, PhD, is a behavioral science researcher at the National Center for Injury Prevention and Control, Centers for Disease Control and Prevention. He is a former professor at San Diego State University, California, where he also served as project-associate to the Childhood Injury Prevention Resource Center. As a member of the National Committee on Injury Prevention and Control, he was cochair of the program implementation and evaluation group, helped author *Injury Prevention: Meeting the Challenge* (1989), and contributed to *EPIC,* a national injury control curriculum (EDC, 1990).

He has been a member of the Centers for Disease Control and Prevention's Expert Advisory Panel, which developed the injury section of the *National*

Adolescent Student Health Survey; participated on the Injury Advisory panel for the *Youth Risk Behavior Survey* instrument (Department of Adolescent and School Health); and was consultant for injury questions on the *National Health Interview Survey.* He contributed to both the injury control Year 2000 Objectives for the Nation and CDC's National Agenda for Injury Control for the 1990s.

Murray L. Vincent, EdD, CHES, is a professor of health promotion and education in the School of Public Health at the University of South Carolina. He has taught sexuality education to groups ranging from preadolescents to the elderly. He has authored numerous articles and book chapters on health education topics, with particular emphasis on sexuality behaviors. He is known nationally as the principal investigator and originator of the South Carolina School/Community Sexual Risk Reduction Model, which documented the efficacy of education in reducing teen pregnancies. This model is now being replicated in four Kansas communities through funding from the Kansas Health Foundation.

A. Sandra Willis, PhD, is an associate professor of psychology at the University of South Carolina, Salkehatchie Campus. Her research interests include health education and human stress, teaching critical thinking skills to college students, and decision-making behaviors among pregnant adolescents. She has delivered research papers and workshops on health psychology, school health education and instructional strategies for high school and college teachers at national and regional conferences. She has worked as a research associate for the Psychological Corporation, writing and editing biomedical entrance examinations. She previously worked as a reproductive health advocate and pregnancy counselor in an urban community-based clinic.

Index

traffic injuries and, 467
American Academy of Pediatrics
(AAP), 73
American Cancer Society (ACS),
630–632, 864
American Lung Association, 632
American School Counselor Associa-
tion (ASCA), 99
American School Food Service
Association, 262

B
behavior, risky, 182–183
adolescent, 269–270
community environment and, 873
data on, 110–111
educational factors, 11
family influence, 688
health factors, 4–5, 56, 58
HIV and, 427–430, 433–434
national surveys, 548
prevention, 61, 124
program funding, 624–625, 862
protective factors, 719–720
race and, 675
rates of, 127, 161
research reports, 547–548
school dropouts and, 610
self-esteem factors, 131
solutions, 711
survey, 745–746
tuberculosis and, 438–439
wellness programs and, 237
birth control. *See* contraception

C
Certified Health Education Specialist
(CHES), 38, 842
recertification requirements, 844,
853
CHES. *See* Certified Health Education
Specialist (CHES)
Coalition of National Health Educa-
tion Organizations, 34–36
Code Blue: Uniting for Healthier Youth,
information sources, 128

recommendations, 105–106, 610
community,
ethnic minorities and, 682–683
leaders, 884
needs, 109, 128
community involvement, 111–112,
626
drug use prevention, 354–355
health education support, 872
neighborhood programs, 697–698
policy development and, 755–756
school partnership, 882
sexuality education, 320–322,
322–323
sexuality intervention, 307–308
support, 135
teacher training, 822
See also family involvement
community/school partnership
programs,
cultural diversity, 885
family empowerment, 884–885
guidelines, 883–888
overview, 883–884
problems, 888–892
conferences, 549
Seaside Health Education
Conference, 40–41
teacher training, 802–803
continuing education, 22, 852–853,
856–857
issues, 853–854
overview, 851
contraception, 301–302, 307–308
racial factors, 318–319
rates of use, 317
controversy, 22–23
censorship, 749–754
decision making and, 612
drug use education, 430
instruction planning and, 134
Michigan Model and, 39
preparation for, 755–759
religious issues, 748–749
sex issues, 93
sexuality education, 427–429

effects of, 351
ethnicity factors, 680
family factors, 354
health risks, 4
HIV exposure and, 433–434
HIV risk, 429–430
information sources, 7–8, 127
injury factors, 452
peer education, 724
prevention planning, 124, 125
program funding, 623–624, 650
rates of, 128, 182, 353–354
risk factors, 334–335
school counseling, 217
school dropouts and, 610
school environment, 362–364
student interest in, 126
See also alcohol use; tobacco use
Drug-Free Schools and Communities
Act, 623–624

E
ECS. *See* Education Commission of
the States (ECS)
Education Commission of the States
(ECS), 41–43
education, health. *See* prevention
programs
educators. *See* teachers
elementary level,
counseling, 223–224
health education for, 21
health education requirements, 621
injury deaths, 448
injury prevention curricula, 463
passive learning, 600
peer education, 724
teacher training, 788–789, 811
environment,
cafeteria, 378
protective factors, 719–720
risk-taking behavior and, 873
safety factors, 464–465
school, 89–90, 145–153, 362–364
social, 166–169, 182–183
ethnicity. *See* race and culture

exercise,
current patterns, 155
rates of, 127, 182
See also physical education

F
family involvement,
activities, 698–699
collaborative assignments, 699
communication, 691–692
companion programs, 696
cultural issues, 692
curriculum development, 694–695
curriculum resources, 703–704
education programs, 695–701, 872
examples, 701–704
family centers, 697
family discussions, 700
funding sources, 706
health plans, 700–701
neighborhood programs, 697–698
newsletters for, 698
partnership programs, 885
problems with, 690–692
program success and, 866
reasons for, 687–690
recommendations for, 704–706
school decision making and, 694
school family centers, 697
school health advisory committees,
695
skill demonstration projects,
699–700
strategies, 692–694
teacher training, 822
value of, 875–876
funding. *See* program funding

H
health care,
access issues, 877–878
cost issues, 507–508
funding sources, 67–68
lack, 862
for poor children, 65–66
schools and, 92–94

Volume One, pages 1–544; Volume Two, pages 545–962

The Comprehensive School Health Challenge

importance of, 169–175
teachers as, 90

S
SADD. *See* Students Against Driving Drunk (SADD)
safety issues. *See* injury prevention
school buildings,
    funding for, 625
    safety factors, 150–151, 464–465
school clinics, 65–66, 189–190, 191–193
    role, 209
    services provided, 191
School Health Education Study (SHES), 31–32
school meals programs, 253–254, 375–378
    funding, 623
    lunch program, 96–97, 253, 262–264
    menu planning, 384–385, 388, 390
    nutrition guidelines, 385–389
school nurses, 92, 768
    continuing education needs, 200
    liability risks, 201–202
    nurse practitioners, 198
    nurse-to-student ratio, 199–200
    parental involvement and, 206–207
    prevention services, 209–210
    requirements of, 196–198
    role, 187
    school clinics, 192
school reform,
    assessment, 608–609
    peer education and, 715–717
    restructuring, 593–608
schools,
    crisis in, 5–6
    empowerment, 603–604
    environment, 89–90, 145–153, 288–289, 610
    family centers in, 697
    governmental bureaucracy and, 602–605
    health insurance in, 159–160

health screening program, 200–201
health services in, 91–94, 184–185, 187–193
meals, 97–98
physician services, 196
restructuring, 593–608
safety issues, 148–153
sexuality education, 324–325
wellness programs, 239–240
Seaside Health Education Conference, 40–41, 505–506
secular humanism, 748–749
self-esteem,
    assertiveness, 275–276
    communication skills and, 274–277
    decision-making skills and, 273–274
    drug use prevention, 357
    enhancing, 286–288
    family involvement and, 688–689
    peer education, 718–719, 727
    protective factors, 719–720
    psychosocial theory, 271
    risky behavior and, 131
    school counseling and, 216
    school system and, 597
sexuality education, 64
    community action, 322–323
    community opposition, 320–322
    condom use, 428–429
    contraceptive use, 301–302, 307–308
    controversy, 751–752
    obstacles, 305
    overview, 299–300
    physical development, 131–132
    psychosocial skills, 293–294
    puberty and, 130–131
    resources, 10
    teachers and, 303–305
    timing of instruction, 303
sexually transmitted disease (STD), 4, 61, 434–438, 745
    chlamydia, 435–436
    education about, 64
    genital warts, 436–437

Volume One, pages 1–544; Volume Two, pages 545–962

health education, 768–769,
 770–772
injury prevention training, 462
inservice training, 135–137,
 783–785
institutional accreditation, 840
models for, 790–792
multiculturalism, 811
needs, 775–776
peer helpers, 811
political lobbying, 829
preservice, 14–15, 765–766, 778
program image, 805–806
program implementation, 821–823
programs, 804–808
for public schools, 803
recommendations, 88–89,
 290–291, 607, 874
recruiting teachers, 793–796
reform, 596
research training, 563
scheduling, 787–788
selecting library materials, 827
standards, 9–10
support for, 807
teaching effectiveness, 784–785
training incentives, 794–795
training trainers, 792–793
voluntary health organizations and,
 874–875
teachers,
attitudes of, 785
certification issues, 849–851
classroom researchers and, 823
communication skills, 828–830
community link, 682–683
competencies, 830–831
credentialing, 837–838
credentials of, 806–807
desirable traits, 831
diversity, 831
elementary level, 140–141
empowerment, 599, 603–606
expectations for, 807–808
freedom of, 757
instructional strategies, 821–822

morale, 167–168
multicultural sensitivity, 671–674,
 683–685
national credentialing, 847
professional association membership, 827–828
as resource persons, 827–830
as role models, 90, 102, 138, 140,
 141, 169–175, 249
school environment and, 147–148,
 164–169
school structure and, 597
sexuality education, 303–304
standards for, 607
state credentialing, 848–849
team teaching, 228–233
technique, 280–285
working environment, 606–607
teaching,
accountability, 603–605, 608–609
African Americans, 676
Asians and Pacific Islanders,
 678–680
cooperative, 822
frameworks, 601–602
health education, 766–768
Hispanics, 676
integrated method, 803
multicultural sensitivity and,
 671–674
Native Americans, 676
neighborhood programs, 697–698
parent education, 695–701
peer education, 710–711, 716
psychosocial skills, 280–285,
 292–294
restructured assessment, 608–609
strategies, 809–810
student involvement, 289–290
studies of, 595
team, 825–826
teen pregnancy. *See* pregnancy, teen
tobacco use,
addictive factors, 331–332
American Cancer Society and,
 630–631

Volume One, pages 1–544; Volume Two, pages 545–962

attitudes about, 767
cost of, 237
cultural factors, 335
education about, 64, 342–343, 344–345
ethnicity issues, 680
health effects, 331–334
health insurance costs, 160
health organizations and, 865–867, 876–877
information sources, 7–8, 127
legislation recommendations, 345–346
National Coalition on Smoking and Health, 866
peer education, 724
politics and, 336–337
prevention program funding, 624–625
prevention programs, 631–632
program evaluations, 548–549
rates, 182
reduction programs, 61, 62–63
secondhand smoke, 332–334
social environment and, 173–174
student interest in, 126
tobacco advertising, 338–240

V
violence,
conflict mediation, 481
gang activity, 479–480
health risks, 4

homicide, 154
homicide rates, 180
information sources on, 7–8
overview, 478–483
prevention programs, 64, 482–483
rates of, 127
weapons and, 182, 481

W
weight control, 393–394
current patterns, 155
health insurance costs and, 160–161
need for, 127
interest levels, 126
See also exercise; physical education
wellness,
activities, 243
behavior and, 161
community involvement, 240–241
evaluation, 246–248
goals, 45–46
program funding, 245–246
programs, 235–251
promotion, 101–107
research, 552
risk factors and, 547–548
school counseling and, 215
school environment and, 145
staff and, 241, 243–244
workplace issues, 231–232
See also prevention